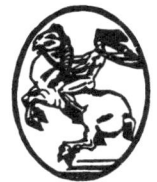

ACTA NEUROCHIRURGICA
SUPPLEMENTUM 28

Proceedings of the 6th European Congress of Neurosurgery

Organized by the
European Association
of Neurosurgical Societies
Paris, July 15–20, 1979

Edited by
J. Brihaye, P. Clarke, F. Loew, J. Overgaard,
E. Pásztor, B. Pertuiset, K. Schürmann, L. Symon

Vol. 1

A. Prognostic Factors in the First Week
of Acute Head Injuries. Implications for Treatment

B. Physiological and Clinical Basis
of Cerebral Reconstructive Vascular Surgery:
Technical Approaches, Including Intravascular
Operations With Critical Assessments of Results

SPRINGER-VERLAG
WIEN GMBH

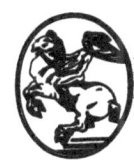

With 85 Figures

ISBN 978-3-7091-4090-1   ISBN 978-3-7091-4088-8 (eBook)
DOI 10.1007/978-3-7091-4088-8

Contents

Forum A
Prognostic Factors in the First Week of Acute Head Injuries. Implications for Treatment

II. Assessment of Outcome

III. Factors Determining Prognosis

a) Prognosis and Series of Patients

Contents VII

IV. How May Prognosis be Influenced by Therapy?

a) Surgical Treatment

Forum B
Physiological and Clinical Basis of Cerebral Reconstructive Vascular Surgery
I. Physiological Aspects

II. Technical Aspects

The Editors

Brihaye, Prof. Dr. J., Clinique Neurochirurgicale, Université Libre de Bruxelles, Rue Héger-Bordet, 1, B-1000 Bruxelles, Belgium.

Clarke, Dr. P. R. R., Middlesbrough General Hospital, Ayresome Green Lane, Middlesbrough, Cleveland, TS5 5AZ, U.K.

Loew, Prof. Dr. F., Neurochirurgische Universitätsklinik, D-6650 Homburg/Saar, Federal Republic of Germany.

Overgaard, J., M.D., Odense University Hospital, DK-5000 Odense, Denmark.

Pásztor, E., M.D., National Institute of Neurosurgery, Amerikai út 57, H-1145 Budapest, Hungary.

Pertuiset, Prof. Dr. B., Université de Paris VI, Groupe Hospitalier Pitié-Salpêtrière, Clinique Neuro-Chirurgicale, 83, Boulevard de l'Hôpital, F-75013 Paris, France.

Schürmann, Prof. Dr. med. Dr. h. c. K., Neurochirurgische Klinik der Johannes Gutenberg-Universität, Langenbeckstrasse 1, D-6500 Mainz, Federal Republic of Germany.

Symon, L., T.D., F.R.C.S., Consultant Neurosurgeon, Gough Cooper Department of Neurological Surgery, The National Hospital, Queen Square, London WC 1N 3 BG, U.K.

Forum A

Prognostic Factors in the First Week of Acute Head Injuries. Implication for Treatment

Acta Neurochirurgica, Suppl. 28, 3—12 (1979)

I. Assessment of Severity of Head Injury During the First Week
a) Basic Clinical Data

Neurochirurgische Universitäts-Klinik Köln
(Direktor: Prof. Dr. med. R. A. Frowein), Federal Republic of Germany

Prognostic Assessment of Coma in Relation to Age

R. A. Frowein

With 5 Figures

Our efforts in contributing to the assessment of posttraumatic coma are based on the increasing number of severe head injuries treated in our clinic in Cologne. There were more than 300 in the last year.

1. Definition

"Severe head injured" are those dying on the day of accident of remaining in coma for more than 24 hours.

"Coma" was defined in Oxford in 1975 (Frowein *et al.* 1976) as an unrousable state of unconsciousness in which the patient's eyes are continuously closed and do not open on command or on receipt of nociceptive stimuli. However, the unconscious patient may respond to nociceptive stimuli with defence movements. Coma comes to an end when the patient opens his eyes.

The coarse-meshed definition of disturbances of consciousness in only the basis for reliable communications. For prognostic assessment one needs two steps:

a) charting of the neurological functions and their disturbances,
b) classification of coma.

2. Charting

One of the best ways to record the course of the most important neurological, psychic, and vegetative functions and their disturbances has been demonstrated by Jennett.

Neurochirurgische Univ.-Klinik Köln
Patient: G. (876/73)   Chr. Name: Ingeborg 14/6/20 Age: 53 yrs

Date 16/8/73		16/8	16/8	16/8	17/8	17/6	18/8	19/8	20/8	21/8	22/8	23/8	24/8	25/8	26/8	27/8	28/8	29/8	30/8	31/8
Time 1645 h		1650	1730	2200	250	810	1700	800	800	800	800	800	800	745	800	800	800	800	755	755	800
Days after		0.005	0.01	0.06	0.10	Op.	1	2	3	4	5	6	7	8	9	10	11	12	13	14	15
Consciousness full	O	O																			
transient syndrome	◑																				
clouding of consc.	◐		◑	◑														◑	◑	◑	◑
unconsciousness	●	●●		●	●	●	●	●	●	●	●	●	●	●	●	●	●	●			
Defence reaction aimed prompt		+	+	+	+																
retarded						+	+	+			++	++	++	+		+	+	+	+	+	+
none									+	+											
Pupils Reaction yes/no		++	++	++	??	++	++	++	00	00	++	++	++	++	++	++	++	++	++	++	++
Diameter: contracted		R=L	R=L	L	L	L	L		L	R=L	L	L	L	L	L	L	L	R=L	R=L	R=L
medium				R	R	R	R	R			R	R	R	R	R	R	R			
dilated																				
Anisocoria				+	+	+	+	+		+										
Pareses Arm R				++	+(+)	++	+		+++	+++	+(+)	+++	+++	+++	++	++(+)	++(+)	+(+)	++(+)	+++	++
L			+	++	+++	++	+		+++	+++	+++	+++	+++	+++	+++	++(+)	++(+)	++	++	++(+)
Leg R				++	++(+)	+(+)			+++	+++	++(+)	++(+)	+(+)	++(+)	+(+)	++(+)	++(+)	++	++
L			+	++	++(+)	+(+)			+++	+++	++(+)	++(+)	+(+)	++(+)	+(+)	++(+)	++	++
Movement spontaneous		+	+	+		(+)	(+)										+	+	+	+
on stimuli				+	+	+	+	+	0	+	+	+	+	+	+	+	+			
Extensor- response A R				E	(E)							E		E	(E)			
L				E	(E)								E	(E)			
L R																		
Respiration: spontaneous		+	+	+																+
intubation				+	+	+	+	+	+	+	+	+	+	+	+	+	+	+	
assisted				+	+	+	+	+	+	+	+	+	+	+	+	+	+	
intermittent				+	+	+	+	+	+	+	+	+	+	+	+	+	
continuous																		
apnea																		
Fundus: normal				+														
Papilloedema				+														
Hemorrhage																		

Fig. 1a. Record form used in Cologne for charting the most important neurological functions in the acute stage after brain damage

In Cologne we use a record form in which the following details are entered (Fig. 1a): the state of consciousness, the defence reaction of the patient, the appearance of paresis of the extremities, and particularly the size and response to light of the pupils as possible indicators of temporal herniation or injury to the midbrain.

From this basis the special, well-known yellow record form of the Berufsgenossenschaften has been developed by Schürmann, Faupel et al., leading to a computer-adjusted syndrome-time diagram.

3. Classification of Coma

For the second step, that is the evaluation of coma syndromes to enable us to arrive at a prognosis, we use the coma classification proposed by Brihaye, Frowein, Lindgren, and Loew in Brussels in 1977 (published in 1978).

Bl. 4	Für den Eigenbedarf

Begleitblatt und Verlaufskontrolle für Schädel-Hirn-Verletzte

(Auszufüllen bei Kopfverletzungen mit Gehirnbeteiligung oder Verdacht auf Gehirnbeteiligung. Die Forderung nach der alsbaldigen Hinzuziehung eines Neurologen bleibt bestehen).

12stellige INr. _____ 5stellige Aufn.-Nr. _____ 3stellige Stat.-Bez. _____

Name _____ Vorname _____ (Geb.-Name) _____

Geb.-Dat. _____ Geb.-Ort _____

Postleitz. _____ Wohnort _____ Straße _____ Nr. _____

Unfalltag _____ Betrieb _____

Kostenträger _____ AkZ _____

(Verdachts-) Diagnose _____

Wichtige Angaben bei Aufnahme (kurz ausfüllen bzw. einkreisen)   **Datum   Zeit**
von wem ?

Hergang des Unfalls / akuten Ereignisses _____

Sofortige Bewußtseinsstörung: nein / ja: A2, A3, A4, B1, B2, B3 (s. Rückseite) ____ ____

                              Dauer ____ sec / min / Std. / Tage / noch ____ ____

Erinnerungslücke: nein / ja / Dauer ____ sec / min / Std. / Tage / noch ____ ____

Blutung: nein / Mund / Nase re/li / Ohr re/li / Wunde wo?   / re / li ____ ____

Liquorfluß: nein / ? /   Nase re/li / Ohr re/li / Wunde wo?   / re / li ____ ____

Andere Verletzung(szeich)en / Begleitkrankheit _____

Nackensteife / Erbrechen / Aspiration ____ ____

Erstversorgung wie ? _____ Wann Tetanusschutz? ____ ____

   durch wen ? _____ Welche Immunisierung? ____

Zugewiesen vom Unfallort / Arzt / Krhs. ____ ____

Eingetroffen zu Fuß / mit PKW / Krankenwagen / NAW / Helikopter ____ ____

Alkohol: nein / ? / ja / (Dauer-) Medikamente: nein / ja ____ ____

Klagen: keine angegeben / (Kopf-) Schmerz / Übelkeit / Schwindel ____ ____

   Gefühlsstörung wo? ____ / andere / re / li ____

Röntgen _____

EEG _____

Wichtige Laborwerte _____ Blutgruppe A/B/0/Rh pos./neg. ____ ____

Therapie vorgeschlagen / erfolgt _____

Sonstiges (z. B. HNO, Augen, Zähne) _____ ____ ____

Weitergeleitet an Dr. _____ / Krhs. ____ ____

                                                                                            b. w.

D (H) 13a (Kopf) Ausgabe 1976   L. Düringshofen, 1000 Berlin 31 ☎ (0 30) 8 91 20 05 — bis Herbst 1976 noch: (0 30) 8 85 20 05

Fig. 1 b

Jahr: 19 / ; Tag und Monat:																					
Zeit:																					
Bewußtsein A1 klar A2 ansprechbar, leicht verlangsamt A3 anrufbar, stark verlangsamt A4 noch erweckbar (auf Schmerz)																					
	r	l	r	l	r	l	r	l	r	l	r	l	r	l	r	l	r	l	r	l
B 1 nicht erweckbar, prompt Reaktion a. Schmerz B 2 nicht erweckbar, träge Reaktion a. Schmerz B 3 nicht erweckbar, keine Reaktion a. Schmerz																					
Streckstarre 1 nein 3 a. Schmerz 5 spontan																					
Lähmung Arm 1 nein 3 partiell 5 total Bein																					
Pupillenweite 1 eng 3 mittel 5 weit																					
Lichtreaktion 1 prompt 3 träge 5 keine																					
Cornealreflex 1 lebhaft 3 schwach 5 erloschen																					
Babinski 1 nein 3 suspekt 5 ja																					
Krampfanfall 1 nein 3 einseitig 5 bds., re-, li-betont																					
Echo mittelständig (M) verlagert nach re / li um	mm		mm		mm		mm		mm		mm		mm		mm		mm		mm	
RR / Schock (S)																					
Puls / Herzstillstand (H)																					
Atmung (alle zutreffenden Zahlen notieren) Frequenz / Atemstillstand (A) 1 spontan 2 intubiert / tracheotomiert 3 beatmet																					
Temp.																					
Sonstiges (alle zutreffenden Zahlen notieren) 1 nein 2 Nackensteife 3 Erbrechen 4 Aspiration																					

am ehesten zutreffende Zahl notieren, auch 2 u. 4

_____ , den _____

Untersucher (Druckbuchst.)

Stempel und Unterschrift

Erläuterungen: Jeder Patient mit Schädel-Hirn-Verletzung bzw. akuter zerebraler Erkrankung benötigt klare Beurteilung, schnelle Diagnose, ordnungsgemäße Kontrolle, unverzügliche Therapie. Genannte Kriterien können dabei entscheidend helfen! Abhängig von der Verlaufsakuität ist fortlaufende Kontrolle nötig. Bei Rücksprache dient der Bogen als Unterlage, bei Verlegung als Begleitblatt, das weiter folgende Vorteile besitzt: es bietet unverzichtbare Merkmale sicherer Beurteilung, beschleunigt die Verlaufsbeobachtung durch graphischen Soforteindruck notenartig einzutragender Zahlen, hilft Verlegungen aussichtsloser oder Bagatell-Fälle zu vermeiden, schult und beteiligt alle beim Versorgungsablauf verantwortlichen Mitarbeiter, gestattet frühestmöglichen Ausblick auf zu erwartende Behinderungen und deren notwendige Rehabilitation, erleichtert spätere Begutachtungsprobleme.

Beim »Bewußtsein« sind mit »A« die nicht Bewußtlosen in ihrer abnehmenden Wachheit beschrieben. »A4« ist der auf starken Schmerz gerade noch Erweckbare, »Bewußtlos« (»B«) ist er, wenn er nicht im geringsten mehr ansprechbar ist, das heißt auch auf starken Schmerz einfachste Befehle nicht ausführt. Die »Reaktion auf Schmerz« dient der feineren Beurteilung des stark Bewußtseinsgestörten. Hiermit und nachfolgend ist die zerebrale Halbseitensymptomatik erfaßt. »Streckstarre« ist wichtigstes Symptom der Mittelhirn-Einklemmung im Tentoriumschlitz: Divergenz der Bulbi, Hyperreflexie, Pyramidenbahnzeichen, Maschinenatmung, Hypertonie, Tachykardie, Hyperthermie, Hyperhidrosis treten hinzu. Längerer Transport verbietet sich meist. Bei »Lähmung« achte man auf Querschnittslähmung, bei reiner Bauchatmung auf Halsmarkläsion! Seitenbetonter »Krampfanfall« ist wichtiges Halbseitensymptom!

Fig. 1b. Record form edited by the Berufsgenossenschaft

Coma I: unconsciousness without any other important neurological disturbances.

Coma II: unconsciousness with additional paresis, fits, and/or pupillary disturbances, especially anisocoria.

Coma III: unconsciousness as in Coma II, but with additional extensor response of at least one extremity. There may also be eye movement disturbances.

Coma IV: unconsciousness with flaccid muscle tone and wide unresponsive pupils, but still with spontaneous breathing.

4. Course of the Coma, and Prognosis

The clinical and prognostic differences between coma stages become clear if we analyse the case histories of 125 severely wounded patients in coma for more than 24 hours (Fig. 2). Differences in, or total lack of, paresis and/or anisocoria or extensor rigidity are taken from the record forms. Here numerous entries of observations are concentrated in that the most serious data are picked out for one day and applied to the above defined stages of coma.

The records of our *surviving patients* show the following: during the comas of one day or more, there might occur coma I, II, or III; but patients who survived the acute stage had in no case remained in coma IV longer than four hours.

The EEG results corresponded with our observations. Analysis was carried out, either by manual counting or by using a Tönnis frequency-interval-analyser (EISA).

The quantitatively dominant frequencies of the daily EEG of every single patient are entered in the diagram. The dominant frequencies of most of our *surviving patients* were within the delta-theta range during the first hours and days; in the following days the dominant frequencies increased; at the end of the period of unconsciousness there was no more delta-activity in the patients over 20 years old.

In the *cases leading to death* (Fig. 3), on the other hand, coma IV as well as coma I-III had occurred, and this was in all age groups.

In conclusion, coma IV, that is primary and long-lasting lack of tone of the extremities and fixed wide pupils, lasting for more than four hours, thus indicates a degree of brain damage that cannot be survived, despite the continuation of spontaneous breathing and despite intensive therapy often practised over several days.

Strikingly favourable, on the other hand, are Bruce's reports of children surviving coma IV for several days, but only assuming that his definition is in accordance with ours.

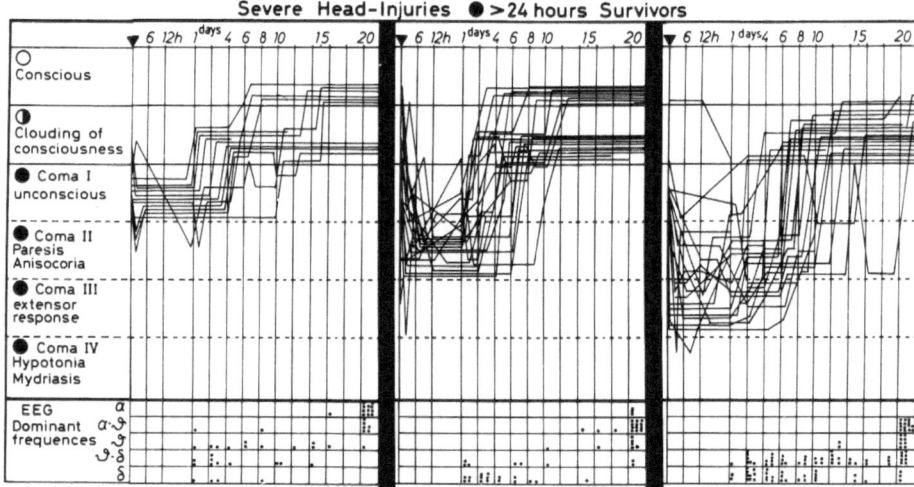

Fig. 2. Individual courses of severely injured patients with coma longer than 24
hours duration. Survivors: practically no comas grade IV

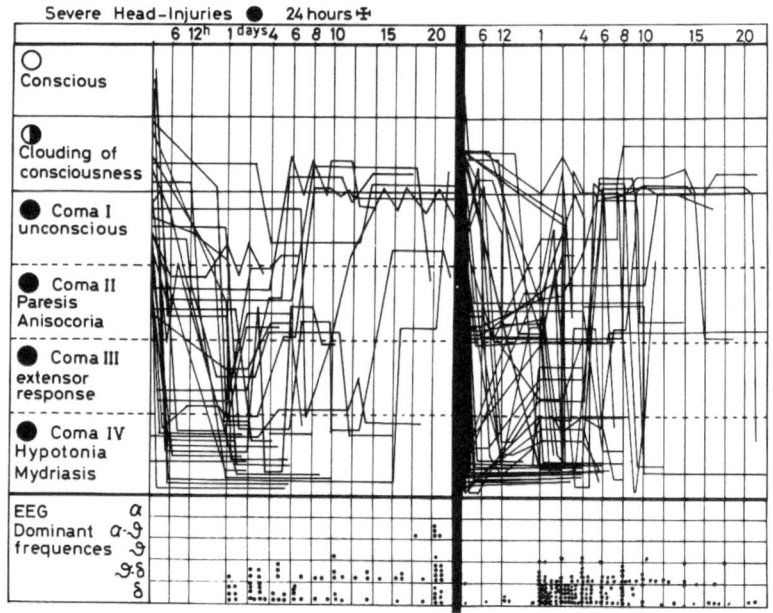

Fig. 3. In the cases leading to death coma IV as well as coma I, II, or III had
occurred, and this in all age groups

In the EEG, most of the patients who died failed to show increase of dominant frequencies.

This means that a very early prognosis and that a prediction of unfavourable outcome, was possible only for those of our patients who remained in coma IV for more than four hours, and this in all age groups.

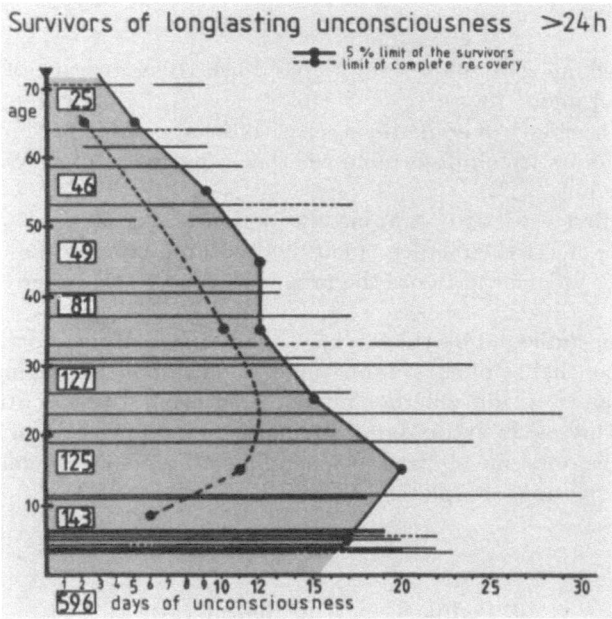

Fig. 4. Limit of 5% for survival after unconsciousness of more than 24 hours duration. 26 cases with unconsciousness exceeding the 5% mark. -.- 5% limit of the survivors; -- -- limit of complete recovery

5. Age

For those patients with long-lasting *coma grade I, II, or III*, the prognostic assessment was possible only after some days, and that in strong correlation with their ages.

During the last years we analysed 1,200 patients with severe craniocerebral injuries, of whom 596 survived a coma I, II, or III lasting more than 24 hours (Fig. 4). In the figure the solid line on the right represents the length of coma that was survived by 95% of each age group. Thus the patients who remained in coma for a longer period

of time had only a 5 % chance of survival. As the figure shows, the 5 %
division line varies according to the age group as follows:

patients over	60 years of age:	5 days
	50–60:	7 days
	30–50:	12 days
	20–30:	15 days
	10–20:	20 days

It is striking that the 5 % limit goes down to an average of 17 days
for children under 10.

Thus, the length of coma together with the age of the patient are the
decisive factors which determine whether a patient will survive brain
damage or not.

In the first week after trauma, for patients over 50 years of age in
coma I, II, or III the chance of survival became minimal (under 5 %),
whereas for younger patients the prognosis is still open after one week
of coma.

The time indicated by the 5 % line is valuable relative information in
so far as the chance of survival becomes so minimal that an individual
decision can be made whether intensive care has to be continued or
stopped. Out of 26 patients surviving a coma longer than the 5 %
decision line only one showed an uncomplicated course in coma I and
ultimately became completely fit for work.

6. Comparison With the Literature

It is not easy to compare our observations with the results published
in the literature, because the data given in relation to duration of coma
and age are rare, and the authors did not always use the same
terminology.

The figures given by Carlsson (1968) for survivors of long-lasting
coma lie in a range far outside our 5 % limit and even outside our
observations of survivors from the longest duration of coma. The
reason for this is that Carlsson, for his definition of the end of coma,
used the beginning of verbal contact and not the time of opening of the
eyes. Similarly, this applies to the results of Philippon (1973), who has
reported the coma duration of 25 young survivors. Only 17 survivors
out of 48 patients of Arnold (1969) are comparable.

Therefore it is desirable that more results might be published, using
the criteria defined in the beginning of the paper.

7. Conclusion

To summarize, I repeat the main definitions:

The severity of post-traumatic brain damage can be defined by the kind and duration of the disturbances of brain function defined as coma. For the assessment of severity and of prognosis in the first week there are two predominant groups of syndromes (Fig. 5).

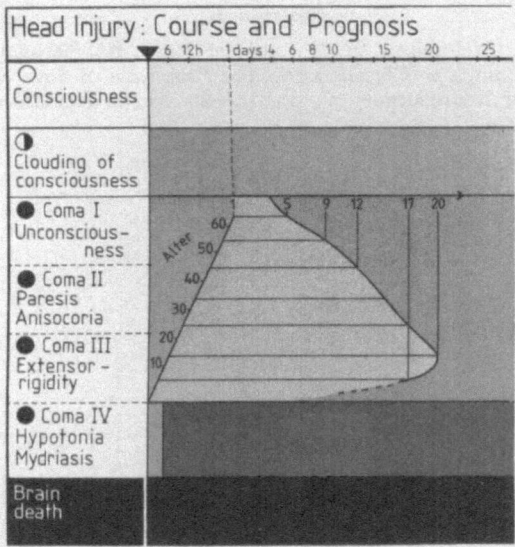

Fig. 5. Elements for assessment of prognosis: grade and duration of coma and patient's age

Patients with acute brain damage, who, despite intensive therapy, remain in coma IV, *i.e.*, with flaccid muscle tone and wide, unresponsive pupils but nevertheless with spontaneous breathing, have an unfavourable prognosis after 4-12 hours, and that in all age groups.

Deviating reports in the literature have to be verified.

For patients in coma I, II, and III the chances of recovery vary considerably depending on age.

The prognosis of survival becomes minimal, that is, it falls below 5%, once the state of coma has lasted 5-20 days, the exact number of days depending on the age of the patient.

For those over 50 years of age the 5% limit has been reached at the end of the first week of coma.

For younger patients an assessment is not possible earlier than after two or three weeks of coma.

Although this classification of cerebral trauma is somewhat crude, it nevertheless conveys, by a clear and distinct definition of syndromes and of intervals, the relative limits of clinically verified prospects of recovery, and therefore may offer an orientation for the length of intensive care.

References

Frowein, R. A., Steinmann, H. W., auf der Haar, K., Terhaag, D., Karimi-Nejad, A., Limits to Classification and Prognosis of Severe Head Injury. Advances in Neurosurgery V, pp. 16—26. Berlin-Heidelberg-New York: Springer. 1978.

Acta Neurochirurgica, Suppl. 28. 13—16 (1979)

Institute of Neurological Sciences, Southern General Hospital,
Glasgow G51 4TF, and University of Glasgow, Scotland

Adding up the Glasgow Coma Score

G. Teasdale, G. Murray, L. Parker, and B. Jennett

With 2 Figures

Since the Glasgow Coma Scale was described[1] a great number of other contres have adopted it, and Langfitt[2] has recommended its widespread use in assessing head injured patients. The scale consists of three separate responses: eye opening (E), verbal (V), and motor responses (M), each classified by a series of grades of responsiveness. Each subdivision of responsiveness can be allocated a number, better grades scoring higher.

The Glasgow Coma Scale

Eye Opening		Best Verbal Response		Best Motor Response	
Spontaneous	4	Orientated	5	Obey commands	6
To Sound	3	Confused	4	Localise	5
To Pain	2	Inappropriate	3	Flexion: normal	4
Never	1	Incomprehensible	2	Flexion: abnormal	3
		None	1	Extension	2
				Nil	1

Whether it is useful, and whether it is valid, to combine the separate scores into some overall measure of responsiveness is considered in this paper.

Relation of Responses to Outcome

The collaborative study[3] has shown that each of the responses at any particular time are closely related to outcome. Table 1 shows the relation between best motor scores at 24 hours and mortality within the first six months after injury. Similar patterns are seen with each response at different times within the first week.

G. Teasdale *et al.*:

Table 1. *Response Score (24 hours best) and Outcome*

Best Motor Response Score	1	2	3	4	5	6
Survival better than vegetative	3%	15%	29%	55%	76%	92%

The three responses tend to relate to each other, particularly when responsiveness is severely depressed in the first few days after injury. For example, a patient whose best motor response is extension will not be speaking and is unlikely to be opening his eyes at this stage. There is thus some redundancy in recording all three items in this circumstance, indicating that a combination of the three results into an overall measure of responsiveness may be accomplished without undue loss of information.

Glasgow Coma Score

The simplest measure is the sum of the three component scores. Fig. 1 shows that the total score is indeed closely related to outcome. Yet, at least in theory, the same total score could be made up in a number of different ways. In practice, and particularly with scores in the lower half of the range during the first week after injury, the overall score proves to result in the majority of cases from one characteristic combination of responses. Even when the same overall score encompasses groups of patients with different component scores, the outcomes of the different groups prove to be similar.

Table 2. *Outcomes for Patients With Coma Score = 8 (24 hour best),*
but Different Eye-Opening Responses

	n	% Surviving
No eye opening (E = 1)	46	76
Eye opening present (E = 2, 3 or 4)	43	72

However, in some patients useful information can be derived from unusual dissociation between the responses: spontaneous eye opening (E = 4) with persisting motor abnormality (M $\leq$ 3) can indicate the likelihood of vegetative survival; and absence of comprehensible verbal response (V $\leq$ 2) in a patient who is alert and obeying commands (E = 4, M = 6) signals aphasia.

Outcome At 6 months

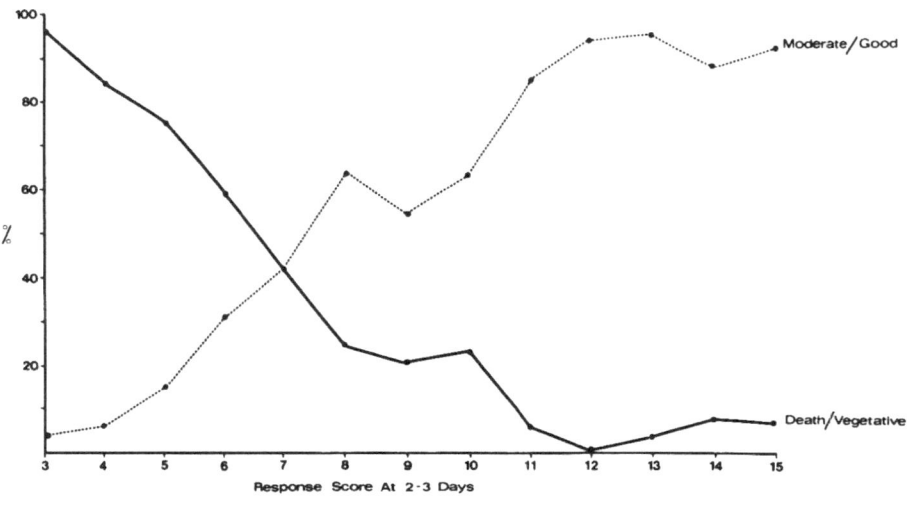

Fig. 1

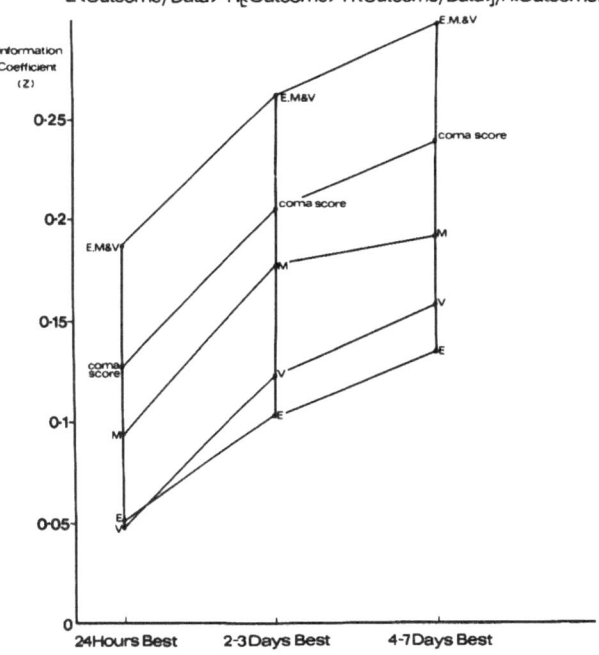

Fig. 2

Information Theoretic Approach

A statistical measure called entropy or uncertainty can be used to calculate the amount of information lost by using the coma score or some subset of the components instead of the three individual results when predicting outcome. An estimate of the average reduction in entropy or uncertainty about outcome when information such as the coma score becomes available is presented as the information influence coefficient. This has a value between 0 and 1; zero indicates that the information does not tell anything about outcome, and 1 means that the information allows perfect prediction of outcome.

Fig. 2 shows that full knowledge of E, M, and V provides the most information about prognosis. On the other hand, the coma sum is much better than any single component alone.

Conclusion

The Coma Score is a useful way of summarizing responsiveness, and can be used as a means of distinguishing broad groups of patients with different severities of brain damage. The loss of information is compensated for by the conceptual simplicity of one number versus three. On the other hand, when describing the state of an individual patient—whether as part of routine clinical monitoring or as a step towards predicting his outcome—it is important to convey the maximum information by considering each response separately.

Indeed, for either of these purposes the Glasgow Coma Scale forms only part of the assessment of head injured patients and should be supplemented by data about pupillary and eye movement disorders, and other signs of damage to the cerebral hemispheres or brainstem.

References

1. Teasdale, G., Jennett, B., Assessment of coma and impaired consciousness. A practical scale. Lancet *11*(1974), 81—84.
2. Langfitt, T. W., Measuring the outcome from head injuries. J. Neurosurg. *48* (1978), 673—678.
3. Jennett, B., Teasdale, G., Galbraith, S., Braakman, R., Avezaat, C., Minderhoud, J., Heiden, J., Kurze, T., Murray, G., Parker, L. (1979). Prognosis in patients with severe head injury. Proceedings of the European Association of Neurosurgical Societies. Paris, July 1979.

Acta Neurochirurgica, Suppl. 28, 17—25 (1979)
© by Springer-Verlag 1979

Service of Neurosurgery and Neuroanaesthesia,
Ciudad Sanitaria Principes de España, Hospitalet, Barcelona, Spain

Protocol for Reception, Management, and Assessment of Head Injuries

F. Isamat, F. Bartumeus, and I. Asins

With 3 Figures

An average of 125 head injuries are seen monthly in our Clinic. 20 % of them have to be hospitalized due to actual or presumptive neurological implications. Traffic accidents are responsible for more than 85 % of these cases.

The use of CT scan, the administration of high dosage of dexamethasone (100 mgm IV at the moment of admission, 48 mgm/day for five days, and progressive gradual withdrawal), and the monitoring of ICP by epidural transducers have spectacularly changed the outcome of these patients.

But, important as all this has been, a standardized HI protocol chart is comprehensive enough for medical and nursing staff, as well as functional for fast assessment of the evolution of any head injury is needed. To the Glasgow protocol on HI we have added a new set of parameters that have clinical as well as statistical value.

The HI Protocol Chart is divided into three sheets: the Reception Chart, the Examination Chart, and the Observation Chart. The Reception Chart (Fig. 1) contains parameters related to respiratory and cardiovascular status, blood analysis, radiology, and standardized dexamethasone therapy. The Examination Chart (Fig. 2) has to be filled with data related to the accident, for biostatistical studies, and the neurological examination and complementary studies. This is the moment when ICP monitoring is established, if the patient belongs to coma II, III or IV group. Only the patients that are fully conscious and have no focal signs, and those that are classified as coma dépassé, are not monitored.

If, on account of the clinical evolution of the HI, the presence of an open wound, or the CT demonstration of a "surgical" lesion, a patient

SERVICIO REGIONAL DE NEUROCIRUGIA	CIUDAD SANITARIA "PRINCIPES DE ESPAÑA"	
PAUTA DE RECEPCION TRAUMATISMOS CRANEOENCEFALICOS		

1. — ESTADO RESPIRATORIO
   (evitar hipoxia e hipercapnia)

    — Administración O₂:
        — sonda nasal .... ☐
        — mascarilla .... ☐

    — Facilitación vías respiratorias:
        — aspiración secreción . ☐
        — tubo Mayo .... ☐
        — intubación { nasal . ☐
                    oral .. ☐
        — traqueostomia .... ☐

    — Tipo de ventilación:
        — espontánea .... ☐
        — asistida .... ☐
        — controlada .... ☐

2. — ESTADO CARDIO-CIRCULATORIO
   (evitar anemia e hipotensión arterial)

    — Fracaso cardíaco ☐

    — Shock periférico:
        — hipovolémico .... ☐
        — neurogénico .... ☐

    — Valoración hemorrágica:
        — cirugía .... ☐
        — trauma .... ☐
        — otros .... ☐

    — Hemorragias:
        — interna .... ☐
        — externa .... ☐

Fig. 1

3. — <u>TRATAMIENTO ANTIEDEMATOSO PRECOZ</u>

    (evitar edema cerebral)

                        — Hiperventilación (p CO_2: 25-30 torr) ☐

                        — Relajantes musculares ☐

                        — Antitérmicos ☐

                        — Anticomiciales ☐

                        — Dexametasona (100 mgr. i. v.) ☐

                        — Manitol 20 % (1 Gr/Kgr/10') ☐

                        — Diuréticos ☐

                        — Analgésicos ☐

                        — Tranquilizantes ☐

                        — Barbitúricos ☐

4. — <u>DIAGNOSTICO PRECOZ LESION EXPANSIVA</u>

    (evacuar hematomas precozmente)

                        — Exploración neurológica (Hoja T. C. E.) ☐

                        — T. A. C. ☐

                        — Angiografía ☐

                        — Ecoencefalograma ☐

                        — EEG ☐

5. — <u>PRUEBAS COMPLEMENTARIAS</u>

                        — Gasometría ☐

                        — Ionograma ☐

                        — Hematocrito ☐

                        — P. V. C. ☐

                        — Medida T. A ☐

                        — Registro P. I. C. ☐

Anestesista Dr.

Neurocirujano Dr.

Fig. 1

HOSPITAL "PRINCIPES DE ESPAÑA"	NEUROSURGICAL REGIONAL SERVICE HOSPITALET - BARCELONA	

EXAMINATION CHART
ON
HEAD INJURIES

	Date	Time	Day
Admission:	/ /		
Accident :	/ /		
Place :			

Blood Pressure   /   Pulse Rate

Respiration { Frecuency   Temp.
           { Type

HISTORY (summary of accident)

CAUSE

TRAFFIC		OTHER		TOXIC FACTORS	
Pedestrian...	☐	Accidental fall.	☐	Alcohol	☐
Driver	☐	Work	☐	Barbiturates	☐
Passanger ..	☐	Agression......	☐	Tranquilizers	☐
- Fronseat ..	☐	Sports.........	☐	Antiepileptics...........	☐
- Backseat..	☐	Suicide	☐	Psycostimulants	☐
Safety belt ..	☐	Gunshot	☐	Others	☐
Helmet	☐				

Vehicle _____ Transport to Hospital _____ Prior { Yes ☐ Where _____
                                                Hosp. care { No ☐

EXTERNAL LESIONS HEAD-FACE

AP   PA   L   R   APICAL

Otorrhagia : Right ☐   Left ☐   **Otorrhea :**   Right ☐   Left ☐

ADITIONAL LESIONS

Fig. 2

NEUROLOGICAL EXAMINATION

PATIENT'S ATTITUDE .... Righthanded ☐ Lefthanded ☐

CONSCIOUS LEVEL (Glasgow coma scale)

A - EYES OPEN

	- Spontaneously	☐
Eyes closed	- To speech	☐
by swelling = C	- To pain	☐
	- None	☐

B - BEST VERBAL RESPONSE

	- Orientated	☐
Endotraqueal tube	- Confused	☐
or traqueostomy	- Inappropiate words	☐
= T	- Incomprehensible sounds	☐
	- None	☐

C - BEST MOTOR RESPONSE

Record the best arm response

- Obey commands ☐
- Localise pain ☐
- Flexion to pain ☐
- Extension to pain ☐
- None ☐

OCULAR EXAMINATION

Fundus { Right .... Left ....

Corneal reflex { R. ☐ (note + or —) { L. ☐

Pupils:

1 - Size {
Isocoria ☐ { Small ☐ Medium ☐ Dilated ☐
Anisocoria ☐ { Right > Left ☐ Left > Right ☐

2 - Reaction { Yes ☐ { Right ☐ Left ☐ No ☐ { Right ☐ Left ☐

OCULAR MOVEMENTS

Normal ☐
Right lat. conjugate gaze ☐
Left lat. conjugate gaze ☐

Lesion {
3.rd Cranial nerve { R. ☐ L. ☐
6.th Cranial nerve { R. ☐ L. ☐

Oculocephalogyric reflex { Absent ☐ Present ☐

Oculovestibular reflex {
Nistagmus ☐
Slow tonic fase to stimulus ☐
Dissociation of conjugate mov. ☐
Complete paralysis ☐

Fig. 2

MOTION

1 - Facial
- Normal ☐
- Paresis ☐
  - Periferic
    - Right ☐
    - Left ☐
  - Central
    - Right ☐
    - Left ☐

2 - LIMBS (Glasgow coma scale)

Arms	R.	L.	Legs	R.	L.
Normal power	☐	☐	Normal power	☐	☐
Mild weakness	☐	☐	Mil weakness	☐	☐
Severe weakness	☐	☐	Severe weakness	☐	☐
Spastic flexion	☐	☐	Extension	☐	☐
Extension	☐	☐	No response	☐	☐
No response	☐	☐			

REFLEXES

Symmetrical and normal ... ☐
Symmetrical and hyperactive ☐
Asymmetrical:

Right Arm............ Left Arm   Babinski
Right Leg............ Left Leg   Right ☐   Left ☐
(Record > or <)

PLAIN X - RAYS

☐ Normal
☐ Fisure ....
☐ Fracture ....

DIAGNOSIS AND PROGNOSIS

COMPLEMENTARY EXAMINATIONS AND/OR TREATMENT

Name Dr.....................

Fig. 2

OTHER EXAMINATIONS

(Record chronologically CT scan, angiography, L. P. EEG, Echo, ICP and emergency analysis)

—
—
—
—
—
—
—
—
—
—
—
—
—
—
—
—
—
—
—

OPERATION

Date and hour ....

Neurosurgeons Drs. ....

OPERATION'S SUMMARY:

Name..

Fig. 2

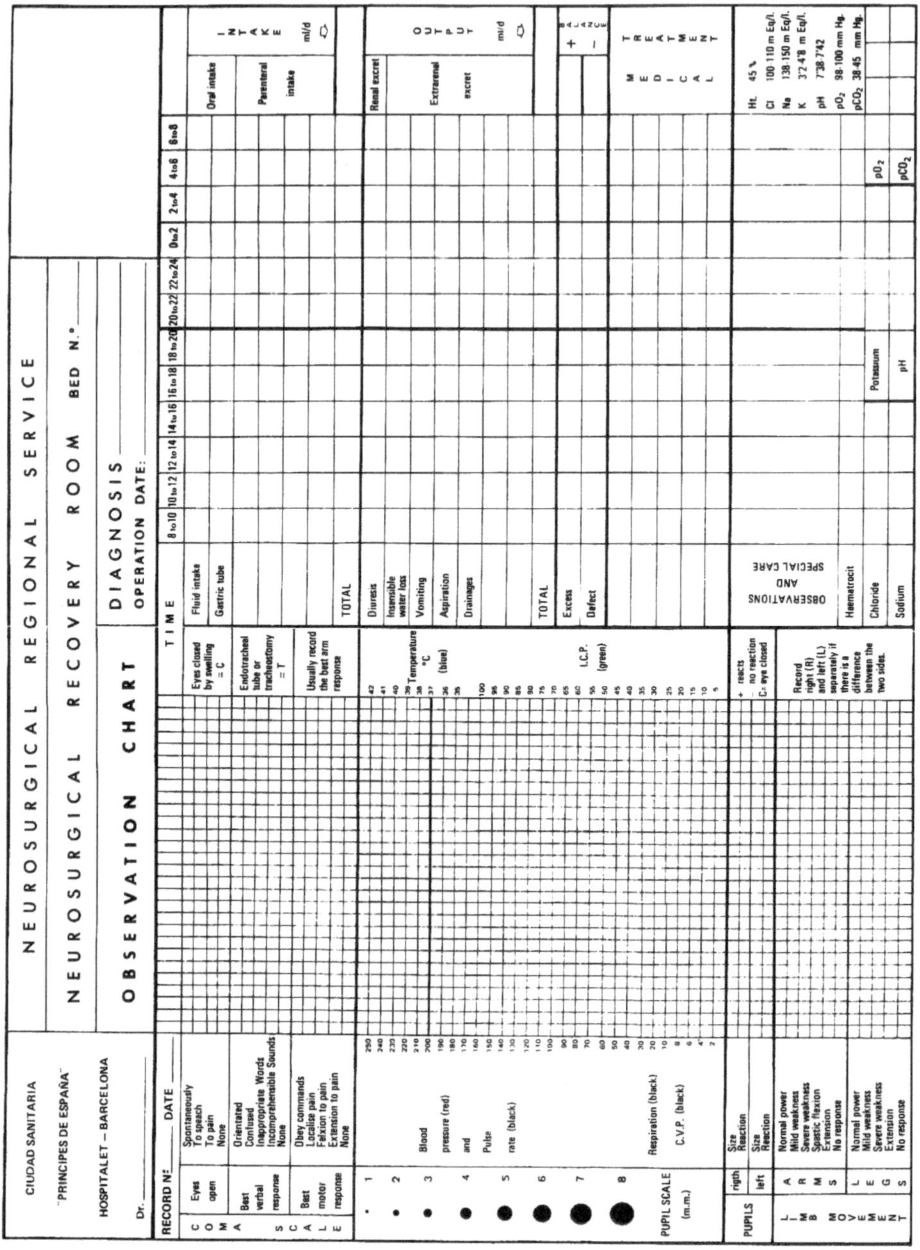
CIUDAD SANITARIA
"PRINCIPES DE ESPAÑA"
HOSPITALET – BARCELONA
Dr.
NEUROSURGICAL REGIONAL SERVICE
NEUROSURGICAL RECOVERY ROOM BED N.°
OBSERVATION CHART
DIAGNOSIS
OPERATION DATE:
RECORD N.º DATE
COMA SCALE
Eyes open
Spontaneously
To speach
To pain
None
Best verbal response
Orientated
Confused
Inappropriate Words
Incomprehensible Sounds
None
Best motor response
Obey commands
Localise pain
Felxion to pain
Extension to pain
None
Eyes closed by swelling = C
Endotracheal tube or tracheostomy = T
Usually record the best arm response
PUPIL SCALE (m.m.)
1 2 3 4 5 6 7 8
Blood pressure (red) and Pulse rate (black)
Respiration (black)
C.V.P. (black)
Temperature °C (blue)
I.C.P. (green)
PUPILS
rigth
left
Size
Reaction
+ reacts
– no reaction
C= eye closed
LIMB MOVEMENT
ARMS
LEGS
Normal power
Mild weakness
Severe weakness
Spastic flexion
Extension
No response
Record right (R) and left (L) separately if there is a difference between the two sides.
TIME
8 to 10
10 to 12
12 to 14
14 to 16
16 to 18
18 to 20
20 to 22
22 to 24
0 to 2
2 to 4
4 to 6
6 to 8
Fluid intake
Gastric tube
TOTAL
Oral intake
Parenteral intake
INTAKE ml/d
Diuresis
Insensible water loss
Vomiting
Aspiration
Drainages
TOTAL
Renal excret
Extrarenal excret
OUTPUT ml/d
Excess
Defect
BALANCE
MEDICAL TREATMENT
OBSERVATIONS AND SPECIAL CARE
Haematrocit
Chloride
Sodium
Potassium
pH
pO2
pCO2
Ht. 45 %
Cl 100-110 m Eq/l.
Na 138-150 m Eq/l.
K 3'2-4'8 m Eq/l.
pH 7'38-7'42
pO2 98-100 mm Hg.
pCO2 38-45 mm Hg.

Fig. 3

needs surgery, he is operated on at once. All patients are then taken to the neurosurgical observation unit where the Observation Chart is used. This Chart (Fig. 3) is similar to the Glasgow Observation Chart of HI, but not only the neurological data and vital signs are recorded, but central venous pressure and ICP values are also incorporated. On the right side of this chart there are recordings of intake and output, medication, nursing observations, and biochemistry.

With this HI Chart the evolution of any patient can be seen at any given moment by any member of the staff.

Acta Neurochirurgica, Suppl. 28, 26—28 (1979)
© by Springer-Verlag 1979

Neurosurgical Clinic, Medical Faculty,
University of Rotterdam, The Netherlands

Eye Movements as a Prognostic Factor

C. J. J. Avezaat, H. J. van den Berge, and R. Braakman

Eye movements, either spontaneous or in reaction to headmovement or caloric stimulation (oculocephalic and vestibuloocular reflexes), emerge from previous studies and from the discriminative analysis of more than 1000 patients contained in the International Data bank (Glasgow, Rotterdam, Groningen, Los Angeles), as a very important prognostic factor which can be obtained by simple bedside observation.

The prognostic value of the various categories of movement differs according to the periods at which they are observed. This means that the prognostic value of absent spontaneous eye movements after 24 hours is not so catastrophic as it is after 7 days. Many of the patients without spontaneous or elicited eye movements in the first 24 hours die, but this is the case for almost all patients without eye movements one week after the start of coma (Table 1).

Table 1. *Outcome After Six Months Related to Vestibuloocular Reactions on Third Day After Onset of Coma Caused by Head Injury*

	Dead	Alive
Unknown	120	246
Absent	52	5
Dysconjugate	34	18 (682 patients)
Conjugate-tonic	59	103
Nystagmus	26	119

Eye movements may have an even more important predictive power in combination with other prognostic factors like EMV-score, pupillary reactions to light etc.

Table 2. *Interrelation Between Vestibuloocular and Oculocephalic Responses Within First Three Days After Coma ($\leq E_1 M_5 V_2$) Caused by Head Injury (1182 Examinations)*

Vestibuloocular	Oculocephalic			
	Absent	Positive minimal react.	Positive conjugate	Fixation
Absent	121	32	11	—
Dysconjugate	19	94	46	3
Conjugate-tonic	16	90	285	24
Nystagmus	4	28	190	219

Table 3. *Interrelation Between Type of Spontaneous Eye Movement and Vestibuloocular Reactions Within First Three Days After Coma ($\leq E_1 M_5 V_2$) Caused by Head Injury*

Vestibuloocular	Spontaneous eye movements				
	Nil	Lateral deviation	Roving dysconjugate	Roving conjugate	Orienting
Absent	127	17	11	6	3
Dysconjugate	74	21	51	10	1
Conjugate-tonic	93	46	101	155	19
Nystagmus	32	18	38	160	171

To take account of missing data a composite score of the three types of eye movement can be made up as a "created eye indicant". Analysis of the data of more than 1000 patients revealed that allocation to four categories of created eye indicant (absent, bad, impaired, and good) is possible and worthwhile. There is a ranked relationship and a statistically significant difference at most periods for good and bad outcome between the four grades.

There is also an interrelation between the three aspects; they are not independent. Some combinations are more common than others (Tables 2 and 3).

The predictive power of eye movements is negatively influenced by antiepileptics and sedative drugs.

The prognostic significance of a certain feature is influenced by its interobserver disagreement. The motor response of the Glasgow Coma

Scale has a low rate of interobserver disagreement, whereas the rate of pupillary reaction is quite acceptable. A formal study of this interobserver disagreement in comatose patients revealed that in all three types of eye movements interobserver disagreement is more than in either motor response, motor pattern or pupillary reaction. This means that sharper definition of the various subcategories is mandatory. Even now however it is hardly conceivable that, in patients not on the respirator or in barbiturate coma, a prediction of outcome is reliably done without taking eye movements into account.

Acta Neurochirurgica, Suppl. 28, 29—34 (1979)
© by Springer-Verlag 1979

Clinic of Neurosurgery* and J. C. U. Hospital of Neurosurgery**,
Iaşi, Romania

The Clinical Criteria in Gravity Assessment of Acute Head Injuries Associated With Coma

V. Dimov* and M. Anghel**

With 2 Figures

In the first few days following severe craniocerebral trauma the classical paraclinical investigative methods of EEG[34], neuroradiological procedures[14] including CT scanning[32,37], and enzyme titration in CSF[13,18,33] have limited use, and sophisticated monitoring of intracranial pressure by computed radiotelemetry[10,15,19,28,38] is available only for a few specialized clinical departments in the world.

For the reasons stated above we have tried to quantify in a prospective study the traumatic coma state and its vital prognosis following a personal scheme which we compared with the Glasgow Coma Scale[20,21,35].

Material and Method

We analysed 48 patients (38 males and ten females, two to eighty years of age) in coma following head injuries admitted between 1 July and November 1978 to the ICU of the Hospital of Neurosurgery, Iaşi, Romania. All these patients fullfilled the criteria for severe head injury designated by the Glasgow group[3], namely unconsciousness for longer than six hours, and inability to obey commands, to utter recognizable words, or to open the eyes. When the injury had occurred more than six hours before admission, only those patients who were still in coma at the time of admission were included[8,23].

Our system is derived from the coma classification in four degrees (Mollaret and Goullon 1959), modified by Arseni (1977), and adding up to a score of 21 points compared to the recent scheme of Jennett et al. (1977) with only 15 points (see Table 1).

We performed carotid angiograms in all cases, and all those who had scores of more than 15 were nasally intubated. Their ventilations were controlled in order to obtain a $P_a CO_2$ of 20-25 torr[12]; all these patients received cortisone derivatives (dexamethasone)[9,26,27], and some of them had cerebral depletive therapy (frosemide or mannitol). They all had antibiotics. We did not measure the intracranial pressure[2,3].

Table 1

Symptom	Degree	Mark
Consciousness	Abolished	1
Vegetative functions	Reduced, modified, reversible	1
	Disturbed and difficult reversible	2
	Severe disturbed, irreversible	3
Deglutition	Labial and bucal stages slow but possible	1
	Labial and bucal stages abolished; pharingeal stage possible	2
	Abolished	3
Protective reflexes	Nonadequat, but prezent	1
	Vanished	2
	Abolished	3
Automatisms	Elementary ones preserved	1
	Abolished	2
Tonus	Eyelid tonus diminished; brain stem hypertonia crysis	1
	Eyelid tonus abolished; segmentary tonus abolished	2
Myotatic and Skin reflexes	Abolished abdominal reflexes. Myotatic reflexes preserved	1
	Abolished	2
Eye reflexes	Cornean reflexes diminished. Slow pupillary reflexes	1
	Abolished cornean reflex. Side or bilateral fixed mydriasis	2
Blinking	Abolished	1
Cough	Difficult	1
	Scarcerly possible or abolished	2

* Normal signs are marked with 0.

Results

Twenty-eight patients were operated upon (see Table 2) with a postoperative mortality rate of 42%. The global mortality rate was 47.8%, and analysed for different age groups it was as follows: 25% in children (2-16 years old), and 64.3% in adults, figures very similar to those found in the literature[4–8, 11, 22, 23, 30, 36].

Our results are presented in Fig. 1 (Glasgow Coma Scale) and Fig. 2 (our own scale).

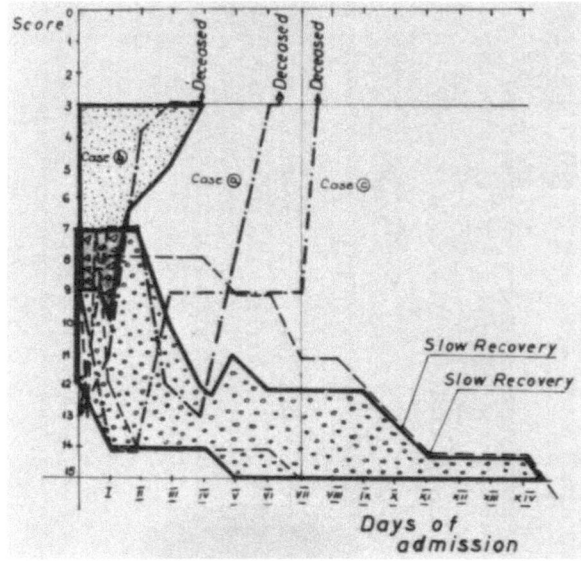

Fig. 1

Table 2

	Age of patients (years)								
Diagnosis	0–10	11–20	21–30	31–40	41–50	51–60	61–70	71–81	Total
Cerebral contusion	6	8	2	2	4			1	23(13)
Epidural haematoma	1		1	2		2	2		8(3)
Subdural haematoma			1		1	3	2	2	9(5)
Cerebral laceration	1				2				3(1)
Intracerebral haematoma	1			1					2(1)
Cerebral wounds		3							3
Total: 48 cases	9	11	4	5	7	5	4	3	48(23)

Number of the patients who died represented by figures in the right bottom corners.

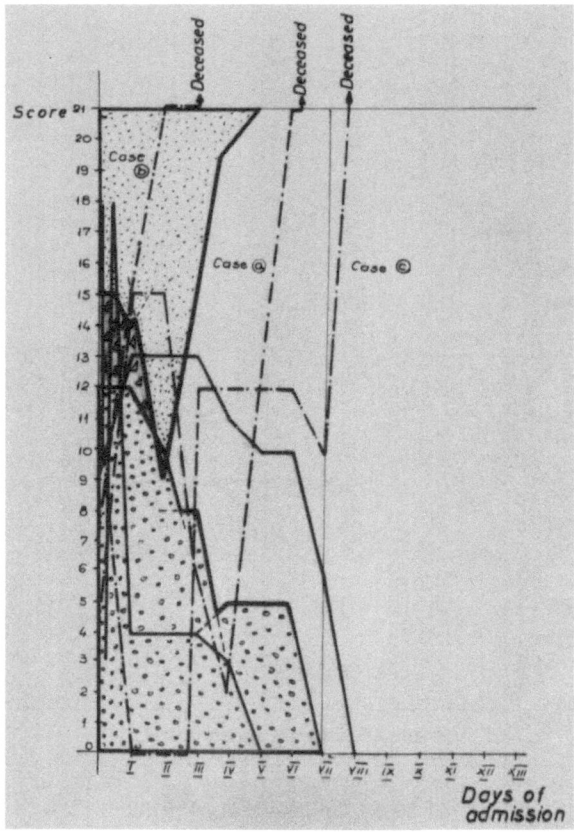

Fig. 2

Discussion

From our scale results all patients having scores more than 15 at admission died in one to five days irrespective of age, sex, technique of operation, interval from the onset of coma until admission (between 5 and 96 hours) and the intensive therapy administered.

All the patients except three with scores between 1 and 12 survived and regained consciousness in a maximum of 7 days following admission (except one patient with a supra and subtentorial brain wound).

The remaining three cases were as follows:

a) A 28-year-old man with a subacute subdural haematoma located parieto-occipitally on the left side and a lacerated wound of the superficial soft tissues located in the same area which was infected (pseudomonas aeruginosa) died because of a suppurative meningoencephalitic postoperative process. His score at admission was 3.

b) A 40-year-old man with a severe and diffuse cerebral contusion. He developed bronchopneumonia on admission and this caused his death. He had a score of 4.

c) A 71-year-old man with a left hemispheric subacute subdural haematoma who, 48 hours after regaining consciousness, again developed coma because of cerebral ventricular collapse and consecutive hydroelectrolyte imbalance which were fatal; score 12[31].

The only case admitted with a score of 13, with an epidural haematoma located in the right temporal area, was operated upon 1 hour 20 minutes after admission and again 8 hours after the first operation. He recovered completely and got back to his previous work.

This presumes that the cases with surgical indications, located in the score range of 12-15 (warning range) can be saved if they are operated upon before the onset of secondary irreversible lesions[16, 17, 24, 25]

From Fig. 1 we can clearly see that the Glasgow Coma Scale is less accurate in the assessment of vital prognosis but seems to be useful in the assessment of functional prognosis of the survivors.

Unfortunately there are not yet published in the literature any data regarding this topic.

Conclusions

1. Our personal scale clearly shows the vital prognosis of head injuries with coma.

2. A few exceptions from the basic prognostic indices are due to some complex factors, the septic complications having the first place.

References

1. Allègre, G. E., et al., Neurochirurgie 19 (1973), 293—294.
2. Auer, L., et al., Neurochirurgie (Stuttg.) 20 (1977), 48—55.
3. Auer, L., et al., Seara Méd. Neurocir. 7 (1978), 117—122.
4. Barge, M., et al., Neurochirurgie (Paris) 23 (1977), 227—238.
5. Becker, D., et al., J. Neurosurg. 47 (1977), 491—503.
6. Bricolo, A., Prolonged posttraumatic coma. Handbook of Clinical Neurology, vol. 24, pp. 699—756 (Vinken, P. J., Bruyn, G. W., eds.). Elsevier. 1976.
7. Bricolo, A., et al., J. Neurosurg. 47 (1977), 680—698.
8. Bruce, D. A., et al., J. Neurosurg. 48 (1978), 679—688.
9. Campan, L., et al., Neurochirurgie (Paris) 20 (1974), 609—616.
10. Collice, M., et al., Neurochirurgie (Paris) 20 (1974), 617—622.

11. Craft, A. W., Head injury in children. Handbook of Clinical Neurology, vol. 23, pp. 445—458 (Vinken, P. J., Bruyn, G. W., eds.). Elsevier. 1975.
12. Enevoldsen, E. M., Jensen, F. T., J. Neurosurg. *48* (1978), 689—703.
13. Fleischer, A. S., *et al.*, J. Neurosurg. *47* (1977), 517—524.
14. Gabrielsen, T. O., Seeger, J. F., Radiodiagnosis of brain injury. Handbook of Clinical Neurology, vol. 23, pp. 239—253 (Vinken, P. J., Bruyn, G. W., eds.). Elsevier. 1975.
15. Gobiet, W., Neurochirurgia (Stuttg.) *20* (1977), 35—47.
16. Hume-Adams, J., The neuropathology of head injuries. Handbook of Clinical Neurology, vol. 23, pp. 35—65 (Vinken, P. J., Bruyn, G. W., eds.). Elsevier. 1975.
17. Hume-Adams, J., *et al.*, Brain *100* (1977), 489—502.
18. Jaklinski, A., *et al.*, Acta Med. Leg. Soc. *20* (1967), 243—244.
19. Janny, P., *et al.*, Neurochirurgie *23* (1977), 187—194.
20. Jennett, B., Prognosis after head injury. Handbook of Clinical Neurology, vol. 24, pp. 669—682 (Vinken, P. J., Bruyn, G. W., eds.). Elsevier. 1976.
21. Jennett, B., *et al.*, J. Neurol. Neurosurg. Psych. *40* (1977), 291—298.
22. Konakhevich, Yu., Sholpo, L. N., Vopr. Neurochir. *3* (1978), 32—36.
23. Langfitt, T. W., J. Neurosurg. *48* (1978), 673—678.
24. Lebedev, V., *et al.*, J. Neuropathol. Psychiat. *78* (1978), 641—64
25. Lindenberg, R., Trauma of meninges and brain. Pathology of nervous system, vol. 2, pp. 1705—1765 (Jeff Minkler, ed.). New York-Düsseldorf-Toronto: McGraw-Hill Book Co.
26. Long, D. M., Maxwell, R. E., Steroids in the treatment of head injury. Handbook of Clinical Neurology, vol. 24, pp. 627—636 (Vinken, P. J., Bruyn, G. W., eds.). Elsevier. 1976.
27. Marshall, L. F., *et al.*, J. Neurosurg. *48* (1978), 169—172.
28. Miller, D. J., *et al.*, J. Neurosurg. *47* (1977), 503—516.
29. Mollaret, P., Goulon, M., Rev. Neurol. (Paris) *101* (1959), 3—15.
30. Muller, G. E., Classification of head injuries. Handbook of Clinical Neurology, vol. 23, pp. 1—22 (Vinken, P. J., Bruyn, G. W., eds.). Elsevier. 1975.
31. Ramamurthi, B., Acute subdural haematomas. Handbook of Clinical Neurology, vol. 24, pp. 275—296 (Vinken, P. J., Bruyn, G. W., eds.). Elsevier. 1976.
32. Richardsin, A., Computerised transverse axial scanning in the management of head injured patients. Handbook of Clinical Neurology, vol. 23, pp. 255—264 (Vinken, P. J., Bruyn, G. W., eds.). Elsevier. 1975.
33. Schuricht, G., Lang, G., Zbl. Neurochir. *39* (1977), 245—252.
34. Stockard, *et al.*, The electroencephalogram in traumatic brain injury. Handbook of Clinical Neurology, vol. 23, pp. 317—367 (Vinken, P. J., Bruyn, G. W., eds.). Elsevier. 1975.
35. Teasdale, G., Jennett, B., Lancet *1* (1974), 81—84.
36. Verjaal, A., Van'T Hooft, F., Comotio and contusio cerebri (cerebral concussion). Handbook of Clinical Neurology, vol. 23, pp. 417—444 (Vinken, P. J., Bruyn, G. W., eds.). Elsevier. 1975.
37. Vigouroux, R. P., *et al.*, Neurochirurgie *22* (1976), 281—291.
38. Zervas, N.-T., *et al.*, J. Neurosurg. *47* (1977), 899—911.
39. Arseni, *et al.*, Semeioļogie Neurochirurgicală. Ed. Med. Bucureşti. 1977.

Acta Neurochirurgica, Suppl. 28, 35—39 (1979)
© by Springer-Verlag 1979

b) Electrophysiological Methods

Department of Neurosurgery, City Hospital of Verona, Italy

Combined Clinical and EEG Examinations for Assessment of Severity of Acute Head Injuries

A. Bricolo, S. Turazzi, and F. Faccioli

Introduction

In the acute stage of head injury, careful clinical examination gives the most reliable assessment of severity of the brain damage and it can detect any changes in conscious level, providing indications both for the practical management and for the ultimate outcome.

Neurophysiological investigations such as EEG and multimodality evoked potentials yield the same results. They are non-invasive procedures, easily performed at the bedside, can be frequently repeated for monitoring, and may be applied to the entire range of head injuries (Ommaya and Gennarelli 1976). Electrical activity is a sensitive index of the physiopathological response of the brain to the impact damage and secondary insults either due to the effect of intracranial ICP and mass lesions, or to systemic alterations like hypoxia and fluid imbalance.

EEG reflects the total amount of CNS dysfunction, whatever the causes, and therefore it can give an early indication of signs of clinical deterioration, which is the basic requirement for the treatment of critically ill patients. Now a days the majority of workers (Greenberg et al. 1977) who deal with neurotraumatology use more advanced techniques derived from EEG. Standard EEG recordings are less used.

In this study we report our large experience of the conventional EEG in neurotraumatology, and discuss the value of combined EEG and clinical patterns in the assessment of severity of head injuries. We also report the preliminary data obtained with continuous EEG monitoring by compressed spectral array, which we think will make EEG procedures more reliable.

3*

Patients and Recording Procedures

During the last ten years, 1600 nonconsecutive comatose patients following head injury, admitted to the intensive care unit of the Neurosurgical Department of Verona, were studied by repeated EEG recordings. Upon admission and periodically thereafter accurate clinical examinations were carried out so that the neurological status at the time of every EEG tracing was known. For practical reasons the neurological signs were grouped into several syndromes (cortico-subcortical, central, midbrain, ponto-bulbar) that indicate different levels of brain dysfunction. EEG recordings were performed at the bedside as soon as possible and repeated frequently over the following days. In addition, 250 patients were studied by continuous EEG monitoring by CSA. The EEG patterns were classified on the basis of our previous experience (Bricolo *et al.* 1973) into four groups: *borderline* (non-reactive diffuse alpha activity); *changeable* (predominant activity in the low frequencies alternating with more organized rhythms in the alpha or higher frequencies); *sleep-like* (evidence of physiological rhythms of sleep); and *slow monotonous* (unreactive slow monotonous activity). Focal abnormalities and epilepsy were not taken into account. The patients' outcome was classified according to the scheme of Jennett and Bond (1975).

Table 1. *Clinical Syndromes, Incidence of Expanding Lesions and Outcome of 1600 Acute Head Injuries Studied by Electroclinical Investigation*

Syndromes	Cases		Expanding lesions		G.R./M.D.		S.D./P.V.		Deaths	
	N.	(%)	N.	(%)	N.	(%)	N.	(%)	N.	(%)
Cortico-subcortical	666	(41.6)	160	(24.0)	452	(67.8)	76	(11.4)	138	(20.6)
Central	506	(31.6)	395	(78.0)	218	(43.0)	84	(16.6)	204	(40.3)
Midbrain	318	(19.9)	191	(60.0)	24	(7.5)	26	(8.1)	268	(84.5)
Ponto-bulbar	110	(6.9)	44	(40.0)	0	(0.0)	6	(5.4)	104	(94.5)
Total group	1600		790	(49.3)	694	(43.4)	192	(12)	714	(44.6)

Results

Table 1 shows the distribution of patients in different neurological syndromes, the incidence of intracranial lesions, and the final outcome. Mortality is significantly low in patients with cortico-subcortical impairment (20.6%), and very high in patients with the clinical pictures of midbrain and ponto-bulbar involvement (84.5 and 94.5%). Central syndrome, which contains patients with initial impairment of upper brain stem, has almost the same mortality rate (40.3%) as the total group (45.6%).

Table 2. *Incidence of EEG Patterns and Clinical Syndromes Related to Mortality Rate in 1600 Acute Head Injuries*

Syndromes	Borderline			Changeable			Sleep-like			Slow-monotonous		
	N.	%	Deaths%	N.	%	Deaths%	N.	%	Deaths%	N.	%	Deaths%
Cortico-subcortical	220	5.6	22.6	1172	29.8	40	2517	64	8.8	23	0.6	63
Central	193	5.6	57.1	1523	44.3	46.4	1186	34.5	27.7	536	15.6	92.8
Midbrain	174	10.9	91.6	508	31.9	75	207	13	63.4	704	44.2	98
Ponto-bulbar	386	55.5	80	67	9.6	81	25	3.6	68	217	31.3	97
9658 Conventional EEG tracings		10	66.6		32	41.3		38	13.3		20	86
250 Continuous EEG monitoring		1.1	77.4		42.6	56		40	16.5		16.3	95

Mortality rate in 1600 patients = 44.6

Individual correlations between EEG findings and clinical syndromes are related to outcome in Table 2. Most frequently a changeable tracing is associated with central or cortico-subcortical syndromes, and slow monotonous tracings to mesencephalic or lower brain stem syndromes, where a changeable EEG is recorded only occasionally. Sleep-like, changeable, and borderline patterns are mostly recorded in cortico-subcortical, central, and lower brain stem dysfunction levels.

As a general rule, EEG patterns are in accordance with the level of neurological dysfunction suggested by the clinical picture. In some cases the electro-clinical correlation allows a more accurate assessment of the situation than the clinical examination alone would do. The presence of both slow monotonous and sleep-like tracings in the central syndrome suggests that in it clinical patterns are grouped in different degrees of severity. Mortality of patients in the central syndrome with slow monotonous EEG is 92.8%, with changeable EEG 46.4%, and with sleep-like EEG 27.7%.

During the acute stage of the traumatic disease the clinical features are more likely to modify than the EEG patterns, but this discrepancy is only apparent because in most cases the more severe status detected by the clinical examination at admission will change to reach the levels of brain dysfunction indicated by the EEG.

The outcome is closely related to EEG patterns, whatever clinical syndrome is associated. Slow monotonous and borderline tracings have the highest mortality rate (86 and 66.6%), changeable and sleep-like the lowest (41.3 and 13.3%). When an EEG pattern persists for several days, it carries further prognostic value. There are some electro-clinical associations of definite prognostic value, unfavourable when a slow monotonous EEG is associated with brain stem and central syndromes, or when a borderline EEG is associated with a ponto-bulbar syndrome. When, instead, sleep-like tracings are associated with cortico-subcortical or central syndromes the prognostic meaning is good. No information is given by the EEG with regard to the degree of recovery.

A comparison of conventional EEG recordings with continuous EEG monitoring shows that the latter is more accurate in detecting any changes in of cerebral electrogenesis.

Final Remarks

Repeated clinical examination combined with serial EEG recordings facilitate the classification of comatose patients into more homogeneous groups and allows a more precise early prognosis.

Furthermore, the neurophysiological study is valuable for the knowledge of the physiopathological processes following trauma, and for developing proper treatment.

References

Bricolo. A., Turella, G., Dalle Ore, G.. Terzian, H.. A proposal for the electroencephalographic evaluation of acute traumatic coma. Electroenceph. clin. Neurophysiol. *34* (1973), 789.

Greenberg, R. P., Becker, D. P., Miller, J. D., Maler, D. J., Evaluation of brain function in severe human head trauma with multimodality evoked potentials. Part 1 and Part 2. J. Neurosurg. *47* (1977), 150—177.

Jennett, B., Bond, M., Assessment of outcome after severe brain damage. A practical scale. Lancet *1* (1975), 480—484.

Ommaya, A. K., Gennarelli, T. A., A physiopathologic basis for noninvasive diagnosis and prognosis of head injury severity. In: Head Injuries, pp. 49—76 (McLaurin, R. L., ed.). Grune and Stratton. 1976.

Acta Neurochirurgica, Suppl. 28, 40—42 (1979)
© by Springer-Verlag 1979

Abteilung für Allgemeine Neurochirurgie of the J. W. Goethe University,
Frankfurt/Main, Federal Republic of Germany

Using the Spectral Analysis of the EEG for Prognosis of Severe Brain Injuries in the First Post-Traumatic Week

W. I. Steudel and J. Krüger

1. Introduction

When assessing the condition of a patient with brain injury the EEG examination is useful[5]. The EEG follow-ups during the first days and weeks after trauma are particularly important. When assessing impaired consciousness the EEG is just as important as other neurological findings and may be used for appraisal of depth and for prognosis of the coma[1]. During the last decade the introduction of computer analysis of the EEG has opened up a new era in EEG applications. Since the mathematics used are principally Fourier analysis and similar spectral methodologies it is particularly suitable for measuring disturbances of basic rhythms.

Based on spectral analysis of the EEG from a group of 50 selected adult patients with severe brain injuries who were unconscious for at least 48 hours after the trauma, we compiled criteria for the prognostic assessment of these patients. In addition, all patients were examined by computer tomography.

2. Methods

2.1. Patients: The study was performed on 50 adults (12 females and 38 males) with severe brain injuries between the ages of 16 and 82 years (median: 40). All patients were admitted within the first 24 hours and were unconscious for at least 48 hours after trauma. Forty-six patients were operated on for at least one haematoma, some being bilateral. There were 18 epidural, 20 subdural, 13 intracerebral haematomas, and 5 extensive depressed fractures. The patients were examined daily with a standard questionnaire according to ten categories of impaired consciousness (see Faupel 1977). The patients were re-examined 6 months after the injury.

2.2. EEG: The EEG was recorded on an 8-channel polygraph on the 1st, 2nd, 3rd, 5th, and 7th days after the incident or the operation. We used frontal (Fp 1-F 3, Fp 2-F 4), temporal (T 3-T 5, T 4-T 6), and parietooccipital (P 3-O 1, P 4-O 2) bipolar leads. In general, the EEG was recorded for 30 minutes, and in some cases for a few hours. The EEG was analysed by a computer on-line. The programme used computed the absolute and relative powers in the standard frequency bands (delta 0.5-3.5 c/sec; theta 3.5-7.5; alpha 7.5-12.5; beta 12.5-32). For further details see references 3 and 4.

2.3. *Computer Tomography:* The examinations were performed with the Siretom I (matrix 128 × 128). All patients were scanned upon admission, and in cases of maintained unconsciousness the scan was repeated every third day. For prognosis the size and distribution of haemorrhages and oedema as well as the extent of midline shift were used.

3. Results

For 40 adult patients with severe brain injuries, we were able to make a survival prognosis during the first post-traumatic week, based on the spectral analysis of the EEG's. Twenty-three of these patients survived, and 17 died. The absolute and relative powers in the standard frequency bands over the parieto-occipital region were used as criteria. Derivations from the frontal or temporal regions do not result in prognostically useful findings. As concerns the absolute and relative powers there are significant differences between the survivors and the non-survivors: the survivors show a significant increase of powers in percentage theta and alpha waves, in particular up to the fifth day. On the other hand, for the patients who died the amplitude of theta and alpha waves decreased. *The best criterion for survival prognosis is an increase of the amplitude in the theta- and alpha-range during the first post-traumatic week.* Computer tomography may be used for appraisal only in certain cases: a midline shift of more than 20 mm, and haemorrhages and oedema in the area of the mesencephalon and the pons resulted in the deaths of all our patients. Oedema and haemorrhages in the areas of the basal ganglia and the corpus callosum do not necessarily mean a fatal prognosis.

For 10 of the 50 patients the above-mentioned criteria could not yield a prognosis during the first post-traumatic week: 4 patients suffered from seizures which could only be suppressed by high doses of barbiturates, and thus could not be included in the evaluation of the EEG during the first week. Five patients showed spindle or alpha activity in the EEG during coma. Therefore, these patients had to be excluded from the assessment during the first post-traumatic week. Another patient had to be considered separately as well, since there was secondary haemorrhage.

4. Comments

According to the literature correct prognosis via EEG is possible with a accuracy of 80 to 99%. The data depend on the type of patients, duration of the period studied, and the severity of the injury. Our results are exactly 80%, although we used spectral analysis of the EEG. It should be emphasized that our patients were comatose for at least 48 hours.

The spectral analysis of the EEG cannot be applied to patients who had to be treated with heavy doses barbiturates during the first week. Comatose patients showing spindle or alpha activity in the EEG (alpha pattern coma) cannot be correctly classified for prognosis. These EEG patterns are given different prognostic values in the literature[1, 6]. In these cases computer tomography does not offer essential additional aid.

Summary

Fifty adult patients with severe brain injuries were examined with the EEG on the 1st, 2nd, 3rd, 5th, and 7th postoperative days. In 40 of these 50 cases a prognosis was given after 7 days as a result of the Fourier analysis of the EEG: 23 patients survived, 17 died. There are significant differences in the EEG's for these two groups: an increase of the absolute and relative amplitudes in the alpha and theta bands for the survivors, and a decrease or no change in the alpha and theta bands for the others, all during the first week. In 10 cases the correct prognosis could not be given: 5 patients showed spindle or alpha activity (alpha pattern coma) in the EEG; 4 cases had to be treated with barbiturates for focal seizures, and one suffered from secondary bleeding. In these cases computer tomography did not yield additional prognostic information.

Conclusion

Patients with severe brain injuries showing an increase of the amplitude in the alpha and theta ranges of Fourier-analysed EEG during the first post-traumatic week will probably survive.

References

1. Arfel, G., Introduction to clinical and EEG studies in coma. In: Handbook of EEG and Clin. Neurophysiology, Vol. 12, pp. 5—23. (Harner, R.. Naquet, R., eds.). Amsterdam: Elsevier. 1975.
2. Faupel, G., Verlaufsbogen, personal communication, 1977.
3. Krüger, J., Steudel, W. I., Schäfer, M., Dolce, G., Cliniconeurological and computer-analysed EEG investigations of patients in coma following operation for cerebral trauma. Adv. Neurosurgery 4 (1977), 230—236.
4. Steudel, W. I., Krüger, J., Using the frequency analysis of the EEG for prognosis in severe brain injuries. Adv. Neurosurgery 5 (1978), 36—43.
5. Stockard, J. J., Bickford, R. G., Aung, M. H., The electroencephalogram in traumatic brain injury. In: Handbook of Clin. Neurology, Vol. 23, pp. 317—367 (Vinken, P. J., Bruyn, G. W., eds.). Amsterdam: Elsevier. 1975.

Acta Neurochirurgica, Suppl. 28, 43—49 (1979)
© by Springer-Verlag 1979

Neurosurgical Clinic, University of Würzburg
(Director: Prof. Dr. K. A. Bushe), Federal Republic of Germany

Prognostic Aspects of Electroclinical and Neuroendocrine Data in Severe Brain Injury*

F. O. Miltner, E. Halves, and K. A. Bushe

With 4 Figures

Introduction

In clinical practice assessment of coma and registration of its development is based successfully upon recording of both the patient's spontaneous activity and the responiveness to external stimulation.

Thus, the investigator able to document neurological status numerically by use of coma classifications.

In more recent investigations emphasis is laid on the conclusion that the various coma classifications ought to be compatible with each other. Attempts were made to attach different results following bioelectrical and/or metabolic studies to coma stages and clinical course in order to get further insight into the nature of the underlying cerebral processes. Some authors used a neurophysiological approach and measured long-term-discontinuous cerebral bioelectrical activity, while other investigators tried to evaluate cerebral event-related-potential shifts.

In comparison to the logical principles of clinical coma classifications we are of the opinion that it is necessary to study cerebral autorhythmic events and cerebral evoked potential patterns. This is completed on the basis of all information available (computed axial tomography, postmortem phathological findings).

This investigation was designed to cast some light upon:

relations of coma level and dynamics of bioelectrical cerebral autorhythms

multimodal evoked response patterns and neurological defects

prognostic value of EEG data in relation to selected coma levels.

* We thank the following companies for kind support and a generous supply of drugs: Merz und Co., Frankfurt, Knoll AG, Ludwigshafen.

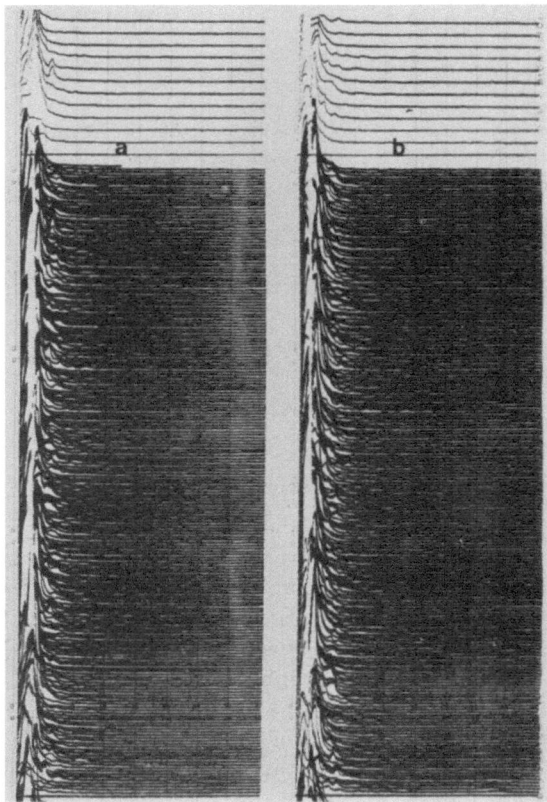

Fig. 1 a, b. Compressed spectral array of spontaneous EEG activity recorded from F 3-C 3 and F 4-C 4 (frequencyband 0.5–16 c/sec). Note: No spontaneous rhythmicity observed, monotonous pattern

Patients and Methods

Our study was performed on 185 patients of both sexes, ages ranging from 22–70 years, and mean body weights of 70.5 kg suffering from severe head-brain injury.

The neurological status differed widely, and allowed differentiation of cases into four categories:

comatose patients with predominant (Coma II) neocortical lesions
neocortical lesions with epileptic seizures
midbrain syndromes (Coma III)
lower brain stem syndromes (Coma IV).

The pathology of the individual cases was verified by localization of lesion sites by computed axial tomography (CAT) and postmortem pathological examination.

In order to register long-term continuous EEG signals in an intensive Care Unit we used the EEG-Trend-Monitoring System of the Schwarzer GmbH. The compressed spectral array allowed the documentation of cerebral autorhythmic events and the responses to iv. application of antiparkinsonian drugs (Biperiden, Amantidine).

Somatosensory evoked potentials (SEP) were recorded bipolarly from points F 3–C 3 and F 4–C 4, nuchal and tympanal, of the Ten-Twenty System. Needle

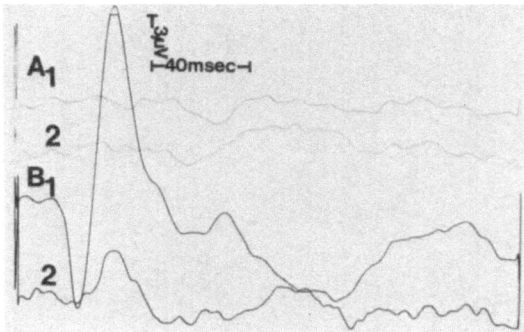

Fig. 2. SEP-pattern of the lower brain stem lesion type A and B stimulation of the left and right median nerve. *1* and *2* records from F3-C3 and F4-C4. Note: Early response only in BI. Functional disturbances of more unilateral extended brain stem structures including lemniscal and extralemniscal systems

electrodes served for stable recordings (5 k Ohm). The bioelectrical cerebral signals were amplified and fed into a four-channel averaging computer. The recording system had a bandpass filter ranging from 0.5–2kc. We averaged routinely 128 responses to stimuli to the median nerves. Sweep durations varied from 40–200 msec.

Results

In our intensive care unit we recorded long-term continuous cerebral autorhythms and somatosensory evoked responses in comatose patients. The bioelectrical cerebral data were correlated with the coma level and neurological development.

Prognostic conclusions were drawn, including clusters of items as follows:

age, coma level, and development,

spontaneous basic rest activity cycle (BRAC),

somatosensory evoked potential pattern (SEP).

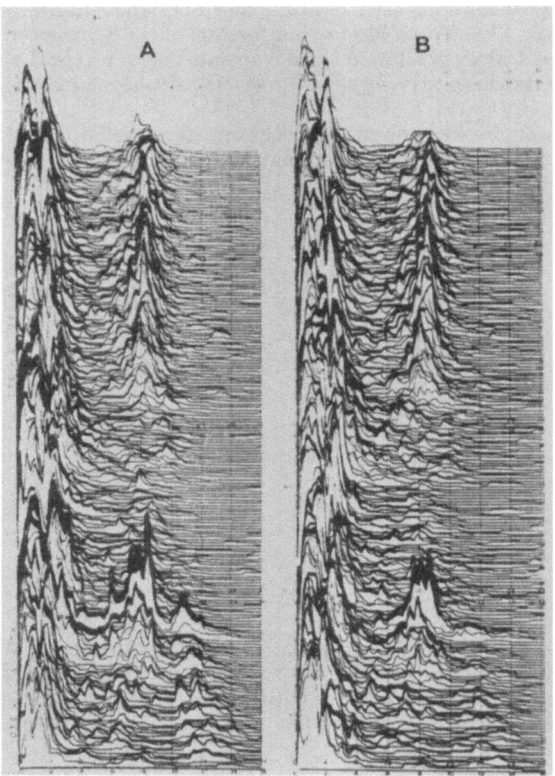

Fig. 3 A, B. EEG-trend analysis (CSA) from F 3-C 3 and F 4 C 4 marked basic rest
activity cycles (BRAC-rhythms)

Clusters Predicting Fatal Outcome

No survivors were found among those patients who showed the
following clusters of items:

1. Age: 22-70, Coma IV, no modulation of cerebral spontaneous
activity, lower brain stem SEP Pattern (Figs. 1 and 2).

2. Age: 50-70, Coma III, no spontaneous or drug-induced modulation
of cerebral activity, higher brainstem lesion pattern in SEP.

3. Age: 60-70, Coma II, epileptic seizure state.

Clusters Predicting Favourable Development

More than 75% of survivors with minor neurological defects and
social reintegration were found among patients showing:

1. Age 20–40, Coma II and III, maintained BRAC-rhythms, hemilateral minor augmented SEP with good augmentation after antiparkinsonian drugs (Figs. 3 and 4).

2. Age 20–40, Coma III, rapid recovery (2 days) after initially disturbed BRAC-rhythms, higher brain stem lesion pattern in SEP, but well augmented (secondary responses (latencies: 200–400 msec).

Varying results were obtained from application of neuroendocrine tests during comas III and IV. In general we found a certain tendency to increase in serum cortisol levels, Human Growth Hormone and Prolactin serum concentrations during the early hospital course.

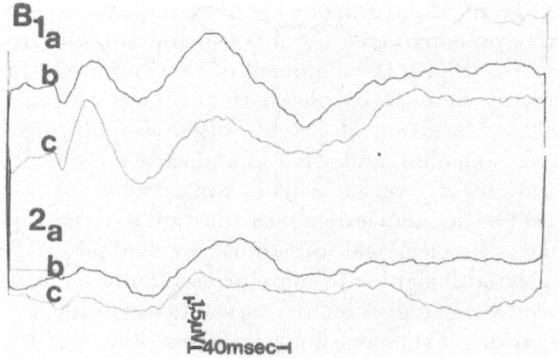

Fig. 4. SEP-pattern variations induced by antiparkinsonian drugs. _1_ and _2_ SEPs after left median nerve stimulation from F 3–C 3 and F 4–C 4. Traces _a, b, c_ at 5 minutes intervalls. Note: Marked augmentation in amplitudes of the primary and secondary complex

Discussion

The electroclinical findings show that it is possible to record cerebral autorhythmic events and cerebral evoked response characteristics under the demands of a neurosurgical intensive care unit. It is necessary to evaluate both bioelectric methods for prognostic statements. Our data are in accord with the published facts of other workers[1, 7–10, 12, 15, 17, 20]. In general we agree with the findings of more recent publications. In detail our conclusions are often contradictory:

1. The employed neurophysiological techniques supplied the medical staff with patterns of additional functional data.

2. The registration of autorhythmic events gives an insight into disturbances of the meso-limbic infradian rhythmic generators.

3. Near field response characteristics to somatosensory stimulation show typical patterns if the symmetric properties of the system are used.

4. Clusters of electro-clinical patterns are valid indicators of the patient's state, and help to differentiate the rough prognosis following the classification of a given coma scale.

Summary

In severe head-brain injury a variety of investigations have been proposed to document a patient's present neurological status, and to record the further clinical development.

Among these methods the value of EEG data in the assessment of coma was restated in more recent publications.

After our experiences with 185 comatose patients we prefer to combine EEG Trend Monitoring by use of a computerized spectral array analysis of spontaneous vigilance changes and somatosensory evoked potential patterns (SEP). Development of coma and final prognosis are, of course, mainly defined by the patients' biographical items (age, constitution, manifestation of chronic diseases following infection or abuse of nicotine, alcohol) and other anamnestic factors (mechanism of trauma, duration of consciousness, appearance of clinical signs characteristic of brain stem lesions). In addition to the complex features described above, bioelectrical data must be evaluated. They lead to more differentiated insight into more or less likely clinical courses.

Fatal outcome was registered in cases of lower brain stem syndrome after a duration longer than one hour. Fatal outcome was documented in old patients after brain lesions when epileptic seizure states occurred. Favourable results were observed with young adults with higher brain stem syndromes and rapid reintegration of infradian cyclic cerebral activity.

References

1. Bricolo, A., Electroencephalography in neurotraumatology. Clin. Electroenceph. 7 (1976), 184—197.
2. Bricolo, A., Rissuto, N., Diagnostic critera for brainstem traumatic lesions. J. Neurosurg. Sci. 20 (1976), 17—32.
3. Brinkmann, R., Cramon, D. von, Schulz, H., The Munich Coma Scale (MCS). J. Neurol. Neurosurg. Psych. int. 39 (1976), 788—793.
4. Domino, E. D., Dren, A. T., Yanamoto, K., Pharmacologic evidence for cholinergic mechanism in neocortical and limbic system (Adey, W. R., Tokinaze, eds.) 27, pp. 237—364. Amsterdam-London-New York: Elsevier. 1967.
5. Frowein, R. A., Classification of coma. Acta Neurochir. (Wien) 34 (1976), 5—10.
6. Frowein, R. A., Terhaag, D., Auf der Haar, K., Früh-Prognose akuter Hirnschädigungen. Acta traumatol. 5 (1975), 203—211 und 291—298.
7. Götte, J., Kubicki, S., Stölzel, R., Klinische Anwendung somato-sensorisch evozierter kortikaler Potentiale. EEG-EMG 4 (1973), 86—96.

8. Greenberg, R. P., Mayer, A. J., Becker, D. P., The prognostic value of evoked potentials in human mechanical head injury. In: Head Injuries. Proceedings of the Second Chicago Symposium on Neural Trauma, pp. 81—88. New York-San Francisco-London: Grune and Stratton. 1976.
9. Harner, R. N., Dorman, R. M., Mechanisms of electro-encephalographic and behavioral changes produces by parenteral L-Dopa. Electroenceph. Clin. Neurophysiol. 27 (1969), 672.
10. Heppner, R., Argyropoulos, G., Lanner, G., Antiocholinergische Behandlung des Schädelhirntraumas. Wschr. Unfallheilk. 76 (1973), 341—358.
11. Hutchison, J. W., Kusske, J. A., Verzeano, M., Cortical and thalamic acticity in the late phases of samotosensory evoked potentials. Electroenceph. clin. Neurophysiol. 45 (1) (1978), 45—51.
12. Jörg, J., Die elektrosensible Diagnostik in der Neurologie. Schriftenreihe Neurologie-Neurology Series. Berlin-Heidelberg-New York: Springer. 1977.
13. Jones, B. E., Bobillier, P., Pin, C., Jouvet, M., The effect of lesions of catecholamine-containing neurons upon monoamine content of the brain and EEG and behavioral waking in the cat. Brain Res. 58 (1973), 157—177.
14. Jouvet, M., The role of monoamines and acetylcholine-containing neurons in the regulation of the sleep-waking cycle. In: Reviews of Physiology 64 (1972), 166—307.
15. Miltner, F., Wickboldt, J., Arousal reactions with unconscious patients elicited by L-dopa, amantadine-HC1 and akineton. In: Advances in Neurosurgery, Vol. 4, p. 6 (Wüllenweber, R., et al., eds.). Berlin-Heidelberg-New York: Springer. 1977.
16. Miltner, F., Wickboldt, J., Effects of anti-Parkinsonian drugs on behavior and EEG of comatose patients. In: Head Injuries. Proceedings on the 28th Annual Meeting of the Deutsche Gesellschaft für Neurochirurgie, pp. 83—87 (Frowein, R. A., Wilcke, O., Karimi-Nejad, A., Brock, M., Klinger, M., eds.). Berlin-Heidelberg-New York: Springer. 1978.
17. Perot Phanor, L., Evoked potentials assessment of patients with neural trauma. In: Head Injuries. Proceedings of the Second Chicago Symposium on Neural Trauma, pp. 77—79 (McLaurin, R. L., ed.). New York-San Francisco-London: Grune and Statton. 1976.
18. Plum, F., Posner, J. B., Diagnosis of stupor and coma, 2. Aufl. New York: Davis. 1972.
19. Teasdale, G., Jennett, B., Assessment and prognosis of coma after head injury. Acta Neurochir. (Wien) 34 (1976), 45—55.
20. Vecht, Ch. J., Van Woerkom, Th. C., Teelken, A. W., Minderhoud, J. M., On the natur of brain-stem disorders in severe head in injured patients. I. Acta Neurochir. (Wien) 34 (1976), 11—21.
21. Williamson, P. D., Goff, W., Allison, T., Somatosensory evoked responses in patients with unilateral cerebral lesions. Electroencephalogr. Clin. Neurophysiol. 28 (1970), 566—575.

Acta Neurochirurgica, Suppl. 28, 50—51 (1979)
© by Springer-Verlag 1979

Medical College of Virginia, Richmond, Virginia, U.S.A.

Early Prognosis After Severe Human Head Injury Utilizing Multimodality Evoked Potentials

R. P. Greenberg, J. D. Miller, and D. P. Becker

Diagnostic studies used to evaluate comatose patients often yield information concerning the anatomical condition, *i.e.*, presence or absence of haematomas, brain displacements etc., not the functional condition of the brain and related structures. For example, a normal cerebral angiogram of computerized axial tomogram may be obtained in patients who succumb to their disease or survive with neurological deficits never detected by these studies. Evoked potentials, on the other hand, like the patients' neurological examination, depend upon neuronal vitality for their realization, and are, therefore, in important method of assessing the functional state of the brain irrespective of the presence or absence of anatomical alterations.

We have recorded multimodality evoked potentials (somatosensory and auditory cortical and brain stem responses as well as visual cortical evoked potentials) in over 200 comatose severe head injury patients. The initial evoked potential evaluation was performed within the first week (mean = day 3) in 87 % of patients. Central nervous system dysfunction in these patients involved focal areas or single neural systems such as the visual, motor, auditory, somesthetic, and/or areas of brain traversed by many neural systems such as the brain stem or cerebral hemispheres. A comparison was made between duration of coma, final outcome and the electrophysiological data.

Results

Three periods of duration of coma, 1-7 days, 8-30 days, over 30 days, were correlated with the brain injury evoked potentials. All patients were unresponsive to verbal commands when studied electrophysiologi-cally. A patient was placed in one of the three duration of coma intervals if he became responsive to verbal commands within that time.

Visual, somatosensory, and auditory near field evoked potentials were significantly associated with duration of coma (p < .05, p < .005, p < .05 respectively). At least 80 % of patients who had either Grade I or II visual, somatosensory, or auditory near-field injury potentials recorded within the first 9 days post-trauma (mean day 3) became responsive within 30 days of injury: specifically, visual evoked potentials 81 % [95 % confidence level (CL), 62 % to 94 % confidence interval (CI)]; somatosensory evoked potentials 84 % (95 % CL, 66 % to 95 % CI); auditory evoked potentials 80 % (95 % CL, 61 % to 92 % CI).

Multimodality evoked brain injury potentials recorded early (mean day 3), and later (mean day 14) in the hospital course were associated with patient outcome. Outcome categories were combined so that good recovery and moderate disability were considered in one group and severe disability, vegetative state, and death in the other. If somatosensory brain injury potentials recorded in this acute period following head trauma were Grade I or II, 90 % of the patients could be expected to have a good recovery or to be only moderately disabled when examined three months or longer after head trauma (95 % CL, 74 % to 97 % CI).

Early prognosis of persistent hemiparesis, retrobulbar visual dysfunction, and persistent auditory dysfunction could also be consistently made.

Multimodality evoked potentials add a new accuracy to early prognosis in severe head injury patients.

Acta Neurochirurgica, Suppl. 28, 52—57 (1979)
© by Springer-Verlag 1979

The Neurosurgical Unit at the Brook General Hospital, Woolwich, England

Heart Rate Studies in Association With Electroencephalography (EEG) as a Means of Assessing the Progress of Head Injuries

B. M. Evans

With 2 Figures

When EEG recordings are taken from patients with head injuries, whilst at the same the ECG and respiration are monitored, striking features are the very marked changes in heart rate (HR) that occur, often accompanying spontaneous changes in the EEG. These changes can be seen even when the respiration is controlled by a ventilator. If such recordings are taken every day following an injury they do not remain constant. During the first few days there is a striking increase in the amount of variation seen and then, later, the variation becomes much less.

These observations suggested the possibility that the HR itself could be used as an indicator of the progress of any individual head injury and might provide information of prognostic value for the eventual outcome.

In order to obtain more detailed information about the beat-to-beat HR changes, head injuries have been observed daily with a Hewlett-Packard cardio-respiratory monitor. This machine, which is an adaptation of the Foetal HR monitor, records the beat-to-beat HR variation from two electrodes on the manubrium sterni, and the apex beat and the respiration by impedance from the apex beat to the right axilla. Such records are easy to obtain at the bedside under adverse conditions. They also have the advantage of being recorded from a site distant from the head, and are completely non-invasive. EEG recordings were taken at intervals in association with these records.

The normal resting HR contains considerable beat-to-beat variation, most of it related to respiration. Other more irregular changes are related to voluntary or involuntary movements, and there are also changes related to the vasomotor and thermoregulatory reflexes[1]. These variations combine to produce a characteristic trace. The variability, which is defined as the difference between the highest and lowest rates recorded, is dependent on age, being much greater in youth than in old age.

The administration of a beta-adrenergic blocking drug (Propanolol 10 mgs i.V.) produces a mean fall in the HR, but does not affect the variability. Atropine 1.2 mg i.V., which blocks the parasympathetic, on the other hand, produces a tachycardia and an almost complete loss of variability. The mean rate therefore depends on both branches of the autonomic nervous system, whereas the variability is dependent on the vagus alone. This observation has been used to determine the presence of autonomic neuropathy in such conditions as diabetes[2] but if the heart and autonomic nerves are intact the same data can be used to provide information about the reflex functioning of the medulla oblongata.

These reflexes produce a predictable pattern of neuronal activity that can be treated in much the same way as the EEG but represents rhythmic changes in the medulla rather than in the cerebral cortex.

Types of Trace Encountered

Although many different types of trace can be seen and are shown in Fig. 1, those which are of importance in head injury are of four types. The sinus arrhythmia type of trace (1a and b) shows continuous sinus pattern that only changes briefly on stimulation. The biphasic trace shows periods of sinus arrhythmia followed abruptly by periods of tachycardia (1c, d, and e). This type of trace shows very high variability, and is usually associated with a biphasic EEG, as described by Bricolo[3]. Bursts of delta activity occur at the same time as the periods of tachycardia. The other two traces show diminished variability. There is a type that shows an almost complete loss of variability with a tachycardia (this will be referred to as atropine like; Fig. 1g), and there is a type that resembles the normal pattern but is of low variability and often shows a tachycardia. This will be called polymorphic, and is shown in Fig. 1h.

These trace types are not peculiar to head injury, they can be seen in any form of acute brain damage, however in head injuries the high variability trace types, like the biphasic pattern, are very common.

Studies on Individual Patients

A total of 145 patients with head injury have been studied over a period of two years. Ten patients, in whom the period of unconsciousness was protracted, have been observed more intensively, and these form the basis of this study.

The group consisted of ten young people from 12-21 years with closed head injuries. They were all unconscious from the time of the injury, and all were examined within six hours. At the time of the first examination two were unresponsive with fixed pupils, and one was unresponsive with weak pupillary reactions to light. The other seven all had reactive pupils. Of these, one had decerebrate and three others weak flexor reactions to stimulation only. The remaining two showed spontaneous flexion movements. The seven patients who were responsive when first seen all deteriorated early, giving rise to anxiety. The flexion movements became decerebrate or decorticate in character, and the level of responsiveness fell. All the group were investigated to exclude collections of blood by CT scan or angiography and, apart from a frontal haematoma in one case, none was found and none required operation.

The final outcome for the group is known. Six made good functional recoveries, one has some intellectual and behavioural disturbance, and three have made poor recoveries with little prospect of caring for themselves. These three last patients were those who were unresponsive with fixed or poorly reacting pupils at the first examination, which is in keeping with the results of many studies in head injury[4,5].

The HR observations on the group were made with daily samples of 20 minutes each. In all but one case, not seen for four days, the first trace was within 48 hours of the injury. In all cases the first trace obtained showed a sinus arrhythmia or biphasic pattern. Sinus arrhythmia traces were only encountered in the first 48 hours, and these records soon changed to show a biphasic pattern with a marked rise in variability that was at its maximum between the second and the sixth day. This change was associated with a change in the clinical state from movement on stimulation only to spontaneous decerebrate spasms. In all but two of the patients the biphasic HR trace was associated with a biphasic EEG pattern. The biphasic appearance persisted for periods which varied from six to twenty-two days and then a further change took place. There was an abrupt fall in the variability and a change in trace pattern so that it became either polymorphic or atropine-like. In all the patients who made a good recovery it was this second change in trace type that was associated with the first clear-cut signs of improvement in the clinical condition such as the appearance of the first purposive movements or the ability to obey simple commands.

Fig. 1. Types of HR trace seen in head injury. *a* sinus arrhythmia pattern, rises of rate only when stimulated, *b* exaggerated sinus arrhythmia, *c* and *d* biphasic pattern, *e* biphasic pattern, patient on ventilator, *f* cyclic pattern, periodic respiration cycles at $1^1/_2$ minutes intervals, *g* Atropine-like, *h* polymorphic with tachycardia, *j* flat trace with cerebral death and isoelectric EEG

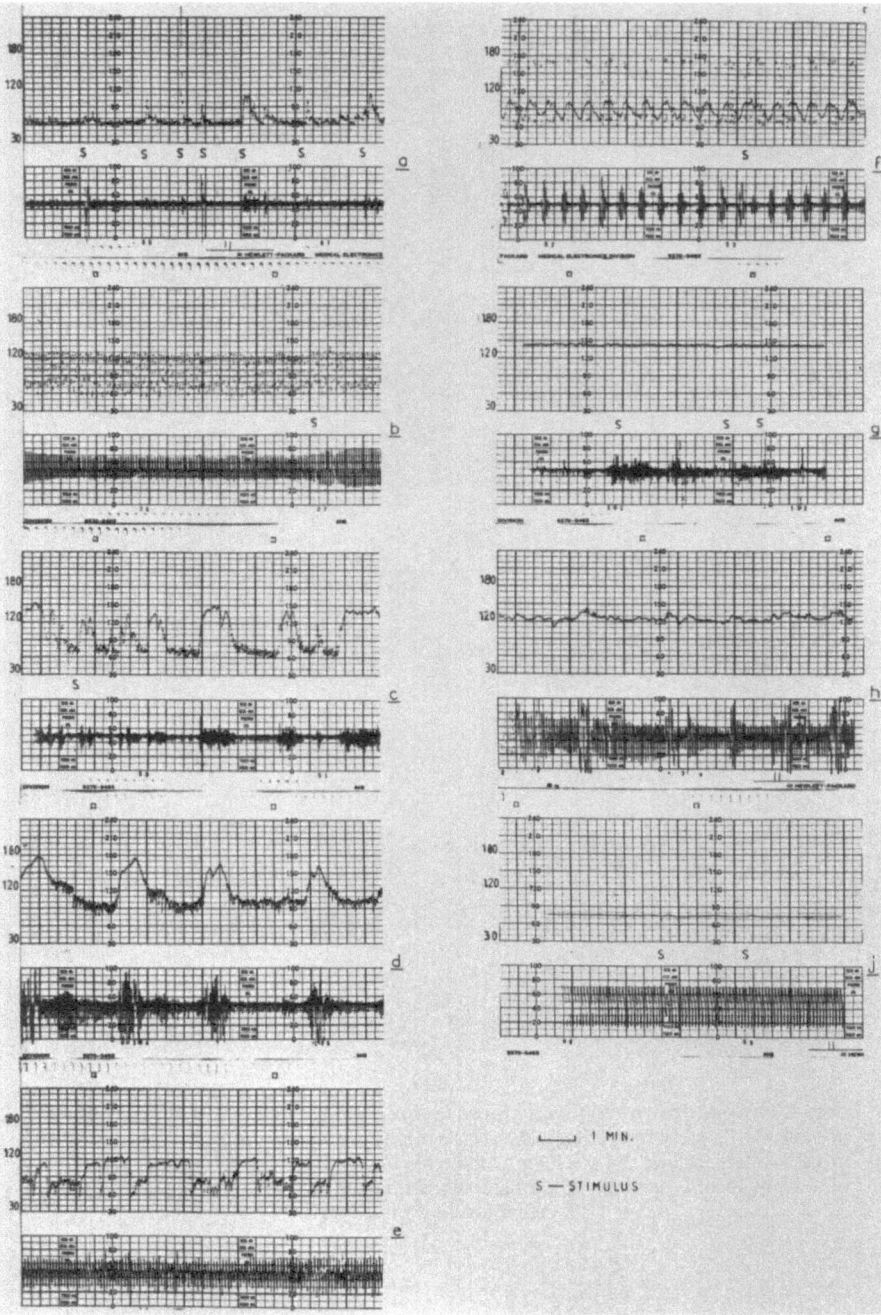

Fig. 1

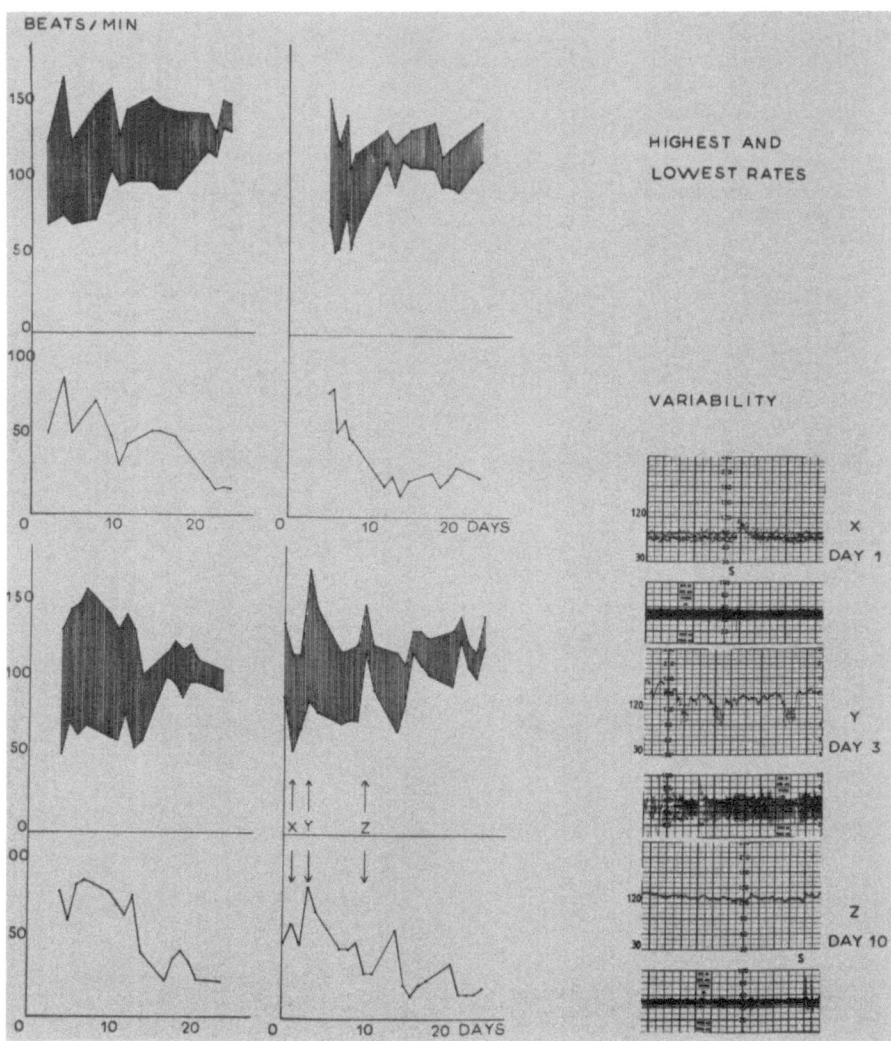

Fig. 2. Graphs drawn from HR traces on four head injuries. *Below*, variability, initially with early rise, then falls. *Above*, highest and lowest rates recorded. Fall in variability associated with a mean tachycardia. HR traces beside graph show evolution in one patient. *X* sinus arrhythmia on day 1, *Y* biphasic on day 3, *Z* Atropine-like on day 10

Fig. 2 shows graphs drawn from the HR findings of four of the patients. The variability, shown at the bottom. after an initial rise, remains high for some days and then falls. The highest and lowest heart rates, shown above, illustrate that the fall in variability is associated with a persisting tachycardia. The HR traces beside one of the graphs show the relevant changes in HR pattern. sinus arrhythmia on day 1, biphasic on day 3, with a rise in variability and the appearance of decerebrate spasms and atropine-like changes on day 10 at which time the patient could obey simple commands. and the variability fell.

A possible explanation of the evolution of the HR pattern and the way in which it follows the clinical state of the patient is that it is related to the resolution of the brain stem dysfunction, and progresses in a caudo-cranial direction from the lower brain stem at the time of the sinus arrhythmia record to the upper brain stem as represented by the biphasic record and finally to the polymorphic or atropine-like trace as the brain stem dysfunction resolves.

These changes can be considered as an additional physical sign which documents the recovery of the patient and has often proved useful in practice. In those patients who clinically might be supposed to have a poor outlook for survival the failure of the HR pattern to progress and establish a good biphasic trace has often been an early sign of deterioration. A good illustration of the usefulness of the observations is the patient from whom the upper left-hand graph was obtained in Fig. 2. This young boy was decerebrate for 22 days with a biphasic trace throughout that time. The change to a polymorphic pattern shortly preceded his clinical improvement, and he has made a fair recovery with some intellectual and behavioural handicap.

There is some indication that the later traces following the establishment of the polymorphic or atropine-like trace will give information about the eventual prospects for a long term recovery.

References

1. Sayers, M., McA., Analysis of heart rate variability. Ergonomics *16* (1973), 1, 17—32.
2. Wheeler, R., Watkins, P. J., Cardiac denervation in diabetes. B.M.J. *4* (1973), 584—586.
3. Bricolo, A., Turella, G., EEG patterns is acute traumatic coma, diagnostic and prognostic value. J. Neurological Sci. *17* (1973), 278—285.
4. Overgaard, J., Christenson, S., Hvid-Hansen, O., *et al.*, Prognosis in head injury based on early clinical examination. Lancet *2* (1973), 631—635.
5. Jennett, B., Prognosis after severe head injury. Clin. Neurosurg. *19* (1972), 200—207.

Acta Neurochirurgica, Suppl. 28, 58—62 (1979)
© by Springer-Verlag 1979

Department of Neurosurgery
(Director: Prof. K. A. Bushe), University of Würzburg, Federal Republic of
Germany

Prognostic Information From EEG and ICP Monitoring After Severe Closed Head Injuries in the Early Post-Traumatic Phase

A Clinical and Experimental Study

O. E. Knoblich and **M. Gaab**

With 2 Figures

Introduction

In conventional EEG recordings, an amplitude flattening and slowing of frequency is found in the first hours after severe enclosed head injuries, without correlation with clouding of consciousness and prognosis. Also, a clinical evaluation does not permit any prognostic statement for the individual case early after trauma. Only by standardized complementation of clinical findings is a better prognostic differentiation possible by use of comparative data calculated by computer from patients from several intensive centres[3].

Since this is an elaborate procedure and since such comparison figures are not available in our catchment area we have compared at an early time after trauma (first 24 hours) computer-supported continuous EEG analysis and intracranial pressure (ICP) measurements with the clinical findings (Glasgow coma scale[3]) and the course in the first four weeks so as to attempt a prognostic evaluation within the first two days.

Since electrical activity of the brain is subject to circadian and ultradian variations in vigilance, the EEG and intracranial pressure after head injury (cold trauma) were first investigated in animal experiments.

Methods

Clinical

In 14 patients with closed head injuries, in whom the ICP was measured (right frontal epidural pressure measurement with miniaturized pressure transducer[1]), the EEG was continuously recorded with bipolar silver needle electrodes fronto-occipitally on both sides and registered on a conventional writer. The power energy was calculated by a computer (FFT, Intertechnique-Plurimat S) in the delta, theta, alpha, and total frequency ranges. The energy spectra were reproduced in arbitrary units.

Experimental

For comparison, right parietal cold trauma of the brain was produced in 50 cats by cooling the intact dura. The epidural pressure and the EEG were measured on both sides. The ventricular pressure was registered by means of catheter after a puncture of the right anterior horn.

Results

Animal Experiments (50 cats)

In the animal experiments, the EEG voltage decreases immediately after trauma with increase in ICP. There is a temporary alpha activation in 50 % of the animals (Figs. 1a, 2), often with a spindle form. A marked slowing of the EEG frequencies is often not noticeable, even later before there is a general flattening (Figs. 1a, 3). The tension can increase again even after hours despite a rising ICP. With a cerebral perfusion pressure (CPP) of 60 mm Hg, the EEG becomes flat, and later isoelectric (Fig. 1b).

Clinical Investigation

Of the 14 patients, four showed a rise in intracranial pressure in the first two days, mostly without delay. The EEG was generally changed severely or to a high degree in these patients only on the second day. In two patients with raised ICP, there was an alpha activation demonstrable for hours. Both survived the first four weeks.

In the other ten patients (Fig. 2a), rises of pressure within the skull were not demonstrable. An alpha activation was present on the first day after trauma in five patients (Fig. 2b). Three of these patients recovered (Fig. 2a). The EEGs of almost all patients were generally changed to a severe or high degree only after 24 hours (Fig. 2a). There were indications of brain stem damage in all cases. With a low clinical

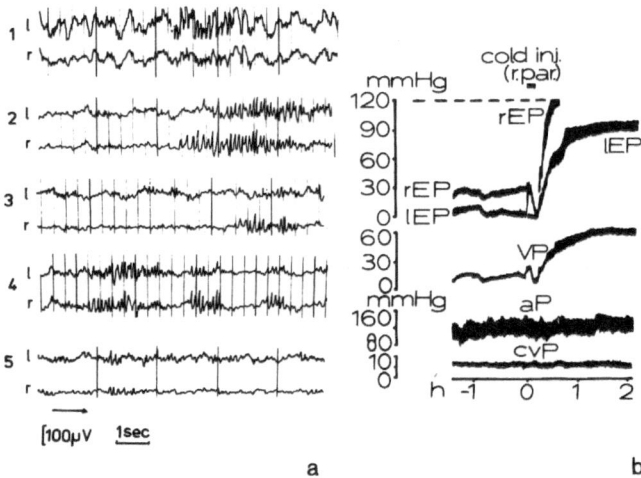

Fig. 1 a, b. Typical course of the EEG recording and ICP before and after right parietal cold trauma to the brain in the cat. a) EEG; *1* Before the cold trauma to the brain. *2* 10 minutes after right parietal trauma, *3* 40 minutes after trauma, *4* 45 minutes after trauma, *5* 2 hours after trauma. Notice the α-activation soon after trauma. b) Before the trauma, left epidural pressure is the same as ventricular pressure, right epidural pressure is slightly rised. After cold trauma to the brain, immediate rise of all brain pressures, especially marked in the case of right epidural pressure. Appreciable pressure gradients CCP = $aP - VP$ after 2 hours at 60 mm Hg. *l* left fronto-occipital, *r* right fronto-occipital, cold inj cold trauma, *r. par.* right parietal, *VP* ventricular pressure, *rEP* right epidural pressure, *aP* arterial blood pressure, *cVP* central venous pressure

score (coma scale) on the first day we found a marked clinical improvement in five of the patients already on the second day. In these cases, high degree EEG-alterations were seen less frequently after 24 hours (Fig. 2a, above). No EEG paroxysms were found.

Discussion

In the early phase after severe closed cranio-cerebral trauma, there is decline of the amplitude of the electrical activity of the brain, most probably due to disturbance of neuronal regulation, rather than direct disturbance of metabolism. In animal experiments a marked diminution of the EEG was demonstrated immediately after trauma, even over the hemisphere which was not directly damaged (diaschisis). A disorder of blood perfusion with concomitant engorgement[2] in the first 24 hours, which does not lead in all cases to a progressive rise in

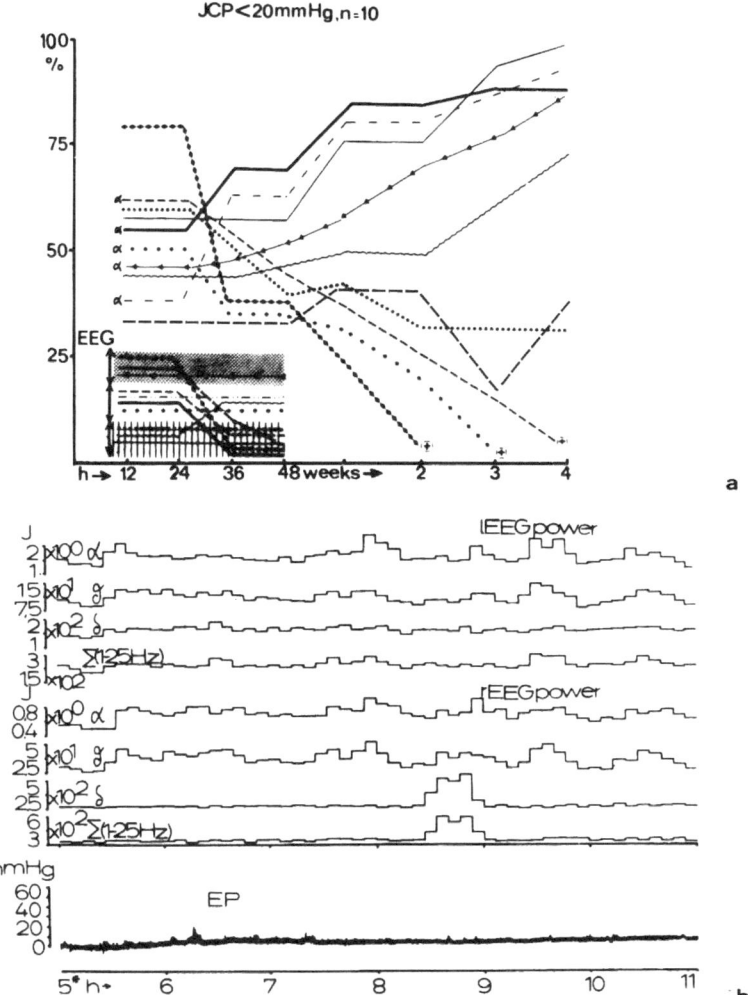

Fig. 2a, b. 4 week clinical course of 10 patients with 48 hours ICP measurement soon after severe trauma (without pressure elevation). Conventional and computer-supported (patient --- in Fig. 2a) EEG investigation of the first two days. a) No correlation between clinical evaluation of the first 36 hours and EEG investigation of the first 24 hours and the later course. Markedly more frequent high grade general EEG alteration on the second day in patients with poor clinical outcome. Two of the patients died showing an acute deterioration of the electrical activity of the brain on the second day. b) A rise in the ICP in this patient (----) is lacking. The EEG power is much lower on the right. Early alpha activation on both sides. Over the right hemisphere after 8 hours, appreciable increase of total power and the intensity of the delta band for 1 hour. ICP intracranial pressure, % clinical severity, α patients with activation in the alpha region, ± patients who died, grey-dotted moderate, white severe, streched high degree alteration in EEG, EP epidural pressure, l left EEG power, r right EEG power

intracranial pressure and brain oedema can reduce the reliability of the EEG and the possibility of the clinical evaluation on the first day.

The alpha activation to be observed in 50 % of the cases on the first day was regarded by us as a stress symptom. It possibly reflects preservation of the functional efficiency of mesencephalic and diencephalic centers. In patients, the severity of the general EEG changes on the second day are more comparable with the clinical finding and later outcome. A more precise statement will be possible after further studies in which computer-supported continuous EEG registration is to be given preference. A single EEG recording is not sufficient. Prognostic conclusions cannot be made from measurement of ICP unless a critical cerebral perfusion pressure is exceeded. In animal experiments, when the cerebral perfusion pressure fell under 60-50 mm Hg only those animals regularly survive, that were adequately treated in time.

Summary

Neither the EEG investigations on the first post-traumatic day after severe enclosed brain injury nor evaluation of the clinical finding on the first day permit a prognosis. Measurement of intracranial pressure is necessary for monitoring of intracranial complications, but can only make a contribution to prognosis when a critical intracranial pressure is reached. There is a slight correlation between the severity of the EEG alteration and the later outcome on the second day. If an alpha EEG is found on the first day, the prognosis in all cases is not so poor as assumed by other authors[4].

References

1. Dietrich, K., Gaab, M., Knoblich, O. E., Schupp, J., Ott, B., A new miniaturized system for monitoring the epidural pressure in children and adults. Neuropädiatrie 8 (1977), 21—28.
2. Jennett, B., Clinical brain swelling, oedema or engorgement (Glasgow). Symposium on Brain Edema, 28th Sept. (1978), Rotterdam.
3. Jennett, B., Outcome after coma due to head injury. Excerpta Medica No. 427, p. 256 (1977).
4. Vignaendra, V., Wilkas, R. J., Copass, M. K., Chatrian, G. E., Electroencephalographic rhythms of alpha frequency in comatose patients after cardiopulmonary arrest. Neurology 24 (1974), 582—588.

Acta Neurochirurgica, Suppl. 28, 63—65 (1979)
© by Springer-Verlag 1979

Neurosurgical University Clinic, Groningen, The Netherlands

Symptoms of Temporal Lobe Contusions in the Early Period Post-Trauma

J. M. Minderhoud

With 3 Figures

In head-injured patients local lesions, especially of the fronto-temporal region, can play an important role in the outcome. The mental sequelae caused by these kinds of lesions can be a severe handicap in the rehabilitation of these patients.

As was found in a pilot study a correlation is present between long lasting confusion, disorientation and behaviour disturbances after regaining consciousness, and the amount of mental sequelae later on.

In a study of 139 head-injured patients with a duration of unconsciousness for more than 24 hours three groups of patients were recognized. These were: a group of patients with confusion and disorientation for a long period (> 9 days) after regaining consciousness (n = 50); a group of patients without this period of long lasting confusion (n = 45), and a group with a moderate period of confusion only (4-9 days).

These groups were made based on the clinical impression and on the time period between the moment the motor score of the Glasgow coma scale had returned to normal (M = 6) and the moment a normal verbal score (V = 5) could be scored.

Significant differences were found between the first and the second groups. The first group, for which the term temporal lobe contusion was used, differed from the second one;

a) the course of recovery in the early days after trauma as scored the Glasgow coma scale predicted a better outcome than was actually found at six months after trauma (Fig. 1);

b) the majority of the patients in this group had local slow wave activity on the electroencephalogram in the left temporal region;

c) a large number of mental sequelae were present at six months

E. M. V. Score at:	G. R.	M. D.$_{(t)}$	M. D.$_{(c)}$
Admission	10.5	8.3	5.2
24 H Best	11.3	9.9	5.4
2–4 D Best	12.7	11.4	6.0
5–7 D Best	13.4	12.6	6.9

Fig. 1. Outcome at six month posttrauma. G. R. good recovery; M. D. moderate disability; $_{(t)}$ temporal lobe contusion; $_{(c)}$ diffuse contusion

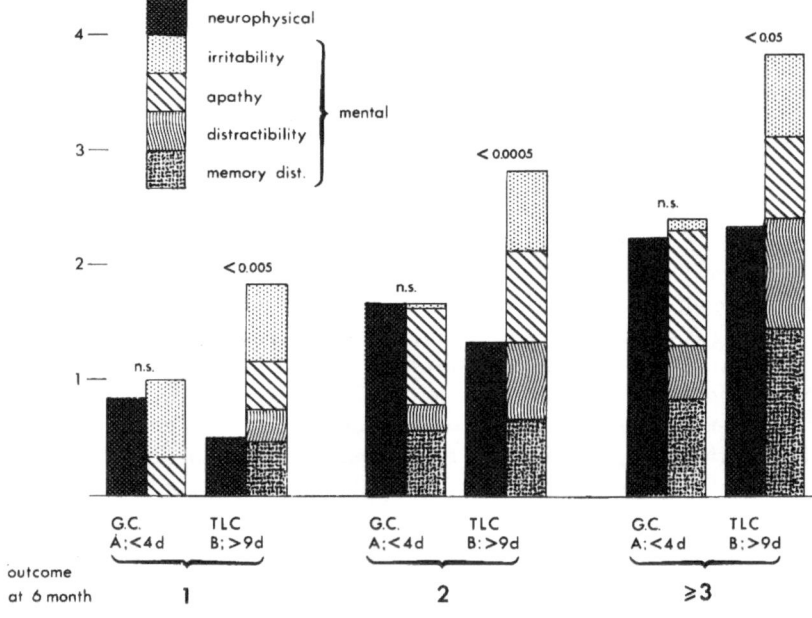

Fig. 2. Neurophysical and mental sequelae in patients with a good recovery (1), a moderate disability (2) or a severe disability (> 3) at six month after trauma. G.C. general contusion, T.L.C. temporal lobe contusion

after trauma, causing the relatively poor outcome of these patients (Fig. 2).

Electro-encephalographic recordings made in the first week after trauma, could detect this kind of lesion even during coma, because of the predictive values of the local slow wave activity in the left temporal region and, to a lesser degree, of diffuse slowing on the right side

If EEG shows slow wave activity	The patient has a general contusion	Temporal lobe contuison
1. Left parieto-temporal	3	23
2. Right-sided diffuse	3	8
	6 (6.3 %)	31 (32.6 %)
3. Any other place	39 (41.0 %)	19 (20.1 %)

Fig. 3

(Fig. 3). The differences between patients with a co-called temporal lobe contusion and those with more diffuse contusions were very clear in the group with a moderate disability at six month after trauma. The major difference was caused by memory disturbances and by irritability and tendency to agression, while in patients with a diffuse contusion a larger amount of inactivity was found (Fig. 3).

Acta Neurochirurgica, Suppl. 28, 66—69 (1979)
© by Springer-Verlag 1979

c) Intracranial Pressure, Cerebral Blood Flow, and
Computerized Tomography

Neurochirurgische Universitätsklinik, Köln,
Federal Republic of Germany

Significance of Intracranial Pressure and Neurological Deficit as Prognostic Factors in Acute Severe Brain Lesions

K. E. Richard and R. A. Frowein

With 2 Figures

Until now efforts to obtain an early prognosis in patients with acute traumatic brain lesions have been mainly based on the neurological condition and on metabolic parameters such as blood gases and acid-base values. Moreover during recent years long-term intracranial pressure measurement has become a predominant clinical topic. The significance of intracranial pressure increase with regard to the prognosis of patients with acute brain lesions, however, has until now been insufficiently assessed.

Material and Methods

In 231 patients with acute brain lesions the mean ventricular fluid pressure (VFP x̄) was calculated from continuous one day pressure curves. Repeatedly during one day the state of consciousness and the neurological global function (level of consciousness, state of responsiveness, pupillary reactions, motor functions, state of tonus, respiration) were examined. These parameters as well as the ages of the patients (infants as well as teenagers—0-19 years; young adults of 20-39 years; older adults of over 40 years) were compared with the outcome (survival; early death *i.e.* up to the 14th day; later death *i.e.* after the 14th post-traumatic/operative day).

Results

1. *Age* (Fig. 1).

In the range of pressure values not pathologically elevated (VFP x̄ 0-20 mm Hg) 88 per cent of the infants and youths, 79 per cent of the young adults, and 54 per cent of the older adults survived.

State of Consciousness, Ventricular Fluid Pressure,
Age of Patients, and Prognosis [231 patients]

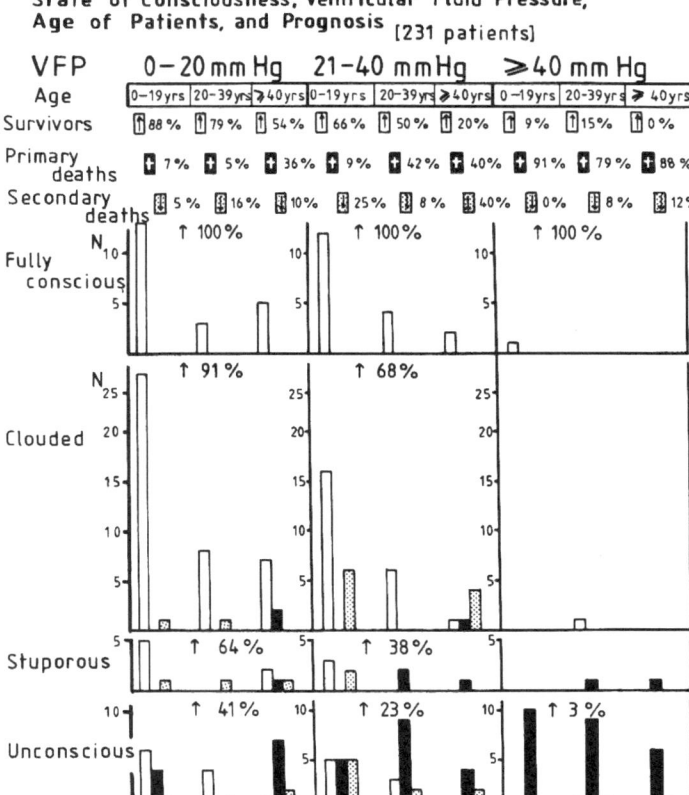

Fig. 1

In the higher ranges of VFP x̄ the survival rate decreased and in the older adults with very high pressure values above 40 mm Hg survival rate dropped to 0 per cent.

2. *Age of the patients and level of consciousness* (Fig. 1).

All of the patients with full consciousness as well as most of the clouded patients survived (white columns).

Pressures more than 40 mm Hg in these cases were measured in only two patients.

Most of the stuporous as well as of the unconscious patients died (black and grey columns).

With increasing disturbance of consciousness and increasing VFP x̄ the percentage of the survivors dropped from 100 to 3 per cent.

3. As to the relation of *intracranial pressure and neurological global function* in general the same trend of decreasing survival rates can be observed, both in the direction of increasing neurological disturbances and increasing intracranial pressure (Fig. 1). The influence of age was also evident in these cases. With very severe neurological deficit (unconsciousness with hyperextension movements and disturbed

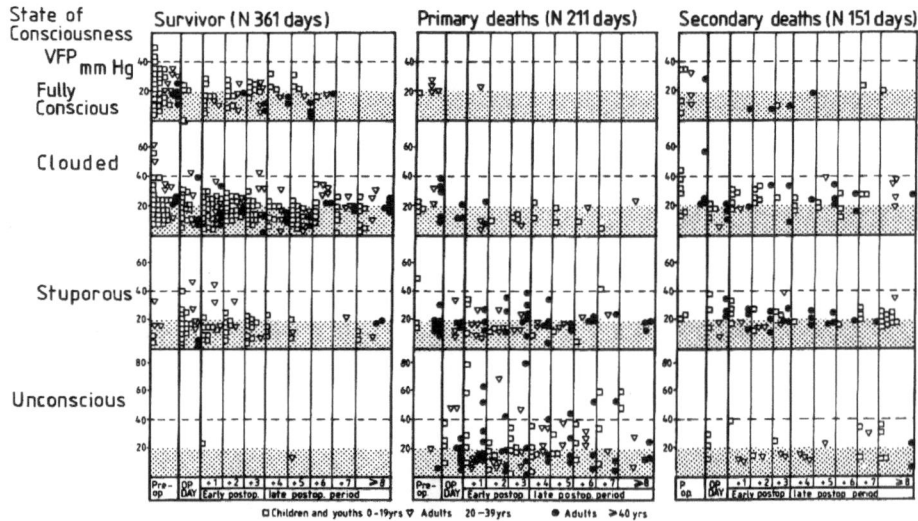

Fig. 2

pupillary reactions) no adult patient with a VFP $\bar{x}$ more than 20 mm Hg survived.

4. *Significance of disturbed state of consciousness or of disturbance of global neurological functions with regard to the time factor* (Fig. 2).

In the early post-traumatic/operative course VFP $\bar{x}$ values scattered considerably and with no relation to the state of consciousness, mostly in those patients who died in the early course. No patient with a VFP $\bar{x}$ above 40 mm Hg survived except for one child.

In the further course all patients with lasting unconsciousness and a VFP $\bar{x}$ higher than 20 mm Hg always died.

High grade neurological disturbances were only survived when the VFP $\bar{x}$ decreased to a level of 20 mm Hg until the 4th day.

Conclusion

Pressure increases appearing first of all under treatment are an expression of the decompensated regulation of intracranial volume. In this regard they are an indirect sign of the basic brain lesion. On the other hand intracranial pressure increases turned out to be a negative prognostic factor in cases of a severe brain lesion.

Further experiences must show whether the survival rate of the patients with severe brain lesions essentially improves after normalization of intracranial pressure, as early as possible.

Acta Neurochirurgica, Suppl. 28, 70—73 (1979)
© by Springer-Verlag 1979

Neurosurgical Department, C. S. "1° de Octobre", Madrid, Spain

Prognostic Value of the Intracranial Pressure Levels During the Acute Phase of Severe Head Injuries

R. D. Lobato, J. J. Rivas, J. M. Portillo, L. Velasco,
F. Cordobes, J. Esparza, and E. Lamas

Introduction

Intracranial pressure (ICP) continuous monitoring after severe craniocerebral trauma seems to be a valuable technique in order to improve the therapeutic management of the patients[5,7,10]. Nevertheless its value in predicting the ultimate outcome of the individual patient remains controversial. Some authors have found a good correlation between ICP levels and outcome[1,7,10,11] while others deny this correlation[2,5,6,9]. These discrepancies may be explained in part by the heterogeneous clinicopathological groups of patients included in some series.

In this paper we analyze the reliability of the ICP levels in predicting the final outcome of 53 patients suffering severe head injuries.

Briefly, patients in this series have been separated into two groups. One group is formed by patients who received emergency craniotomies in order to evacuate intracranial mass lesions. The other group includes those patients presenting diffuse brain damage (the so-called primary brain stem contusion). ICP monitoring was achieved during the acute phase (3-7 days) of the disease in every patient.

Correlation between the initial ICP levels and outcome in these two groups of patients will be discussed.

Material and Methods

This study is based on the records of 53 patients (12 women and 41 men) with ages ranging from 3 to 68 years (average 32.1 years) admitted in a comatose state after suffering severe blunt head injuries. Eleven patients also had relevant traumatic injuries in other parts of the body. Thirty-nine patients showed decerebrate or decorticate postures (posturing), while 14 had purposeful or semipurposeful reactions to pain stimulation (not posturing).

Patients appearing arreflexic and apnoeic on admission, those receiving delayed surgery, and those others dying of medical causes have been not included in this series.

All the 53 patients had cerebral angiography or CT scan studies on admission. In 35 cases showing expanding lesions ICP monitoring was started immediately after the emergency craniotomy. In cases showing no apparent operable lesions ICP was also monitored soon after diagnosis. In most cases intraventricular fluid pressure was measured by means of a polyethylene catheter placed in the right frontal ventricular horn. In ten cases ICP was measured epidurally by means of a fibre-optic sensor (Ladd system). In five cases a subarachnoid screw was employed. In many patients CSF Volume/ Pressure relationships were estimated sequentially according to current techniques[8]. In a few cases the CSF and blood lactate levels were measured. Some patients had arterial pressure continuous recordings, this parameter being periodically measured for short intervals in the remaining patients.

Standardized neurosurgical care has been applied in this series. All patients received dexamethasone 4-8 mg every 6 hours for 3-4 days, this dosage being progressively reduced. Patients were intubated and artificially ventilated for variable periods (rate 11-14 minutes, tidal 12-15 cc/kg). Most of them were hyperventilated because of raised ICP. Arterial pCO_2 was kept between 26-32 mm Hg and pO_2 above 75 mm Hg. If ICP remained elevated despite surgery and hyperventilation, then ventricular fluid drainage, when feasible, or hyperosmolar solutions or both were employed; as a rule mannitol has been used in doses of 0.3 g/kg body weight injected as a bolus.

Outcome of patients in our practice is classified according to the scale of Jennett and Bond[4], but for simplicity we will use here the broad categories of Functional survival versus Vegetative-Dead.

Results and Comments

The final outcomes of our patients in relation to the anatomical diagnosis, the presence or absence of posturing, and the ICP levels is reflected in Table 1. We did not measure ICP before surgery in the group of patients with space-occupying lesions, but postoperative ICP monitoring represents in our experience an important aid both for improving the management and for predicting the final outcome in these patients. In fact, as may be appreciated from Table 1, patients showing sustained intracranial hypertension (ICP > 40 mm Hg) after surgical descompressions had a poorer outcome than those showing normal ICP levels, the difference being statistically significant (p < 0.05). On the other hand, ICP levels seem to have also a predictive power in patients with diffuse brain damage. All patients with this diagnosis in our series showed uni- or bilateral posturing, and only 28 % of those having normal ICP died, while 87 % of those with ICP levels higher than 40 mm Hg also died, the difference being statistically significant (p < 0.05).

Impaired CO_2 response of the cerebral blood flow has been found in patients showing severe brain damage after head injuries[3], and

Table 1. *Relationship Between Cerebral Lesion, Motor Responses*, ICP Levels, and Outcome*

Diagnosis	Mean ICP (mm Hg)			Total
	0–20	20–40	> 40	
Intracranial mass lesions				
Epidural haematoma	$4\left(\dfrac{3\vert1}{0\vert0}\right)$	$0\left(\dfrac{0\vert0}{0\vert0}\right)$	$1\left(\dfrac{0\vert0}{1\vert0}\right)$	$5\left(\dfrac{3\vert1}{1\vert0}\right)$
Subdural haematoma	$4\left(\dfrac{1\vert2}{1\vert0}\right)$	$1\left(\dfrac{1\vert0}{0\vert0}\right)$	$2\left(\dfrac{0\vert1}{1\vert0}\right)$	$7\left(\dfrac{2\vert3}{2\vert0}\right)$
Cerebral contusion	$8\left(\dfrac{2\vert4}{2\vert0}\right)$	$6\left(\dfrac{1\vert3}{0\vert2}\right)$	$9\left(\dfrac{1\vert1}{7\vert0}\right)$	$23\left(\dfrac{4\vert8}{9\vert2}\right)$
Diffuse brain lesion	$7\left(\dfrac{5\vert0}{2\vert0}\right)$	$10\left(\dfrac{2\vert0}{1\vert0}\right)$	$8\left(\dfrac{1\vert0}{7\vert0}\right)$	$18\left(\dfrac{8\vert0}{10\vert0}\right)$
Total	$23\left(\dfrac{11\vert7}{5\vert0}\right)$	$10\left(\dfrac{4\vert3}{1\vert2}\right)$	$20\left(\dfrac{2\vert2}{16\vert0}\right)$	$53\left(\dfrac{17\vert12}{22\vert\ 2}\right)$

* Motor responses at admission.

Key: Functional survival $\left(\dfrac{-\vert-}{-\vert-}\right)$
Vegetative died

Posturing   Not posturing

defective autoregulation may contribute to maintain intracranial hypertension in such cases. In this sense we have observed that the response of ICP to increased hypocapnia (ICP fall after increased hyperventilation) was usually better in patients who survive than in those who died. An explanation for this fact could be that patients responding to hypocapnia had a relatively greater amount of healthy brain tissue than those who did not respond or who scarcely responded.

In our experience estimation of the CSF Volume/Pressure relationships is useful in predicting decompensations of the intracranial dynamics but has no prognostic value by itself.

In conclusion we believe that ICP levels found during the acute phase of severe head injuries provide predictive power for outcome.

References

1. Becker, D. P., Vries, J. K., Sakalas, R., et al., Early prognosis in head injury based on motor posturing, oculocephalic reflexes and intracranial pressure. In Head Injuries (McLaurin, R. L., ed.), pp. 27—30. New York: Grune Stratton, Inc. 1976.
2. Bruce, D. A., Langfitt, T. W., Miller, J. D., et al., Regional cerebral blood flow intracranial pressure and brain metabolism in comatose patients. J. Neurosurg. 38 (1973), 131—144.
3. Envoldsen, E. M., Jensen, F. T., Autoregulation and CO_2 responses of cerebral-blood flow in patients with acute severe head injury. J. Neurosurg. 48 (1978), 689—703.
4. Jennett, B., Bond, M., Assessment of outcome after severe brain damage. A practical scale. Lancet 1 (1975), 480—484.
5. Jennett, B., Johnston, I. H., The uses of intracranial pressure monitoring in clinical management. In Intracranial Pressure (Brock, M., Dietz, H., eds.), pp. 353—356. Berlin-Heidelberg-New York: Springer. 1972.
6. Johnston, I. H., Johnston, J. A., Jennett, B., Intracranial pressure changes following head injury. Lancet 2 (1970), 433—436.
7. Miller, J. D., Becker, D. P., Ward, J. D., et al., Significance of intracranial hypertension in severe head injury. J. Neurosurg. 47 (1977), 503—516.
8. Miller, J. D., Garibi, J., Pickard, J. D., Induced changes of cerebrospinal fluid volume. Arch. Neurol. 28 (1973), 265—269.
9. Tindall, G. T., Fleischer, A. S., Intracranial pressure monitoring and prognosis in closed head injury. In Head Injuries (McLaurin, R. L., ed.), pp. 31—34. New York: Grune Stratton, Inc. 1976.
10. Troupp, H., Intraventricular pressure in patients with severe brain injuries. J. Trauma 7 (1967), 875—883.
11. Vapalahti, M., Troupp, H., Prognosis for patients with severe brain injuries. Brit. Med. J. 3 (1971), 404—407.

Acta Neurochirurgica, Suppl. 28, 74—77 (1979)

Department of Neurotraumatology, Central Department for Emergencies, and Intensive Therapy in the General Hospital of Friedrichshain, Berlin (Medical superintendent: OMR Prof. Dr. sc. med. Scheidler)

The Prognostic Value of Intracranial Pressure Monitoring After Severe Head Injuries

H. Feldmann, G. Klages, F. Gärtner, and J. Scharfenberg

With 2 Figures

Common experiences prove the measuring of brain pressure after severe head injuries to be useful in the treatment of brain swelling. The measurement of brain pressure in correlation with the initial and with later post-traumatic neurological examinations during the first seven days after an accident makes possible some statements about prognosis and survival.

Material

On the basis of a series of 38 patients the practical use of ICP long-term monitoring in severe head injuries is analysed. All our patients suffered from a severe disorder in consciousness with no eye-opening or verbal responses, as described in the Glasgow Coma Scale of 1977. They only showed motor responses.

The 38 patients were between 6 weeks and 80 years old (on an average 35 years of age). Twenty-six were male, the other 12 were female. Thirty patients were the victims of traffic accidents. Eight had been injured in other ways.

Table 1 illustrates the distribution of complications after head injuries. Three out of 38 patients suffered from an epidural haematoma. 7 from an subdural haematoma, and 28 from an intracerebral mass lesion or other diffuse brain damage. The best prognosis was with epidural and subdural haematomas. A high percentage of patients with diffuse brain damage died.

In all patients the intracranial pressure was monitored through a polyethylene intraventricular or subarachnoid catheter, inserted in the operating theatre. The patients who suffered from diffuse brain damage had intraventricular catheters, whereas in the surgically treated patients the catheter was placed in the subarachnoid space on the side of the surgical intervention.

Table 1. *Outcome After Severe Head Injuries*

	Number of patients	Outcome				
		Good recovery	Moderate disability	Severe disability	Persistent veget. rate	Death
Epidural haematoma	3	2	—	—	—	1
Subdural haematoma	7	1	1	4	—	1
Intracerebral mass lesion	16	1	2	1	2	10
Diffuse brain injury	12	1	1	3	1	6
Total (per cent)	38	5 = 13.2	4 = 10.5	8 = 21.1	3 = 7.9	18 = 47.4

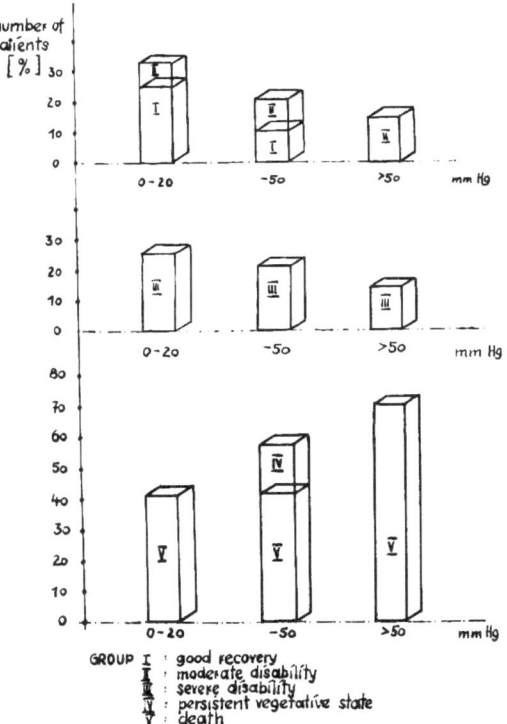

Fig. 1. Outcome from severe head injuries related to course of intracranial pressure during monitoring

Results

Figure 1 shows the outcome from severe head injuries. related to the course of intracranial pressure during monitoring. There is a clear correlation between the level of the pressure and the outcome.

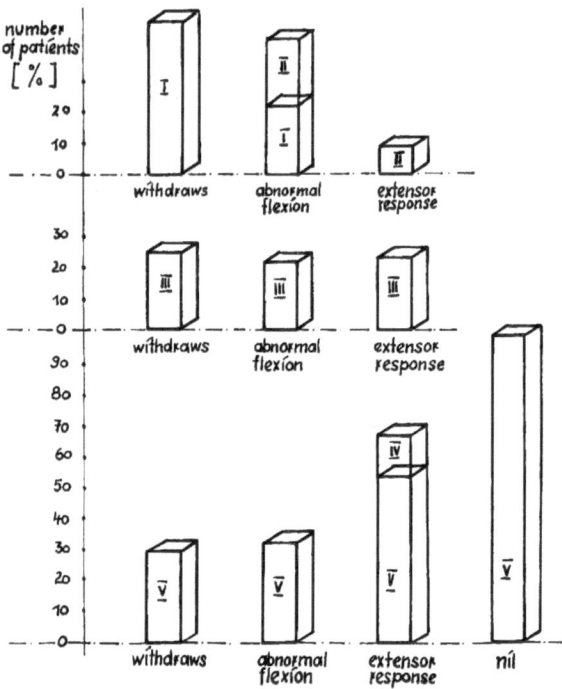

Fig. 2. Best motor response by admission (Glasgow Coma Scale) and outcome (all patients without eye opening and verbal response)

In the group of patients with brain pressure exceeding 50 mm Hg more than 70% died. Intracerebral pressure (ICP) ranging from 20 mm Hg to 50 mm Hg occurred in patients with intracranial mass lesions and diffuse brain injuries and also in patients with space-claiming haematomas. In this group the mortality amounted to 50%. In the group with a good recovery most patients showed an ICP below 20 mm Hg.

It may be considered to be an accident that all patients with a persistent vegetative syndrome were found in the group with a brain pressure ranging from 20 to 50 mm Hg. In the second and third groups with moderate and severe disability, it is impossible to detect a direct association between the level of brain pressure and outcome.

A relative reliable symptom for a poor outcome seems to be the appearance of Lundberg-waves A. They developed in seven of our cases. There were a lethal issue in four patients and a severe disability in two cases; one patient remained moderately disabled.

Figure 2 shows the relationship between the neurological status and the outcome. The level of unconsciousness assessed by the motor responses (withdrawals, abnormal flexion, or extensor response) correlates with the poor outcome. The early appearance of extensor response is a bad symptom and is often (in more than 50%) connected with a lethal issue.

In the last group with a mortality rate of 100% there were patients who had no motor responses at the first neurological examination.

Summary

ICP monitoring appears not to be essential for the prognosis of head injury patients, but it may be of some clinical value in association with the neurological status and other clinical data.

The results of ICP measurement show that a high level in brain pressure and the poor outcome have a better correlation with one another than a lower level of brain pressure and a good recovery.

Acta Neurochirurgica, Suppl. 28, 78—84 (1979)
© by Springer-Verlag 1979

Departments of Surgical Neurology and Neuropathology*,
University of Edinburgh, Scotland

Prognostic Signs During Continuous Monitoring of the Ventricular Fluid Pressure in Patients With Severe Brain Injury

S. A. Tsementzis, A. Gordon*, and F. J. Gillingham

With 2 Figures

Introduction

Continuous monitoring of the intracranial pressure (ICP) may be of value in the prognosis of severe brain damage. High pressures have been recorded in those severe brain injuries in which the ICP has been measured, and neurosurgeons have stressed the close relationship between the level of intracranial hypertension and clinical deterioration (Lundberg et al. 1965, Vapalhati and Troupp 1971, Jorgensen 1973). There are, however, examples in the literature of patients with very severe head injuries with a normal ICP (Jennett and Johnston 1972). In other words, while the absolute level of ICP may be indicative of severe brain damage, it cannot alone be used as a prognostic criterion.

Our experience suggests that fluctuations in the level of the ICP and the amplitude and frequency response of the cerebral pulse may be reliable indicators of changes in cerebrovascular haemodynamics; in particular, the morphology of the tracings may provide incontrovertible evidence of arrest of cerebral circulation. Changes in the diastolic blood pressure and the ventricular CSF volume may also be of prognostic significance.

Material and Methods

Thirty cases with severe brain damage due to either a closed head injury or cerebrovascular accident were studied. Eleven of them, eight males and three females, aged 12 to 48 years, died; they developed changes of their ventricular fluid pressure (VFP) wave form which, characteristically, differed from those seen in the nineteen cases who survived their primary injury.

In this paper we compare the findings in these two groups, directing attention particularly to the non-survivors.

The method used for the measurement of the VFP was that of Lundberg (1960). A catheter was inserted into the right lateral ventricle, and its extracranial end was connected through a rigid tube to a Bell and Howell pressure transducer. The VFP was displayed at constant amplification by a paper recorder (Bryans, 2800) for a period of 3 to 8 days.

Results

I. Survivor Group

In nine cases we observed plateau waves which attained a maximum value of 90 mm Hg. The amplitude and rate of the cerebral pulse was increased during the development of each such wave. At the end of each, the VFP wave form regained its preplateau appearance as regards its absolute value, amplitude, and frequency.

The increase in the heart rate and in both the systolic and diastolic arterial pressures recorded was also restored to normal levels at the end of each plateau wave.

Withdrawal of a few millilitres of CSF is known to reduce the VFP more effectively than any dehydrating agent or drug. In addition to the recording system we, therefore, set up a drainage system so that when the VFP was dangerously increased ventricular CSF could drain intermittently into a flask sited 15 cm above the patient's head. Towards the end of each plateau wave a few drops of CSF drained into the flask, whereas prior to the development of an A wave CSF did not drain.

II. Non-survivor Group

During continous recording of the VFP all of these patients showed a moderate to high resting pressure and several A waves, the plateau level of which varied from 80 to 110 mm Hg (ct 90 mm Hg). In each of these cases, after a run of A waves, the VFP fell to a level below the previous elevated interplateau levels, and the frequency and amplitude of its oscillations was slightly reduced. This fall progressed over a period of 1-6 hours, and then gradually the pressure rose to an even higher interplateau level than previously. The elevated pressure was maintained; no more plateau waves occurred and the patient was clinically dead (Figs. 1a, b, c). The oscillations and the amplitude of the cerebral pulse showed a progressive reduction and never recovered their preplateau appearance.

Later recording showed two different patterns of VFP tracing: a) Cerebral pulsation disappears and the now flat VFP tracing drops to a negative value; weak pulsations are temporarily restored by injection

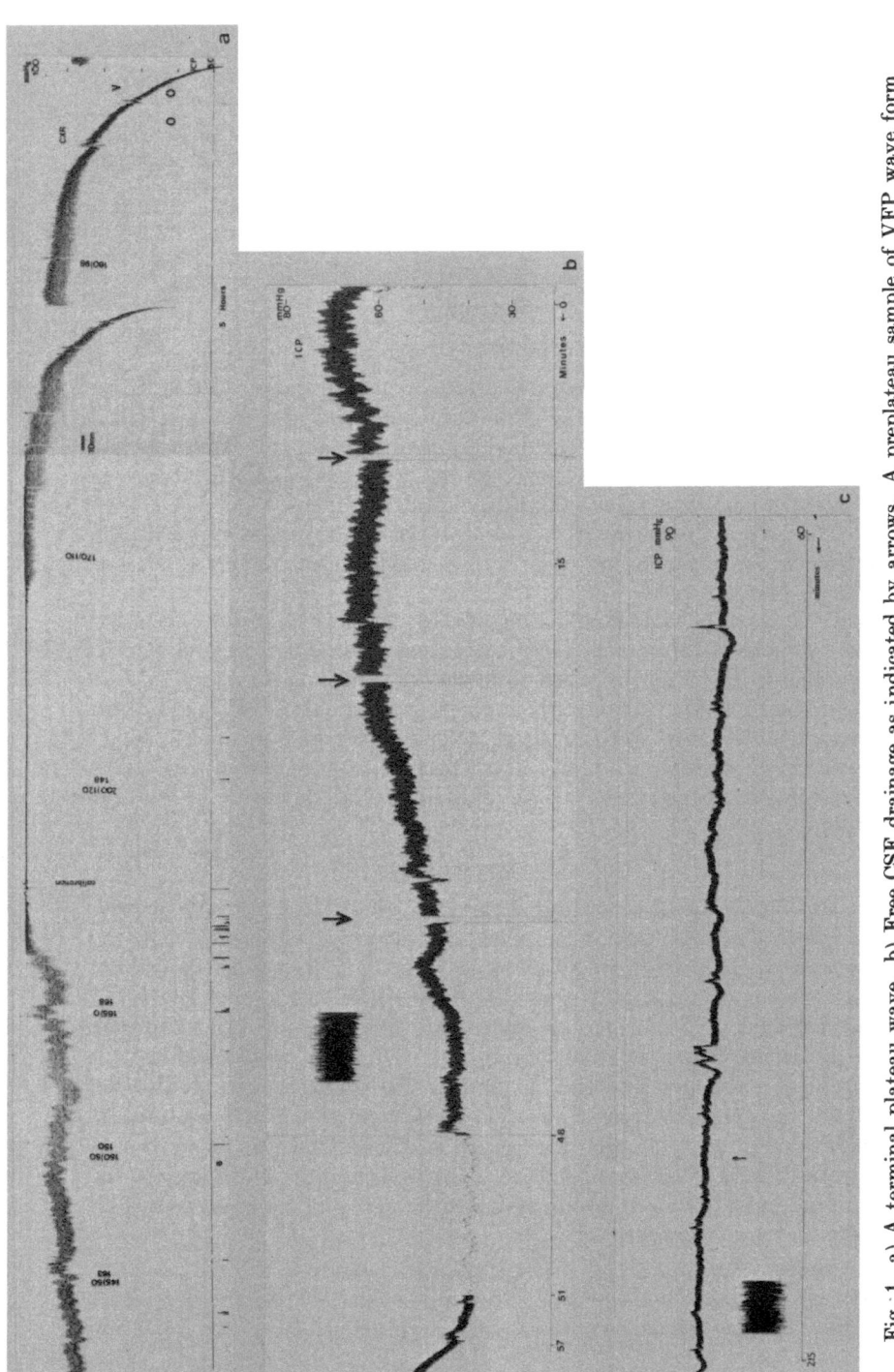

Fig. 1. a) A terminal plateau wave. b) Free CSF drainage as indicated by arrows. A preplateau sample of VFP wave form above tracing on the left. c) Arrow below trace shows time of compression of the external jugular veins. A preplateau sample of VFP wave form on the left bottom

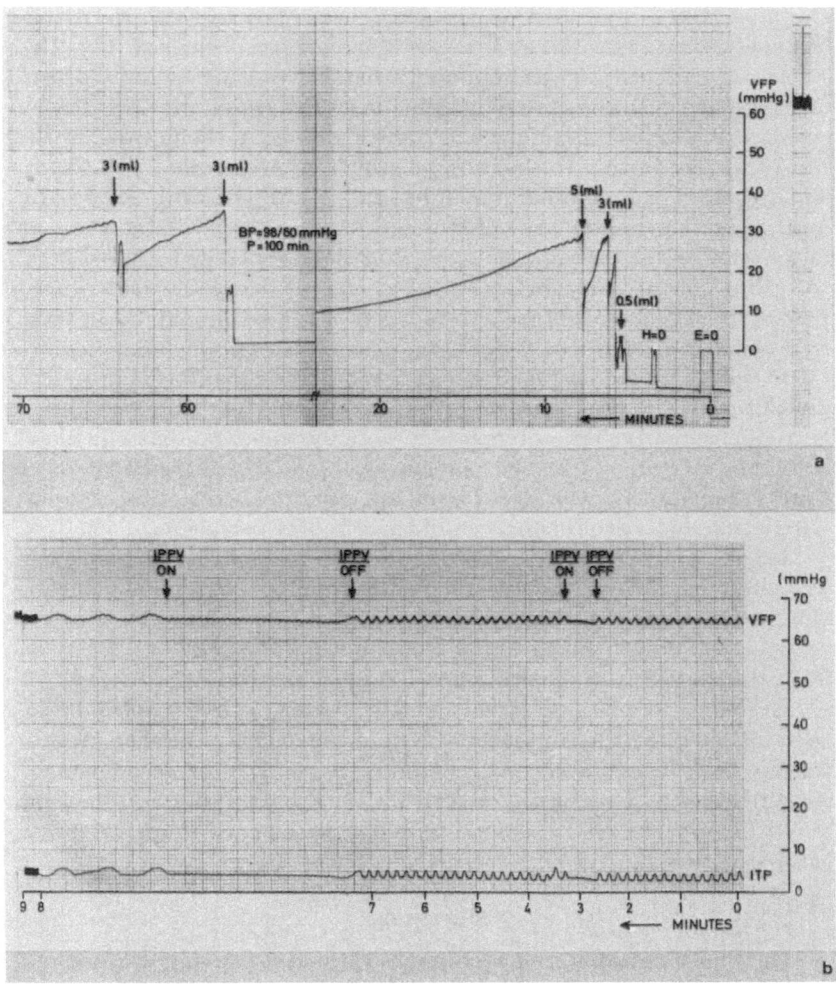

Fig. 2. a) Disappearance of cerebral pulsations. b) Ventricular pulsations are locked in phase with the respiratory (ITP) excursions; when ventilator (IPPV) is switched off the previously masked shallow Hering-Traube-Mayer waves are seen at a subnormal frequency. (*E* Electronic zero, *H* hydraulic zero)

of a few ml of water into the ventricle (Fig. 2a). b) The ventricular pulsations are locked in phase with the respiratory excursions; when the ventilator is switched off the previously masked shallow Hering-Traube-Mayer waves are observed at a subnormal frequency (Fig. 2b).

In one patient who was kept on mechanical ventilation for two days after he developed the above changes the VFP was not altered either by compression of both jugular veins or by a change in the position of the head from the resting to the upright (which induced some 30° flexion). The injection of a minimal amount of saline into the ventricle rapidly and greatly increased the VFP without altering the frequency and amplitude of the cerebral pulse, in complete contrast with the VFP recordings of the survivor group. The cerebral perfusion was assessed before, during, and after the development of the terminal plateau wave by subtraction of the ICP from the mean systemic arterial pressure (MSAP). As we see in Fig. 1a, a representative recording, during the development and the initial stage of the plateau level the increased ICP is compensated for by an increase in both systolic and diastolic blood pressure. At the end of the plateau level, the MSAP is equal to or slightly greater than the ICP, producing, severe slowing of the cerebral circulation and virtual cessation of the cerebral perfusion.

Interestingly enough, towards the end of the ultimate plateau wave we could not detect the diastolic pressure by sphygmomanometer, whereas the systolic was easily registered. A low diastolic pressure reappeared later in the declining phase of the VFP (Fig. 1a). Later on both the systolic and diastolic pressures became significantly low.

In five patients we observed a small amount of CSF (4 to 10 drops) to drain into the flask immediately after each of the earlier plateau waves, but the later plateau complexes were not so accompanied. Administration of mannitol or glycerol at this stage did not alter the VFP. Finally, the characteristic terminal plateau wave appeared and the patient died.

Discussion

The CSF pulsations are synchronous with the arterial pulse, and are modified by respiration. Most workers accept that the pulsation is arterial in origin and this is thought by some to be transmitted from the basal and spinal arteries (Antoni 1946, Dunbar et al. 1966) and by others from the ventricular choroid plexuses (Bering 1955). The amplitude and the frequency of the cerebral pulse may be altered by variations in the ICP (Ryder et al. 1952).

Cerebral pulsations are normally damped by the operation of those mechanisms which tend to prevent the ICP from rising, namely CSF displacement, reduction or cessation of CSF production, or reduction of intracranial blood volume as a result of change in cerebral vasomotor tone. Progressive elevation of the ICP results in sequential exhaustion of these compensatory mechanisms. Damping of the CSF pulsation being thus abolished, its amplitude increases and the wave form comes to resemble that of the arterial pulse.

This sequence of events is commonly seen during the development of plateau waves. These are thought to be produced by rapid reversible increases in the cerebral blood volume, but intermittent blockage of the CSF pathways or alterations in the water exchange into the brain tissue have also been incriminated (Lundberg 1960). Our patients, all of whom had prolonged intracranial hypertension, most probably had lost some of their buffering capacity. It has been reported that during intracranial hypertension the CSF volume is the first to be lost, initially by displacement into the spinal subarachnoid space and secondly by diminished production directly due to the increased ICP (Shapiro 1974). Sudden blockage of the CSF pathways produces a relatively small and gradual elevation of the VFP. In order to account for cyclic alterations in brain volume by means of water exchange one would have to postulate a rapidly reversible mechanism whose existence is, in general, denied.

The development of A waves, therefore, would appear to be due to reversible changes in cerebral blood volume which are mediated by the vasomotor tone, an argument which is reinforced by the progressive loss of ventricular CSF and the major haemodynamic changes that occur during and after the last A complex. Compensatory mechanisms are to some extent preserved during all except the terminal complex. When VFP exceeds some critical level the elevation of the MSAP is no longer effective.

We are unable to explain the disappearance of the radial diastolic pressure towards the end of the ultimate plateau complex or its reappearance. Direct measurement of the systemic arterial pressure may provide evidence as regards these changes in the diastolic pressure during a terminal plateau wave.

Reactive hyperaemia following a period of intracranial hypertension is a phenomenon known since the experimental work of Forbes and Nason (1935) and today is well accepted. This, we think, may be the explanation of the CSF drainage following a plateau wave. We suggest that such hyperaemia increases the intracranial volume in the recovery phase of the A wave. Initially, this is compensated for by the displacement of CSF, as long as this is available; its disappearance means the loss of an important compensatory factor, and further increases in ICP would be buffered only by adjustments of the brain blood volume. The brain blood volume can, of course, accommodate to

6*

intracranial hypertension but only to a limited extent and for a limited period of time. As the occurrence of this phenomenon implies a certain integrity of the compensatory mechanisms for intracranial hypertension its restriction to the survivor group is not unexpected.

Synopsis

1. The presence of CSF in cases with intracranial hypertension is a favourable prognostic sign; its absence is indicative of a progressive and potentially lethal intracranial hypertension.

2. A series of characteristic changes in the absolute value of the VFP as well as in the amplitude and rate of the cerebral pulse can provide reliable evidence of the integrity of the cerebral circulation.

3. Short-lasting disappearance of the diastolic pressure towards the end of the ultimate plateau wave and subsequent significant lowering of both the systolic and diastolic pressures is an additional bad prognostic sign.

References

Antoni, N., Pressure curves from the CSF. Acta med. scand. (suppl.) *170* (1946), 431—462.
Bering, E. A., Choroid plexus and arterial pulsation of CSF. Demonstration of the choroid plexuses as a CSF pump. AMA Arch. Neurol. Psychiat. *73* (1955), 165—172.
Dunbar, H. S., Guthrie, T. H., Karpell, B., A study of the CSF pulse wave. Arch. Neurol. *14* (1966), 624—630.
Forbes, H. S., Nason, G. I., Cerebral circulation; vascular responses to hypertonic solutions and withdrawal of CSF. Arch. Neurol. Psychiat. (Chic.) *34* (1935), 533—547.
Jennett, B., Johnston, I. H., The use of ICP monitoring in clinical management. In: ICP. Experimental and Clinical Aspects. (Brock and Dietz, eds.), pp. 353—356. Berlin-Heidelberg-New York: Springer. 1972.
Jorgensen, P. B., Clinical deterioration prior to brain death related to progressive intracranial hypertension. Acta Neurochir. (Wien) *28* (1973), 29—40.
Lundberg, N., Continuous recording and control of ventricular fluid pressure in Neurosurgical practice. Acta Psychiat. Scand. *36* (suppl. 149), (1960), 1—191.
Lundberg, N., Troupp, H., Lorin, H., Continuous recording of the ventricular fluid pressure in patients with severe acute traumatic brain injury. J. Neurosurg. *22* (1965), 581—590.
Ryder, H. W., Espey, F. W., Kimbell, F. D., Posenauer, A., Podolsky, B., Evans, J. P., Modification of effect of cerebral blood flow on the CSF pressure by variations in the craniospinal blood volume. AMA Arch. Neurol. Psychiat. *68* (1952), 170—174.
Shapiro, H., Anaesthesia, intensive care and the Neurosurgical patient. In 25th Annual refresher course lectures, October 12-13, 1974, Annual meeting of the American Society of Anaesthesiologists. Ed. in U.S.A., pp. 212: 1—13.
Vapalahti, M., Troupp, H., Prognosis for patients with severe brain injuries. Brit. med. J. *3* (1971), 404—407.

Acta Neurochirurgica, Suppl. 28, 85 (1979)
© by Springer-Verlag 1979

Neurosurgical Clinic of the Municipal Hospital Nordstadt,
Hannover, Federal Republic of Germany

CT, EEG, and ICP Recordings During Intensive Care of Acute Head Injuries

M. Samii, K. von Wild, H. Baumann, K.-D. Lerch,
J.-R. Moringlane, and A. Sepehrnia

Experience has demonstrated that CT is superior to any other technique in the diagnosis of acute head injuries and in the follow-up as well. CT allows an accurate evaluation of the contributary role of cerebral oedema in production of the mass effects associated with intracranial haematomas, hygromas, and contusions (Lanksch, New, and Scott).

The EEG examination is of great value in assessing brain function during post-traumatic coma, as has been shown by many authors, e.g. Bergamasco, Bergamini, Bricolo, Lorenzoni, and von Wild). Concurrently with the alteration of consciousness, the EEG also shows changes and at the same time the EEG is affected by the other effects of trauma upon the brain.

Continuous monitoring of intracranial pressure (ICP) during intensive care of head injuries has become a generally accepted method (e.g. Brock and Dietz, Reulen, and Schürmann).

The possibility of polygraphic recordings during intensive care allows for an exact and more detailed examination of the brain function and better judgement of prognosis.

In our unit we recorded CT, ICP, and EEG in 20 patients with acute head injuries after operation and in nonoperated patients as well at 1, 2, 3, 4, and 7 days after trauma. CT records with the aid of an EMI 1010 Scanner, and intraventricular or epidural measurement with the aid of a Setham SP 50 transducer and Hellige equipment were also made. The EEG recordings were taken from the scalp, and were analyzed visually and automatically. Using FFT on a BIO 16-computer, a power spectrum was calculated every 4 s for the frequencies of 0–32 Hz with a resolution of 0.25 Hz. The EEG segments analyzed were 160 s long and free of artefacts. All data were correlated with the neurological findings according to the Glasgow coma scale. Results will be demonstrated.

Acta Neurochirurgica, Suppl. 28, 86—88 (1979)

Medical College of Virginia, Richmond, Virginia, U.S.A.

CT Scan, ICP and Early Neurological Evaluation in the Prognosis of Severe Head Injury

J. Douglas Miller, S. K. Gudeman, P. R. S. Kishore, and D. P. Becker

The prognostic value of careful neurological evaluation using standard terminology performed serially over 72 hours in patients with head injuries of designated severity has been shown by Jennett and his colleagues. The growing use of muscle relaxants with artificial ventilation and the increasing interest in the use of induced barbiturate coma reduces the opportunity for serial neurological evaluations over an extended period. Furthermore, there is a need to identify at the earliest possible stage those patients in whom a particularly poor outcome is to be expected, because it is in this group that newer and perhaps riskier therapies are justified. Inclusion of patients in whom a better outcome is to be expected may yield a falsely optimistic view of a test therapy. One solution is to wait for a certain period of time to ascertain that the head injury is serious. This has the disadvantage that it may delay application of therapy to a point where no treatment can be effective because neurological deterioration has become irreversible.

In previous studies we have evaluated ICP monitoring and CT scanning separately to find those features associated with a poor outcome. In this study we assess the value of combining information on the CT scan with ICP data using very simple classifications.

Patients and Methods

We studied 74 patients with closed head injury whose coma score after resuscitation was at or below E2, M5, V2 on the Glasgow Coma Scale. For our data analysis we selected the coma score obtained in the emergency room. We excluded patients who on CT scan had a purely extracerebral mass lesion (41) and classified the CT scan appearances in the 74 patients as a) normal, b) diffuse brain swelling (small or absent ventricles with the shift of midline structures), c) contusion (intraparenchymal lesions of increased density) or

d) mixed (extracerebral lesion plus contusion). ICP was classified normal if it remained below 20 mm Hg or abnormal if it rose about 20 mm Hg during the first three days from injury (in virtually all cases if ICP increased it did so within the first six hours). Outcome of patients was classified using the 5 point scale of Jennett and Bond.

Results

In these 74 patients, two-thirds of whom had EMV scores of 3-7 on admission to the emergency room, there was a poor outcome (severely disabled or dead) in 36 % overall. Poor outcome was less frequent (15 %) in those who showed normal CT scan or diffuse swelling only than in those who had intraparenchymal lesions of increased density (64 % poor outcome—$\chi^2 = 18.94$; P < 0.001). Intracranial hypertension was more frequent in those patients with contusions on CT scan (57 % incidence) than in those with diffuse swelling or normal CT scans (17 % incidence—$\chi^2 = 13.16$; P > 0.001).

Table 1

Outcome	CT scan normal or diffuse swelling		CT scan contusion or mixed lesions	
	GR/MD	SD/Dead	GR/MD	SD/Dead
ICP normal	30 (88 %)	4 (12 %)	10 (71 %)	4 (29 %)
ICP increased	5 (71 %)	2 (28 %)	2 (11 %)	17 (89 %)
	$\chi^2 = 1.31$; n. s.		$\chi^2 = 12.92$; P < 0.001	

Table 2

Outcome	CT scan normal or diffuse swelling		CT scan contusion or mixed lesions	
	GR/MD	SD/Dead	GR/MD	SD/Dead
Coma score on admission				
3/4	0 (0 %)	3 (100 %)	1 (11 %)	8 (89 %)
5/6/7	18 (86 %)	3 (14 %)	8 (50 %)	8 (50 %)
8/9/10	15 (100 %)	9 (0 %)	4 (57 %)	3 (43 %)
11	2 (100 %)	9 (0 %)	0 (0 %)	1 (100 %)

When this information was combined for its significance for outcome it emerged that in patients whose CT scan was normal or showed only diffuse swelling the presence of raised ICP did not influence outcome, whereas in those patients with cerebral contusions there was a strong correlation between raised ICP and a poor outcome (Table 1).

When the value of the coma score obtained in the emergency room was assessed the opposite conclusion was drawn. In those patients with a CT scan showing diffuse swelling or normality poor outcomes were related closely to a low coma score, while in patients with cerebral contusions the coma score on admission was unrelated to outcome (Table 2).

Comment and Conclusions

In patients who arrive comatose at hospital following a head injury or who deteriorate to this state the CT scan permits rapid division of patients into groups which have a different outcome and different incidence of raised ICP. If the CT scan shows normal appearances or only diffuse swelling ICP is usually normal, most patients do well and poor outcomes can be predicted by a low coma score on admission. (It must be borne in mind that this study excludes patients with acute epidural and subdural haematoma unassociated with intraparenchymal contusion haemorrhage.) If the CT scan shows intraparenchymal lesions of increased density there is a 50% chance that the patient will have intracranial hypertension (if there is also an extra-axial mass this rises to 75%). If ICP is normal most patients do well, if ICP is elevated most do badly whether or not surgical decompression is employed. In this group of patients initial coma score does not add to the prediction of a poor outcome.

References

1. Miller, J. D., Becker, D. P., Ward, J. D., Sullivan, H. G., Adams, W. E., Rosner, M. J., Significance of intracranial hypertension in severe head injury. J. Neurosurg. *47* (1977), 503—516.
2. Sweet, R. C., Miller, J. D., Lipper, M., Kishore, P., Becker, D. P., The significance of bilateral abnormalities on the CT scan in patients with severe head injury. Neurosurgery *3* (1978), 16—21.

Acta Neurochirurgica, Suppl. 28, 89—92 (1979)
© by Springer-Verlag 1979

Département d'anesthésiologie de La Pitié (Pr. Ag. P. Viars)*
and Clinique neurochirurgicale de La Pitié (Pr. B. Pertuiset)**

Post-Traumatic Acute Rise of ICP
Related to Subclinical Epileptic Seizures

J. P. Marienne*, G. Robert**, and E. Bagnat*

With 2 Figures

Monitoring of intracranial pressure (ICP) is a routine procedure after severe head injuries. In non-surgical lesions, uncontrolled intracranial hypertension gives a very poor prognosis. The relations between the ICP's high level and épileptic seizures, though not very often reported in severe head injuries, seem interesting from a practical therapeutic point of view.

Case Report

A sixteen-years-old girl was admitted to La Pitié Neurosurgical Clinic two hours after a severe head injury responsible for immediate loss of consciousness. She was then in deep coma with non-reactive dilated pupils on both sides, and signs of bilateral decerebration.

The CAT scan (Fig. 1) showed a diencephalic lesion associated with left temporal and right parietal haemorrhagic contusions. The lateral ventricules were collapsed. A subdural screw was inserted in order to monitor the ICP.

The initial treatment was the following:

controlled ventilation,

dexamethasone (96 mg the first day, and decreasing doses the following days),

25% mannitol infusion (50 ml during 5 minutes) when ICP was above 15 mm Hg,

Phenobarbitone (0.3 g a day),

Laevomepromazine (0.15 g a day).

During the first 48 hours, symptoms of autonomic dysfunction became evident. The ICP was controlled at a mean level of 20 mm Hg, but tracheal aspiration raised the ICP up to 40 mm Hg.

On the third day, the ICP mean level raised slowly, with poor response to mannitol infusion.

On the fourth day, peaks of intracranial hypertension (50 mm Hg) occurred spontaneously every 15 minutes. The repetition of this phenomenon was striking. The mannitol was able to lower the ICP mean level, but was not able to remove the peaks.

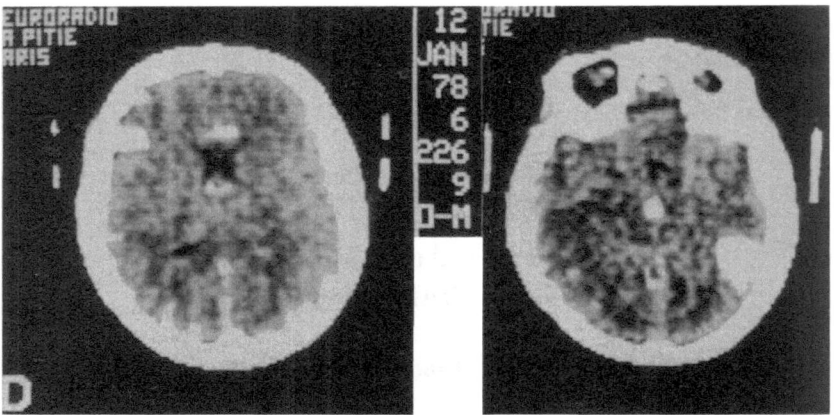

Fig. 1

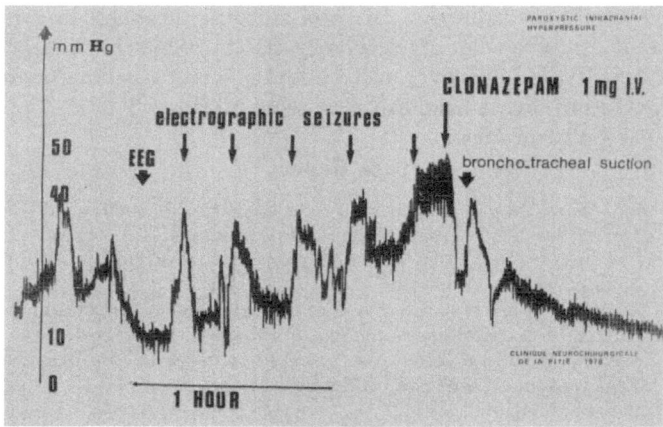

Fig. 2

A simultaneous EEG recording was performed with evidence of typical electrical seizures, but the patient exhibited no clinical signs. The seizures started twenty seconds before the ICP rise, and lasted for three minutes. After intravenous bolus of clonazepam (1 mg) both the paroxysmal ICP rise and the electrical seizure vanished (Fig. 2).

Discussion

1. The paroxysmal increase of ICP is related to epileptic seizures for the two following reasons:

The chronology of the two phenomena is always the same, the electrical seizure starting 20 seconds before the ICP rise. After the end of the seizure, the ICP decreases in a few minutes and returns to the mean level.

The epileptic seizure cannot be secondary to intracranial hypertension because of this chronology, and because the mannitol, when lowering the ICP mean level from 40 to 20 mm Hg is unable to remove the peaks of ICP.

2. The manometric accident noticed during the evolution of the seizure cannot be related to epilepsy because our patient was then absolutely quiet, and there were no respiratory or haemodynamic changes.

A direct effect upon brain metabolism is the best hypothesis. Following the work of Penfield *et al.* Ingvar demonstrated that there was a considerable increase in cortical blood flow (CBF) 15 to 20 seconds after the beginning of an epileptic fit. This delay is strikingly similar to what we have noticed between the seizure and the paroxysmal intracranial hypertension. Even a small increase in CBF can raise promptly the ICP from 20 to 40 mm Hg.

Conclusion

Even when there is no clinical epileptic seizure and even when the patient is given phenobarbitone 0.3 g a day, the evidence of ICP paroxysmal rise must lead to a simultaneous recording of ICP and EEG. Specific treatment will then be very effective in reducing the ICP.

Summary

The authors report a case of post-traumatic intracranial hypertension with ICP paroxysmal rise related to subclinical epileptic seizures. The interest of detecting such a phenomenon is emphasized from a practical therapeutic point of view.

References

Ingvar, D. J., Regional cerebral blood flow in focal cortical epilepsy. Stroke *4* (1973), 359—360.

Levante, E., George, B., Thurel, Cl., Thiebault, J. B., In Goulon-Rapin: Réanimation et medecine d'urgence, pp. 80—91, 1974.

Munari, C., Calbucci, F., Benericetti, E., Dall'Olio, W., Versari, P., Registratione poligrafica di due grisi convulsive secondariamente generalizzati: correlazioni con la pressione endocrania. Riv. Neurologia *46* (1976), 471—481.

Penfield, W., von Santha, K., Cipriani, A., Cerebral blood flow during induced epileptiform seizures in animal and man. J. Neurophysiol. *2* (1939), 257—267.

Plum, F., Posner, J. B., Troy, B., Cerebral metabolic and circulation responses to induced convulsions in animals. Arch. Neurol. *18* (1968), 1—13.

Shapiro, H. M., Intracranial hypertension. Anaesthesiology *43* (1975), 445—472.

Acta Neurochirurgica, Suppl. 28, 93—95 (1979)
© by Springer-Verlag 1979

d) Other Laboratory Findings

Gough Cooper Department of Neurological Surgery, National Hospital, London,
and Institute of Neurological Sciences, Southern General Hospital, Glasgow, Scotland

Serum Myelin Basic Protein, Clinical Responsiveness, and Outcome of Severe Head Injury

D. G. Thomas, L. Rabow, and G. Teasdale

Myelin basic protein (MBP) can be detected in the blood of headinjured patients. The level varies with different kinds on injury, and correlated with outcome in 157 patients with injuries of all degrees of severity[1]. This paper reports the results in patients with injuries of a certain minimum severity (defined as one followed by coma for at least six hours and who were included in the international collaborative study[2]).

Methods

Serum MBP was measured by disequilibrium radioimmunoassay[3]. We have compared the highest level recorded during the first week after injury with outcome at six months and with patients' best level of responsiveness (as assessed by the Glasgow Coma Score[4]), 2-3 days after the onset of coma.

Results

The level of serum MBP was higher in patients who died or who were vegetative or severely disabled survivors than in the group making moderate or good recoveries (Table 1).

Also, the level of serum MBP was higher in patients with a coma score of 7 or less (2-3 day best score), compared with those with higher scores (Table 2). Responsiveness, as assessed by the coma score, also relates to outcome so that we have compared serum MBP level and outcome within each of the two clinical groups (Table 3). The mean levels differ but this is not significant in the less responsive group, in which the levels are widely scattered and few patients recover.

Table 1. *Outcome and Serum Myelin Basic Protein Level*
(highest within 1 week of injury)

Outcome	n	Serum MBP ng/ml mean + S.D.
Dead/Veg/Severe	36	60.8 ± 73.4
Moderate/Good	27	41.5 ± 27.3

$t = 2.08 \quad P < 0.05$

Table 2. *Glasgow Coma Score (2-3 day best) and Serum Myelin Basic Protein Level*
(highest within 1 week of injury)

Coma Score	n	Serum MBP ng/ml mean + S.D.
3-7	34	60.5 ± 41.2
> 8	29	42.7 ± 27.4

$t = 2.00 \quad P < 0.05$

Table 3. *Outcome Responsiveness and Serum Myelin Basic Protein Level*

Coma score			Serum MBP ng/ml mean + S.D.
3-7	Dead/Vegetative/Severe	28	63.3 ± 46.5
	Moderate/Good	6	49.5 ± 16.2*
> 8	Dead/Vegetative/Severe	8	51.8 ± 8.8
	Moderate/Good	21	44.3 ± 25.6**

  * NS.
 ** Significant at 45 % level, Wilcoxon Test.

Conclusion

This preliminary study shows that serum MBP levels in the first week after severe head injury were higher in patients who failed to recover; they were also high in patients with depressed responsiveness. More extensive studies are needed to discover whether determination of serum MBP levels can add to prognosis based on clinical criteria and also whether the biochemical test can be used as a reference to validate clinical observations from different sources.

Acknowledgements

We gratefully acknowledge our collaborators Dr. J. W. Palfreyman and Dr. J. G. Ratcliffe, Radioimmunoassay Unit, Department of Biochemistry, Royal Infirmary, Glasgow.

References

1. Thomas, D. G. T., Palfreyman, J. W., Ratcliffe, J. G., Serum myelin basic protein assay in diagnosis and prognosis of patients with head injury. Lancet *1* (1978), 113—115.
2. Jennett, B., Teasdale, G., Galbraith, S., Braakman, R., Avezaat, C., Minderhoud, J., Heiden, J., Kurze, T., Murray, G., Parker, L., Prognosis in patients with severe head injury. Proceedings of the European Association of Neurosurgical Societies. Paris, July 1979.
3. Palfreyman, J. W., Thomas, D. G., Ratcliffe, J. G., Radioimmunoassay of human myelin basic protein in tissue extract, cerebrospinal fluid and serum and its clinical application to patients with head injury. Clinica Chimica Acta *82* (1978), 259—270.
4. Teasdale, G., Murray, G., Parker, L., Jennett, B., Adding up the Glasgow Coma Score. Proceedings of the European Association of Neurosurgical Societies. Paris, July 1979.

Acta Neurochirurgica, Suppl. 28, 96—97 (1979)
© by Springer-Verlag 1979

Department of Neurology and Neurosurgery and Cerebrovascular Research
Laboratory,
Faculty of Medicine, State University of Tartu, Estonia, U.S.S.R.

The Significance of Cerebral
and Systemic Disseminated Intravascular Coagulation
in Early Prognosis of Brain Injury

A. Tikk and U. Noormaa

The main aim of the present investigation is to resolve the dynamics of local cerebral and systemic coagulation disorders, and to evaluate their significance in early prognosis of brain injury. The investigation was carried out in 92 patients with brain injury as follows: 10 patients with brain concussion and slight brain contusion, 12 patients with moderate brain contusion, 34 patients with severe brain contusion together with great neurological deficit, and 36 patients with fatal brain contusion, 24 of whom died in the first week of illness and 12 stayed in an apallic state and died some months or some years after brain injury. Platelet counts, intravascular platelet aggregation, fibrinogen concentration, paracoagulation tests for soluble fibrin, whole blood fibrinolytic activity (FA), electrocoagulography (EC), and thromboelastography (TEG) in systemic venous and arterial as well as in cerebral venous blood were performed. The data were compared with controls.

The results show that haemostatic disorders in cerebral venous blood prevailed over those of the systemic circulation. Hence, in the first week after brain injury the platelet count fell more in cerebral venous blood than in systemic venous and arterial blood. Severe thrombocytopaenia in fatal cases correlated well with the increased number of circulating platelet aggregates. Statistically significant arteriovenous difference in fibrinogen occurred only due to the fall of fibrinogen concentration in cerebral venous blood. At the end of the first week the fibrinogen concentration normalized only in the survivors; it fell in the blood of the systemic circulation of fatal cases. The remarkable increase of soluble fibrin in 4-7 days after brain injury showed intensive fibrinogen catabolism, especially in nonsurvivors. At the same time, FA increased, relatively more in cerebral venous blood as compared with systemic, also in nonsurvivors versus survivors. EC and TEG studies showed phasic changes in haemostasis: hypercoagulation, hypocoagulation, and hypocoagulation with increased FA. In severe brain injury remarkable hypocoagulation and very high FA, especially in cerebral venous blood, correlated well with the fatal outcome.

A good relation was found between haemostatic abnormalities and severity of disorders of consciousness in brain injury. According to our results, there was only a slight hypercoagulable shift, transitory fall in platelet count, and an increased platelet aggregability in cerebral venous blood samples in patients with clear consciousness in the first days after brain injury, which normalized at the end of the first week of trauma. In patients in stupor the above mentioned disorders lasted up to the end of the first week. The comatose patients, on the contrary, showed from the first hours of illness severe thrombocytopaenia, an increased number of circulating platelet aggregates, a progressive fall of fibrinogen concentration, and concomitant increase in soluble fibrin with significant hypocoagulation and intensive fibrinolysis, more pronounced in cerebral venous blood samples as compared with systemic ones. The dynamics of haemostatic disorders was especially characteristic of lethal cases of brain injury.

Hence, the present investigation demonstrated dynamic coagulation and fibrinolytic activity disorders, described in the literature as disseminated intravascular coagulation—DIC (McKay 1965). Frequent appearance of isolated disorders of haemostasis in cerebral venous blood (hypercoagulation, consumption coagulopathy, and hypocoagulation with increased fibrinolysis) formed the basis for diagnosis of local cerebral disseminated intravascular coagulation. But it should be mentioned that, in cases of severe brain injury with cerebral DIC, general systemic DIC occurred also. This leads to severe disorders of microcirculation and dysfunction of almost all organs of the body. It is possible, that DIC accounts for the main risk factors, limiting the possibility for recovery after brain injury because of cerebro-circulatory impairment, causing cerebral anoxia and cerebral oedema, respiratory distress syndrome, and haemorrhagic complications. A relationship between the severity of disseminated intravascular coagulation and recovery from brain injury was revealed. This allows us to evaluate the severity of disseminated intravascular coagulation, which occurs in the first week after brain injury, as an early prognostic criterion for brain injured patients. It therefore remains to be shown whether the early and intensive treatment of increased intravascular coagulation and platelet aggregation is an efficient treatment for brain injury.

Acta Neurochirurgica, Suppl. 28, 98—102 (1979)
© by Springer-Verlag 1979

Neurosurgical Centre, Zwolle, The Netherlands

Disseminated Intravascular Coagulation Related to Outcome in Head Injury

W. Pondaag

Summary

In 46 head-injured patients coagulation studies were performed immediately after admission. In 76 % of all cases signs of disseminated intravascular coagulation (DIC) were found. DIC was related to the severity of the injury and outcome. It is suggested that DIC may be used as an important parameter in assessing craniocerebral trauma.

In a previous report it was stated that disseminated intravascular coagulation (DIC) is met frequently in head-injured patients (2.5-15.3 %), and is associated with a more severe grade of injury and an increased mortality[4]. This paper explores in more detail the relationship between outcome after head-injury and signs of DIC, as detected by laboratory studies performed in the first few hours after injury.

Clinical Material and Methods

As soon as possible after admission for head injury blood gas analysis and coagulation studies were performed in 46 patients, as a part of the complete work-up for assessing the severity of the injury and planning of treatment.

Blood pH was determined according to the Astrup method.

The blood coagulation studies included (normal values and units, not repeated again, between brackets): thrombocytes (100-350 10^9/L), fibrinogen (2-4 g/L), thrombin time (TT) (20-25 seconds), factor V (80-100 %), fibrin/fibrinogen degradation products (FDP) (negative), ethanol gelation test (EGT) (negative). For the purpose of this study grades of DIC were defined:

DIC —: coagulation profile completely within normal values.

DIC ± : a few parameters abnormal, but no one exceeding following limits: thrombocytes 66, fibrinogen 1.3, TT 37.5, factor V 60, FDP 10-20 µg/ml, EGT dubious positive.

Table 1. *Relations Between DIC, Coma-Score and Outcome*

Column I: † < 48 hours; II: † < 1 week; III: † > 1 week.
IV: persistent vegetative or severely disabled state; V: recovery

Table 1 a

	Coma score 3/4	Coma score 5/6/7	Coma score > 7
DIC +	19	4	3
DIC +	3	3	3
DIC —	2	4	5

n = 46, χ^2-test: p > 0.05

Table 1 b

	I	II	III	IV	V
DIC +	13	0	3	1	9
DIC ±	1	1	0	0	7
DIC —	0	0	1	1	9

n = 46, χ^2-test, mortality vs survival, :p < 0.01

Table 1 c

	I	II	III	IV	V
Coma-score 3/4*	12 11 DIC + 1 DIC ±	0	3 3 DIC +	2 1 DIC +	7 4 DIC + 2 DIC ±
Coma-score 5-7	1 1 DIC +	0	1 1 DIC +	0	9 3 DIC + 3 DIC ±
Coma-score > 7	1 1 DIC +	1 1 DIC ±	0	0	0 2 DIC + 2 DIC ±

n = 46, χ^2-test, mortality vs survival, :p < 0.01

* All patients (5) with score 3 died within 48 hours.

DIC + : fibrinogen < 1.3 and FDP > 40 µg/ml, or if FDP positive but less, then EGT positive.

Also classified DIC + were 3 patients with profiles respectively: 1. fibrinogen 2.2, but FDP > 80, EGT dubious positive, 2. FDP negative, but fibrinogen 0.97, factor V 66, EGT dubious positive, 3. fibrinogen 2.0, but FDP 20, factor V 58, EGT positive.

In assessing the neurological status patients were scored using a responsiveness scale, known as the Glasgow coma scale[3].

According to the suggestion of Cooper and Clark[2] an outcome-index. defined as the sum of the % deaths and the % patients surviving in a persistent vegetative or severely disabled state, divided by the % patients, scored 3 or 4 at admission, was calculated.

Results

Of the 46 patients studied, 32 (70%) were male. The mean age was 26.3 years (range 4-73 years). The younger age classes predominated: 0-9 years 11 (24%), 10-19 years 13 (28%). All injuries were caused by traffic or domestic accidents, there were no missile injuries. In 70% of the patients skull fractures were seen, and in 17% a haematoma was found. In 39% there were also extracranial lesions, mostly fractures of the lower extremities. Twenty-four (52%) patients scored 3/4 on the coma scale, 11 (24%) scored 5/6/7, 11 (24%) scored 8 and more. Therapy was not strictly standardized. Hyperventilation and high dose steroid therapy was instituted in both 22% of the patients, osmo-therapy was seldom, and then only in a very limited way, used. In these 46 patients in comparable groups no significant influence of therapy on outcome could be detected. The total mortality was 41%, 14 patients dying within 48 hours, 1 patient dying within one week, and 4 patients dying after one week. Two (4%) patients survived in a persistent vegetative and severely disabled state.

The outcome index for the whole group was $46\%/52\% = 0.86$, but was strongly influenced by age:

   0-10 years (mean age 7.3, range 4-10) outcome-index 0.57
   0-15 years (mean age 9.6, range 4-14) outcome-index 0.71
   > 11 years (mean age 33.7, range 13-73) outcome-index 1.00
   > 15 years (mean age 36.0, range 16-73) outcome-index 1.13

DIC + was found in 26 (56%) patients, DIC ± in 9 (20%), DIC — in 11 (24%) patients. DIC + and ± was evenly distributed in all age groups. Detailed relationships between DIC, coma-scale scores and outcome are given in Table 1a, b, c. Individual parameters are compared for the group of early deaths and the group of survivors in Table 2a, b, c. Note that in one death the EGT was not available, and in one survivor the FDP. Relations between blood pH and outcome are given in Table 3.

Discussion

It needs no discussion to state that it is very important to be able as soon as possible and in a reliable way to assess in a head-injured patient the degree of severity of the lesion and prognosis, especially when considering in a patient at risk, aggressive management (ICP

Table 2. *Relations Between Individual Parameters of DIC and Early Mortality and Recovery*
Legend for columns see Table 1

Table 2 a

	I	V	
Thrombocytes	158 ± 18 (SE)	200 ± 10.39	t-test: p < 0.05
Fibrinogen	1.24 ± 0.27	2.14 ± 0.19	t-test: p < 0.01
Factor V	49 ± 5.96	75 ± 4.98	t-test: p < 0.01

Table 2 b

	I	V
FDP positive	0	13
FDP negative	15	9

$n = 37$, χ^2-test: $p < 0.001$

Table 2 c

	I	V
EGT —	6	14
dubious	4	7
+	4	2

$n = 37$, χ^2-test: NS

Table 3. *Relation Between pH and Outcome*
Legend for columns see Table 1

	I	II	III	IV	V
pH > 7.50	3	0	0	0	3
	3 DIC +				2 DIC +
pH < 7.30	5	0	0	1	0
	5 DIC +			1 DIC —	

monitoring, hyperventilation, highdose steroid therapy etc.). There is ample information in the literature on efforts to relate the neurological status to outcome, using neurological signs of different aspects (responsiveness, motor pattern, pupil reactions etc.). However, due to the specific characteristics of neuronal physiology, it is often difficult, and sometimes impossible, to state if a certain neurological deficit is reversible or not, before a longer period of observation has elapsed, or outcome is factually known. Therefore a search for non-neurological parameters with predictive value regarding outcome of head-injury is of some interest.

The clinical DIC-syndrome with fulminating course, characterized by multiple organ failure and overt haemorrhagic tendency, is rarely encountered in neurosurgical patients. But DIC is in fact a basic pathological mechanism found in most diverse pathological states. DIC* is well known to be associated with trauma and shock, the latter defined as impairment of tissue perfusion on the microcirculatory level, and occurs frequently, related to the degree of severity of the injury in head-injured patients, as this and the previous study indicate, and as has also been reported recently by others[4, 1, 5]. The blood pH is related to outcome by its correlation with DIC via metabolic acidosis. From the data of this study a flow diagram could be constructed with following elements:

1. pH < 7.30 and DIC + → all patients will die.

2. pH < 7.30 and DIC — → ? survival in persistent vegetative state?

3. pH > 7.30 and DIC — → all patients should survive, mortality is dependent upon the risk of complications of prolonged coma and aggressive care, especially in the elderly, and is in a way reflecting the standard of intensive care.

4. pH > 7.30 and DIC + → patients are at risk; with score 3 they will die, with score 5 or more they should survive.

In the 14 patients of this study, with coma-scale score 4, DIC + or ±, and pH above 7.30, no significant relationship could be detected between outcome and age, hyperventilation, and high-dose steroid therapy respectively. In the future, proposed new therapies should be validated in this group.

References

1. Auer, L., Disturbances of the coagulatory system in patients with severe cerebral trauma. Acta Neurochir. (Wien) *43* (1978), 51—59.
2. Cooper, P. R., Clark, K., Outcome index for head-injured patients (Letter). J. Neurosurg. *49* (1978), 777.
3. Jennett, B., Teasdale, G., Galbraith, S., *et al.*, Severe head injuries in three countries. J. Neurol. Neurosurg. Psychiat. *40* (1977), 291—298.
4. Pondaag, W., Disseminated intravascular coagulation in head-injured patients. In: Advances in Neurosurgery, vol. 6, pp. 159—163 (Wüllenweber, R., Wenker, H., Brock, M., Klinger, M., eds.). Berlin-Heidelberg-New York: Springer. 1978.
5. Sande, J. J. v. d., Veltkamp, J. J., Boekhout-Mussert, R. J., *et al.*, Head injury and coagulation disorders. J. Neurosurg. *49* (1978), 357—365.

---

* As a state of latent consumption coagulopathy.

Acta Neurochirurgica, Suppl. 28, 103—107 (1979)
© by Springer-Verlag 1979

National Institute of Traumatology,
Department of Neurosurgery, Budapest, Hungary

Prognostic Significance of the Changes in the Carbohydrate Metabolism in Severe Head Injury

T. Pentelényi, L. Kammerer, F. Péter, M. Fekete,
L. Korányi, M. Stützel, G. Veress, and A. Bezzegh

With 1 Figure

This is quite a new development in neurosurgery for assessing severity of head injury or predicting outcome following severe head injury during the first week with the help of endocrine data.

Our team made a long-range research on the topic Disturbances of the carbohydrate metabolism and the endocrine system in non-diabetic brain injured patients. Our aim was to state what kind of endocrine changes closely related to the carbohydrate metabolism are caused by brain injuries.

The examinations were done in 130 patients of the National Institute of Traumatology, Budapest during the last five years. Serial examinations were performed in the non-diabetic brain-injured patients and in the chest-, abdomen- and limb-injured or polytraumatised control patients. From the day of injury we determined daily the fasting blood glucose, serum insulin, cortisol, growth hormone, plasma glucagon, norepinephrine, and epinephrine levels up to the recovery or to the death of the patients.

The results were compared with the neurological and pathological changes determining the severity of brain injury.

Data were analysed by computer. There are a lot of very important details concerning the method of this research but it is impossible to deal with them in such a short paper.

Results, Statements

1. There are well-defined differences between the changes of the fasting blood glucose level of *brain-injured patients* and *control patients.*

2. In the clinical neurological picture the *state of consciousness* seems

to be correlated with the fasting blood glucose level. Coma caused by
brain injury is accompanied by elevation of blood glucose level, clearing
of consciousness by normalization of it. There is quantitative
correlation between the severity of the disturbance of consciousness
and the degree of hyperglycaemia: the deeper the coma the higher and
wider is the fasting blood glucose range.

3. In the background of the blood sugar changes we found
simultaneous alterations of the basal plasma levels of numerous
hormones. Thus, the most important hormone levels controling
carbohydrate metabolism show special alterations, too. The hormonal
state of hyperglycaemia caused by severe brain injury is characterized
by very low basal insulin level, extremly high glucagon and cortisol
levels, moderate elevation in the catecholamine levels, and very high or
decreased growth hormone level—depending on the time of examination after injury.

4. According to the changes of the various endocrine parameters
four periods can be differentiated during the post-traumatic course:
first two days, 3-7. days, second week, third week. In the patients in
various states of consciousness (Fischgold-Matis: clear consciousness,
coma stages 1, 2, 3, 4) different changes can be seen in the plasma levels
of every parameter. Till the third week the average values of fasting
blood glucose measurement in the coma 3 patients differ significantly
from those measured in the patients in all other states of consciousness.
Similar results can be seen in the various hormonal changes.

5. We constructed a *head injury classifying system* by which we could
clarify connections between the changes of the *endocrine system, state of
consciousness*, and *pathological course*. According to the endocrine
changes *four types* of brain-injured patients could be separated. The
typical features of each type were mathematically verified, and now
they are illustrated in schematic figures. For example *blood glucose*
(Fig. 1).

In the *first type*—recovered patients—elevated fasting glucose level
was found in comatose state. Together with the improvement of the
state of consciousness the normalization of glucose level was observed.
If the patient went into deeper coma again blood glucose was elevated
too; if consciousness appeared the glucose level was normal again.

The most seriously injured patients belonged to the *second type*:
they died in 48 hours. The fasting blood glucose level was very high, in
most cases above 200 mg per cent.

In the *third type* the lethally injured patients were alive for 1-2
weeks. During this period big fluctuations of the basal glucose level
could be demonstrated beside unchanged deep coma.

In the patients of the *fourth type* there was a temporary

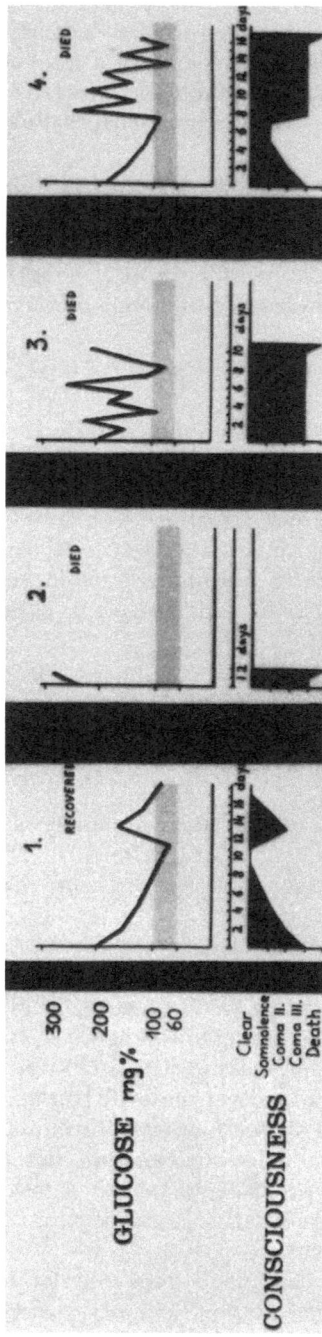

Fig. 1. Four types of changes of fasting blood glucose in head-injured patients

improvement in the state of consciousness with a decrease of the high glucose level during the first days; but because of a fatal complication deep coma and a rapid elevation of the glucose level were observed. In the next period permanent deep coma was seen with gradual decreasing of blood glucose.

Similar characteristic changes were identified in the different types concerning also the basal plasma levels of the various hormones mentioned above.

Up to this point these are new pathophysiological data in connection with severe brain injuries. But some of them have also prognostic significance.

From the point of view of *Assessment of severity of head injury during the first week:*

Changes indicating severe brain injury in a non-diabetic comatose patient are

1. Fasting hyperglycaemia above 180 mg per cent.
2. Decreased, constantly low basal insulin level.
3. Very high serum cortisol level (above 60–70 µg/100 ml).
4. Extremly high basal growth hormone level in the first day (above 10–15 ng/ml) but constantly low unchanged level from the 2nd day.
5. Very high basal plasma glucagon level (above 2000 pg/ml).
6. With glucose loading there is a good insulin reaction but there is a so-called paradox answer in the growth hormone level.

From the point of view of *Assessment of outcome following severe head injury:*

We can predict fatal outcome on the basis of endocrine alterations as follows—in the state of coma stage 2 or 3:

1. Fasting hyperglycaemia above 240 mg per cent, mainly in the first day.
2. Bouncing fasting blood glucose level (between 100 and 400 mg per cent) during the first week, changing day by day.
3. In spite of high and fluctuating blood glucose, deeply depressed and unchanged basal insulin level during the first week.
4. Extremly high cortisol level of above 100 µg/100 ml.
5. Decreased plasma epinephrine level under 0.1 ng/ml.

We stress that these changes are not factors determining prognosis since they are not causes of death—but we can determine fatal prognosis in advance in the presence of these signs. They are irreversible consequences of a severe pathological process which results in death.

As a practical conclusion we can advise the regular following of fasting blood glucose. This seems to be the most simple and most informative test among the examinations mentioned above. Its regular performance once a day can be assured even in comatose brain-injured patients.

References

1. Pentelényi, T., Characteristics of head and brain injuries in diabetic patients. Book of the Fifth European Neurosurgical Congress. EANS, p. 189. Oxford 1975.
2. Pentelényi, T., Kammerer, L., Changes in the blood glucose after head injury and its prognostic significance. Injury *8* (1977), 264.
3. Pentelényi, T., Kammerer, L., Blood glucose reflects outcome in head injury. Medical Monitor *2* (1977), 9, 14.
4. Pentelényi, T., Kammerer, L., Stützel, M., Balázsi, I., Alterations of the basal serum insulin and blood glucose in brain injured patients. Injury, in press.
5. Pentelényi, T., Kammerer, L., Stützel, M., Péter, F., Alterations in the basal blood glucose, serum IRI, corticosteroid and growth hormone levels in brain injured patients. J. Neurosurg. Sci., in press.

Acta Neurochirurgica, Suppl. 28, 108—112 (1979)

Department of Neurosurgery, Department of Neurology,
and Department of Clinical Chemistry, University Hospital, Linköping,
Sweden

CK_{BB}-Isoenzymes as a Sign of Cerebral Injury

L. Rabow and **G. Hedman**

With 2 Figures

Summary

CK_{BB}-isoenzymes in serum and CSF have been shown to be raised in patients after head injury with objective signs of damaged brain tissues (contusio cerebri), but not in the absence of these signs (commotio cerebri).

It has been shown earlier by us[6, 7] and by others[3, 4, 8] that the anodal LD-isoenzymes, preferably measured by HBD-activity[2], are released into the blood stream after head trauma with damage of cerebral tissues, and also that a correlation exists between the enzyme activity in serum and the patients' outcome[5]. The LD-isoenzymes or HBD are, however, not brain specific, and they also occur in comparatively high levels in normal serum, which makes diagnostic conclusions uncertain in some cases, especially in patients with multiple trauma. Furthermore, as the same isoenzymes are abundant in red blood corpuscles, LD-measurements in CSF are difficult or impossible to evaluate after a brain injury. Creatine Kinase, CK, on the other hand, has three isoenzymes, CK_{MM}, CK_{MB}, and CK_{BB}, the last of which is almost brain specific. It cannot normally be shown in serum, nor does it occur in the erythrocytes. The clinical usefulness of this isoenzyme has, however, been hindered until recently by methodological difficulties. But Somer et al.[9] and later Maas[2], both using electrophoretic separation of the CK isoenzymes, have shown increased activities in serum and CSF respectively, after experimental brain injury, the former also in a few patients with head injury. Bell et al.[1] have measured CK_{BB} activity in serum and CSF by radioimmunoassay in 61 patients with various neurological disorders and found statistically significant elevations in the serum after acute cerebrovascular accidents, and in some patients with severe head trauma. The aim of this study was to test the value of CK$_{BB}$-measurements in the evaluation of the degree of parenchymatous brain damage after a head injury.

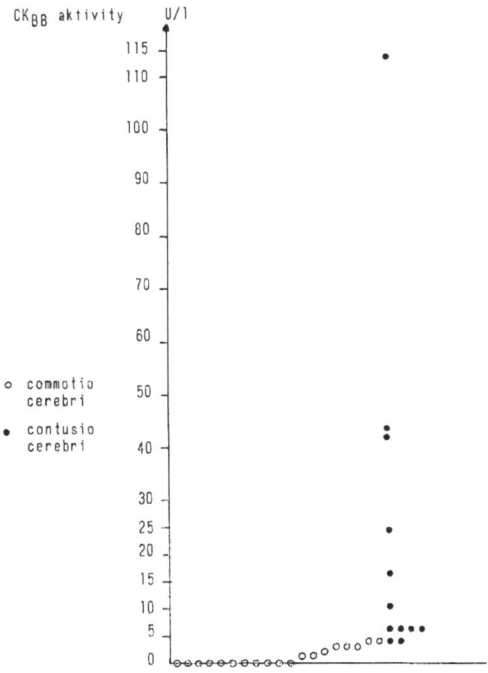

Fig. 1. CK$_{BB}$-activity in serum after head injury

Material and Methods

Two consecutive series of patients admitted to hospital after head injury were studied; 19 patients with a mild injury (commotio cerebri)—defined as a period of unconsciousness not exceeding ten minutes, no focal neurological signs, and no seizures—and 12 patients who were shown by neuroradiology or operation to have a cerebral contusion/laceration. Samples were drawn at admission, on the first morning after the trauma, and on one of the following two days. In 10 of the concussion patients and in 5 of the contusion patients CSF samples were also available within 24 hours after the trauma. CK-isoenzymes were separated by ion exchange using diethylaminoetylsephadex columns and a three step chloride ion eluation*. Measurements were made

---

* Kit commercially available from Worthington Corporation.

spectrophotometrically on the NADH-NAD system at 340 nm and 30 °C. LD
and HBD were measured as described earlier[2]. Most samples were analysed
within a few hours, and the rest were stored at — 20°, for not more than a week.

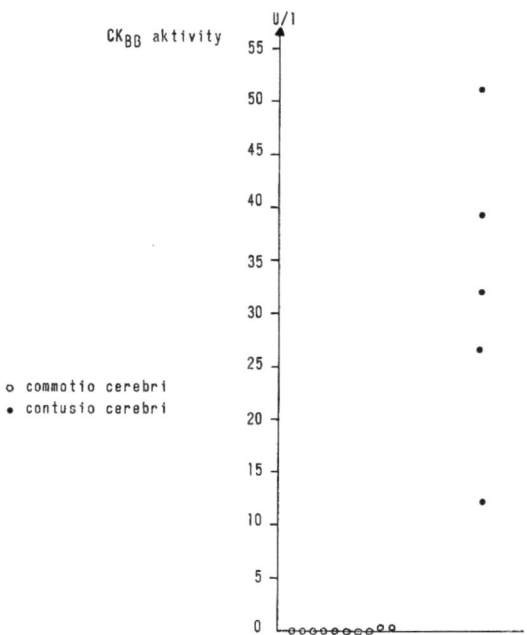

Fig. 2. CK_{BB}-activity in CSF after head injury

Results

The results of the CK_{BB}-measurements—maximum values within
24 hours—are shown in Figs. 1 and 2. The highest CK_{BB}-activity in
serum in any concussion patient was 4.0 U (2 patients) whereas the
lowest value in the contusion group was 4.2 U. In more than 50% of the
concussion patients there was no measurable CK_{BB}-activity in serum at
all. No CK_{BB} activity could be shown in CSF from concussion patients,
while CSF from the contusion patients, showed very high levels. S-
HBD was within normal limits in all the concussion patients, and
significantly raised in all but one of the contusion patients. S-LD total
was significantly raised in 6 (30%) of the concussion patients and in all
the contusion patients. CK_{MM}, finally, was raised in most patients from
both groups.

Discussion

As, obviously, a head trauma with concussion does not cause any raised CK_{BB} activity—in fact in most cases no detectable activity at all—it seems that even a very low CK_{BB}-activity in serum or CSF after a head trauma is a sign of at least some injury to the cerebral parenchyma. Although all our patients with a cerebral contusion/laceration showed increased CK_{BB}-activity in serum, the series is a rather small one, and so it could still be possible that small injuries can occur without such increase. The maximum CK_{BB}-activity invariably occurred within 24 hours after trauma, and as the activity seems to be able to change considerably within a very short time[2], it is of great importance to get the samples for analysis as early as possible after the injury, and also to get at least two samples within the first 24 hours in order to make a reliable decision whether the brain is injured or not. It is interesting to note that, whereas there was never any detectable CK_{MM}- or CK_{MB}-activity in CSF from the concussion patients, CK_{MM}-activity was comparatively high in the CSF from patients with parenchymatous brain injury—this CK-fraction probably emanating from the traumatic subarachnoid bleeding. For the same reason HBD (and LD) was also raised in CSF from patients with brain contusion. Consequently, after intracranial aneurysmal surgery, LD, HBD, and CK_{MM}, but not CK_{BB} or CK_{MB} were increased in the CSF.

If CK_{BB}-activity in serum, as we believe it does, reflects the amount of damaged brain tissues, then a correlation with outcome would be most probable. This study will continue with the purpose of answering that question.

References

1. Bell, R. D., Rosenberg, R. N., Ting, R., Mukherjee, A., Stone, M. J., Willerson, J., Creatine kinase BB isoenzyme levels by radioimmunoassays in patients with neurological disease. Ann. Neurol. 3 (1978).
2. Maas, A. I. R., Cerebrospinal fluid enzymes in acute brain injury. Thesis. Rotterdam 1977.
3. Rao, C. J., Shukla, P. K., Mohanty, S., Reddy, Y. J. V., Predictive value of serum lactate dehydrogenase in head injury. J. Neurol. Neurosurg. Psychiat. 41 (1978), 948—953.
4. Lindblom, U., Aberg, B., The pattern of S-LDH isoenzymes and S-GOT after traumatic brain injury. Scand. J. Rehab. Med. 4 (1972), 61—72.
5. Rabow, L., Isoenzymes of lactic dehydrogenase as a prognosticon in patients with contusion cerebri. Ibid. 90—92.
6. Rabow, L., Hebbe, B., Lieden, G., Enzyme analysis for evaluating acute head injury. Acta Chir. Scand. 137 (1971), 1240—1244.
7. Rabow, L., Tibbling, G., Serum activities of HBD and the isoenzymes of LD as an index of traumatic brain injury. Acta Neurochir. (Wien) 37 (1977), 245—261.

8. Thomas, D. G. T., Rowan, T. D., Lactic dehydrogenase in head injury. Injury 7 (1976), 258—262.
9. Somer, H., Kaste, M., Troupp, H., Konttinen, Brain creatine kinase in blood after acute brain injury. J. Neurol. Neurosurg. Psychiat. *38* (1975), 572—576.

Acta Neurochirurgica, Suppl. 28, 113—114 (1979)

Department of Anaesthesiology (Prof. H. Reinhold) and
Neurosurgical Intensive Care Unit (Prof. J. Brihaye),
Institut Bordet, Bruxelles, Belgique

Disturbances of the Carbohydrate Metabolism in Acute Head Trauma

Th. Deloof, J. Berre, F. Genette, A. Van de Steene,
and E. Mouawad

The controlled study of the carbohydrate metabolism in 281 head injuries has allowed us to judge the frequency of hyperglycaemia among injured people (E. Mouawad 1973).

We have been able to establish a narrow correlation between the extent of hyperglycaemia and the seriousness of the cerebral lesions: thus from a group of patients whose glycaemia was greater than 300 mg %, there was a mortality of 89%. These data confirm the views put forward previously by P. Fossati (1968).

By titrating the growth hormone, cortisol, and insulin in the blood we were able to verify that the increase of the glycaemia in the head injured patients resulted in the first place in a reaction linked with stress, as Allison (1967, 1968, 1969) has already written: there are increase of hormones antagonistic to insulin and inhibition of insulin secretion by the catecholamines (Porte et al. 1966, 1967). The direct action of cranial trauma on the hypothalamic structures is retained (King and McLaurin 1970).

In our experience, the treatment of this post-traumatic pseudo-diabetes should at first be symptomatic and involve insulin therapy and rehydration. At the same time, the treatment should not be pursued energetically as is the case in hyperglycaemic diabetic coma; in particular, rehydration would be more prudent, taking into consideration the cerebral pathology which necessitates a restriction of water, or at least a normovolaemia. At the same time, the insulin therapy should be moderate, a level of glycaemia of 150/200 mg % being for us an acceptable comprise. Indeed, a too sudden or too brutal lowering of the glycaemia induces a hypo-osmolarity of the blood which facilitates or maintains cerebral oedema.

Besides the specific insulin treatment, we have stated that the treatment of the cerebral lesion itself could lower the hyperglycaemia, with the reduction of brain oedema (E. Mouawad 1974). In order to do this we have used systematic mechanical ventilation for eight years (normoventilation or slight hyperventilation) associated with other conventional medications: osmotherapy, hormonotherapy (dexamethasone), diuretics, sedative medication, and continuous monitoring of intracranial pressure.

In Conclusion

The measure of the amount of blood glucose in the injured patients is a valuable biological parameter for the diagnosis of the lesional gravity and for the outcome.

Acta Neurochirurgica, Suppl. 28, 115—119 (1979)
© by Springer-Verlag 1979

Neurosurgical Clinic of the University of Würzburg
(Dir. Prof. Dr. K.-A. Bushe), Federal Republic of Germany

The Prognostic Value of Osmolality Within the First Week of Sustaining Head Injury

M. Gaab, H. A. Trost, and K. W. Pflughaupt

With 2 Figures

Introduction

On sustaining severe brain damage, there generally follow disturbances of metabolic regulation. The latter is a central function of the
diencephalon[10] and brain stem[7]. Thus several groups have monitored
various blood metabolites e.g. hyperglycaemia[12], azotaemia[2], lactate-
pyruvate[8], proteins[2, 4] and lipids[3] with regard to prognosis after head
injury. However, though mentioned[2, 12], blood and CSF osmolality
have not been systematically investigated despite the known role of the
diencephalon in osmoregulation[13, 15]. We therefore investigated the
course of blood and CSF osmolalities, correlating them with clinical and
other biochemical data.

Methods

In patients with severe head injury i.e. coma (without opening eyes during
the first 24 hours)[11], the course of blood osmolality was cryoscopically*
measured daily. In addition, 18 serum values including Na^+, K^+, Cl^-, Ca^{++},
glucose, urea, uric acid, creatinine, total proteins, albumin and various enzymes
were measured by autoanalyser. In patients without elevated ICP[5] and
without intracranial space occupation/midline shift in CT-scan, the same values
were analysed in lumbar CSF.

The clinical status was registered twice daily using a modified Glasgow
coma scale[11]; without verbal response due to intubation but including pupillary
reaction, the values (scores) varied between 3 and 17 (Fig. 2). The daily water
balance and urine specific gravity were measured. All patients evaluated,
received the same basic therapy. Patients with renal failure (oligo/anuria,
creatinine > 2 mg > 12 hours before death), those with > 24 hours diabetes

---

* Knauer osmometer.

8*

insipidus and those undergoing osmotherapy, were excluded. Of the remaining 78 patients, 58 survived and 20 died, all of whom were examined pathologically.

The data were statistically evaluated and compared (t-Test survivors/non-survivors; regression analysis of laboratory data).

Results

In all survivors, the osmolality values returned to normal (281–297 mosm/kg) within 14 days of the injury. No increase in levels was observed at any time in one group; the second group showed transient elevations of up to 330 mosm spontaneously, mostly between 2 to 6 days after trauma (Fig. 1). These periods were associated with unconsciousness or unresponsiveness. The mean osmolality of the survivors during the first week, was 300 ± 22 mosm/kg ($\bar{x} \pm$ SD).

In the 20 non-survivors, the mean osmolality of 342 ± 31 mosm/kg during the first week was significantly higher ($p < 0.001$). The values of survivors/non-survivors are plotted against time in Fig. 1. As can be seen, no survivor had a mosm/kg value above 340, and no patient with ≥ 335 mosm/kg over a period of > 3 days survived. These values in non-survivors were unresponsive to treatment.

Osmolalities ≥ 340 mosm/kg were always associated with a comatose state. The time course of clinical status, osmolality, serum glucose, and serum sodium are correlated in Fig. 2. The mean glucose (279 ± 157) and sodium (145 ± 9.7) of non-survivors was significantly ($p < 0.01$) elevated as compared to the survivors (glucose 148 ± 83 mg/dl, Na^+ 140 ± 5.5 mval/l). Hyperglycaemia and azotaemia are associated with elevated osmolality, but regression analysis did not reveal any significant correlation coefficient between osmolality and any isolated serum value.

Lumbar CSF osmolality, obtained from 3 non-survivors, followed the plasma value, but with some delay, as is shown in the following table (1 Pat.):

Days after injury	1	2	3	4	
Plasma osmolality	373	402	380	392	mosm/kg
CSF osmolality	355	377	373	386	

Pathological examination revealed severe structural damage or softening in the hypothalamic area, but secondary changes after brain death must also be considered.

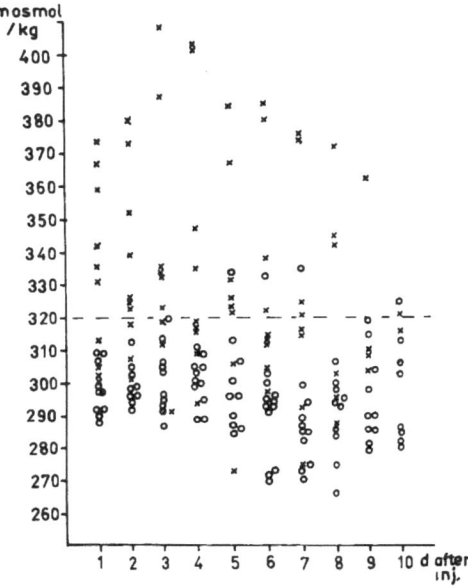

Fig. 1. Blood osmolality plotted against days. o = survivors, x = non-survivors

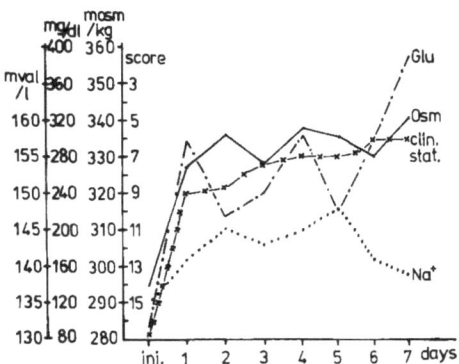

Fig. 2. Non-surviving patients during the first week of injury. Course of clinical status (values obtained according to mod. Glasgow coma scale ranged between 3 and 17), plasma osmolality Osm (mosm/kg), glucose glu (mg/dl), and sodium Na^+ (mval/l)

Discussion

As EEG and ICP measurements do not alone provide a definitive prognosis[3, 11, 14] within the first week of sustaining injury, laboratory values of prognostic relevance should be sought. Blood data, in contrast to CSF, are readily obtained without endangering the patient—daily blood analysis is standard in intensive care. However, the regulation of these blood parameters is maintained by various organs including the brain, whereas osmoregulation, provided that renal function is preserved, resides in the hypothalamus[13, 15] where most osmo-receptors are found. Our data suggests that blood osmolality measurements should be considered in further attempts to find a reliable method of survival-estimation in the early stages of acute cerebral disease. This would also enable optimization of neurosurgical and intensive care treatment.

Even regarding osmolality alone, values in excess of 340 mosm/kg over three days would indicate a true osmoregulatory failure as a strong indication of hypothalamic death and consequently predict very low survival chances.

Elevated blood osmolality may also explain persistent coma in these patients, despite normal ICP and CBF, as acute hyperosmolality has been shown to result in unconsciousness[1].

Finally, blood osmolality is of importance in therapy *e.g.* fluid balance and contra-indications to osmotherapy[6].

References

1. Arieff, A. I., Kleeman, C. R., Studies on mechanism of cerebral edema in diabetic coma. J. Clin. Invest. *52* (1973), 571—583.
2. Auer, L., Holzer, H., Tritthart, H., Gell, G., Azotaemia in severe head injury-central dysregulation or renal failure? Acta Neurochir. (Wien) *41* (1978), 355—361.
3. Auer, L., Marth, E., Petek, W., Holzer, H., Gell, G., The prognostic value of biochemical data from blood and CSF: Analysis in patients with severe head injury. In: Frowein, R. A., Wilcke, O., Karimi-Nejad, A., Brock, M., Klinger, M., eds. Advances in Neurosurgery, Vol. 5, Head Injuries-Tumors of the cerebellar region, pp. 132—137. Berlin-Heidelberg-New York: Springer. 1978.
4. Auer, L., Petek, W., Serumproteinveränderungen bei Patienten mit Schädelhirntrauma. Acta Neurochir. (Wien) *33* (1976), 301—309.
5. Gaab, M., Knoblich, O. E., Dietrich, K., Gruss, P., Miniaturized methods of monitoring intracranial pressure in craniocerebral trauma before and after operation. In: Frowein, R. A., Wilcke, O., Karimi-Nejad, A., Brock, M., Klinger, M., eds. Advances in Neurosurgery, Vol. 5, Head Injuries-Tumors of the cerebellar region, pp. 5—11. Berlin-Heidelberg-New York: Springer. 1978.

6. Gaab, M., Pflughaupt, K. W., Ratzka, M., Wodarz, R., Gruss, P., Critical intracranial effects of osmotherapy. In: Wüllenweber, R., Wenker, H., Brocl, M., Klinger, M., eds. Advances in Neurosurgery, Vol. 6, Treatment of Hydrocephalus-Computer Tomography, pp. 193—205. Berlin-Heidelberg-New York: Springer. 1978.
7. Gerstenbrand, F., Lücking, C. H., Die akuten traumatischen Hirnstammschäden. Acta Psychiatr. Nervenkr. *213* (1970), 264—281.
8. Hausdörfer, J., Heller, W., Oldenkott, P., Stolz, I. C., Alterations of metabolism in brain edema following head injury. In: Schürmann, K., Brock, M., Reulen, H. J., Voth, D., eds. Advances in Neurosurgery, Vol. 1, Brain Edema-Cerebello Pontine Angle Tumors, pp. 34—41. Berlin-Heidelberg-New York: Springer. 1973.
9. Hausdörfer, J., Heller, W., Junger, H., Preger, R., Veränderungen des Lipidstoffwechsels nach akuten experimentellen Schädel-Hirn-Traumen. Med. Welt *27* (1976), 426—431.
10. Hess, W. R., Das Zwischenhirn. Syndrome, Lokalisation und Funktionen, 2. Aufl. Basel: Schwabe. 1954.
11. Jennett, B., Bond, M., Assessment of outcome after severe brain damage. Lancet *II* (1975), 480—485.
12. Park, B. E., Meacham, W. F., Netsky, M. G., Nonketotic hyperglycemic coma. Report of neurosurgical cases with a review of mechanisms and treatment. J. Neurosurg. *44* (1976), 409—417.
13. Schmidt-Nielsen, B. M., Mackay, W. C., Comparative physiology of electrolyte and water regulation. In: Morten, M. H., Kleeman, C. R., eds. Clinical disorders of fluid and elctrolyte metabolism, 2. ed., pp. 45—93. New York: McGraw-Hill. 1972.
14. Vapalahti, M., Troupp, H., Prognosis for patients with severe brain injuries. Brit. Med. J. *3* (1971), 404—407.
15. Verney, E. B., The antidiuretic hormone and the factors which determine its release. Proc. roy. Soc. *B 136* (1947), 25—106.

Acta Neurochirurgica, Suppl. 28, 120—123 (1979)

II. Assessment of Outcome

University Department of Neurosurgery,
Pittsburgh, Pennsylvania, U.S.A.

Post-Traumatic Amnesia, Post-Concussional Symptoms, and Accident Neurosis

A. N. Guthkelch

The Glasgow Coma Scale, as developed by Jennett and his colleagues, is of the greatest value in the prediction of the outcome of very severe injuries. In less severe cases, where the problem is one of loss of working time rather than of life or death, where questions of the patient's ability to work may have serious medico-legal as well as purely medical implications, but where the patient's symptoms are largely subjective, a reliable estimate of the likely duration of the patient's disability is no less important.

Long ago Ritchie Russell pointed out that the length of post-traumatic *amnesia* (PTA) in closed head injury patients is of value in predicting the duration of their subsequent disability but it is still not universally accepted. Possibly some workers distrust a parameter which depends entirely on the patient's own statements, but there is a clear relationship between the length of PTA and the frequency of traumatic anosmia, consistent with being proportional to the amount of indirect violence applied to the brain. Moreover, it has recently been pointed out that the PTA tends to be about four times as long as the time taken to return to consciousness as judged by the patient's ability to reply to questions, and this relationship can be used in verification.

Without such a discriminant, it is difficult to make a fair assessment of the symptom-complex comprising headaches (often related to exertion or to posture), giddiness, loss of concentration, insomnia, irritability, and so on which comprise the post-concussional syndrome. This paper summarizes the results of the personal investigation of a consecutive series of 398 head injury cases, almost all sustained either in industrial or in motor vehicle accidents. The patients were all aged

Table 1. *PTA, Anosmia and Length of Absence From Work*

Length of PTA	Percentage incident of anosmia	Percentage of patients returned to work at					Total patients
		1 mo.	2 mos.	4 mos.	6 mos.	12 mos.	
< 1 hour (Mild concussion)	4	38	60	79	88	91	156
1-24 hours (Moderate concussion)	10	13	43	70	84	91	76
1-7 days (Severe concussion)	20	8	22	49	67	84	51
> 7 days (Very severe concussion)	24	—	1	17	27	36	115
						Total	398

between 18 and 60 years, and all were in full-time regular gainful employment at the time of the accident.

Table 1 shows clearly that the longer the period of post-traumatic amnesia, the slower the return to work and the greater the likelihood of prolonged disability. Of course, the post-concussional syndrome is only one cause of disability in these patients, but nearly 40 % of the mildly concussed patients are back at work within a month while those with moderate concussion take rather longer and it is six months before the majority of patients with a PTA lying between one and seven days are working. Very few patients with a PTA of more than seven days return to work within two months and many are still disabled after a year.

We may summarize by saying that the average length of post-concussional symptoms varied between less than a month when the PTA did not exceed one hour, to more than six months when it exceeded seven days.

One must ask why 40 % of patients who have sustained only mild concussion remain disabled for more than four months. Apart from three patients in whom the initial injury led to unexpectedly severe complications, namely carotid artery thrombosis, vertebral artery thrombosis, and meningitis accompanying cerebrospinal fluid fistula respectively, three common factors were identified: 1. Neck injuries were frequently observed especially in the older patients and in those suffering from pre-existing spondylosis. Many such patients had been erroneously regarded as complaining of neurotic headache. 2. Vertigo due to labyrinthine injury was also frequent: in assessing this symptom

A. N. Guthkelch:

Table 2. *Observed and Expected Frequency of Accident Neurosis According to Severity of Injury and Circumstance of Accident*

Frequency of accident neurosis	Severity of concussion				All patients	
	Mild	Moderate	Severe	Very severe		
Observed	13	7	4	3	27	$X^2 = 0.169$
Expected	14	6.7	3.5	2.8		$df = 3$
						$p = .7$

Frequency of neurosis	Occupation				All patiens	
	Non-Manual		Manual			
	Non-industrial	Industrial	Non-industrial	Industrial		
Observed	6	1	3	17	27	$X^2 = 23.52$
Expected	9.57	2.30	8.75	6.38		$df = 3$
						$P < .001$

Hallpike's test was invaluable and it should be more widely used. 3. Psychological disturbances are also important and their frequency after head injury has been widely debated. Some authors have given figures as high as 20 % or even 40 % whereas Symonds has suggested that what appears to be neurosis is caused by the symptoms of organic brain damage in relatively mild form. In this study a distinction was established between reactive depression and anxiety on the one hand and the state of mind that has called Accident Neurosis or Compensation Neurosis on the other. Patients who develop depression or anxiety after a head injury often have a previous history of nervous instability: many have unusually heavy family responsibilities and in some a history of previous injury was elicited. They are often embarrassed to talk of their symptoms and they display the same tendency to recovery which is the rule in non-accident cases. In this series emotional disturbances, as distinct from organic mental syndromes following severe injury, rarely prolonged the subsequent period of disability by more than two or three months whatever the severity of the original injury, causing only a modest shift to the right at each level of Table 1.

So-called Accident Neurosis is quite different. The patient is voluble about his symptoms, which he describes in vague but highly-coloured terms, and he usually exhibits attention-seeking behaviour. There is often a discrepancy between his (or her) performance in the clinic and in the street outside. There is no relationship between the severity of the injury and the ensuing period of absence from work, which continues until it serves no further purpose, *e.g.* because issues of compensation have been finalized. In the present series the total incidence of accident neurosis was 6.8 %, and if one excludes all patients who exhibited permanent disablement of organic origin, one can see that there was a uniform incidence of Accident Neurosis at all levels of brain injury (Table 2) but a highly significant relationship between the frequency of Accident Neurosis and the circumstances of the accident, with a large excess among manual workers sustaining their accidents in an industrial setting. As Miller has said, the exploitation of his injury (enables) the unskilled worker to acquire capital in what he accepts as a ruthlessly acquisitive society.

In summary, it is submitted that a careful investigation of head injury cases can greatly reduce the element of guess-work involved in assessing the validity of subjective complaints such as those of the post-concussional syndrome and of emotional disturbance. These can be and should be distinguished from the uncommon and unpleasant condition which has been euphemistically labelled Accident Neurosis but for which a better and shorter name is Fraud.

Acta Neurochirurgica, Suppl. 28, 124—125 (1979)
© by Springer-Verlag 1979

Institute of Neurological Sciences, Southern General Hospital
and University of Glasgow, Scotland

Burdens Imposed on the Relatives of Those With Severe Brain Damage Due to Injury

M. R. Bond, D. N. Brooks, and W. McKinlay

In recent years workers in several countries have established that the mental sequelae of severe brain injuries handicap the injured person far more than his or her residual physical disabilities, and that close relatives, friends, and employers find that they cause the greater disruptions of family and social life (Bond 1975, Dikman and Reitan 1977, Oddy and Humphrey 1978, Najenson *et al.* 1978). These observations have led to proposals that rehabilitation of severely injured individuals should include far greater attention to the problems caused by mental handicap (Bond and Brooks 1976), a point of view which receives support from the work of Najenson *et al.* (1978) who found that the use of family counselling, in addition to usual rehabilitation practices, significantly improved the adaptation of even the most severely disabled to his or her new social role. In order to determine the optimum time for different rehabilitative techniques it is essential to understand the process of recovery in detail (Bond and Brooks 1967), to have a conceptual model of the stages of recovery (Bond 1978), and to have acceptable methods of assessing outcome (Jennett and Bond 1975). These needs have been partly fulfilled, but greater understanding of the precise effects, at different times during recovery, of disability upon family members is required because the process of adaptation clearly involves both the patient and those caring for him. With this in mind a study of the burden imposed upon family members, and spouses in particular, was started in Glasgow in 1976.

This paper gives information generated by the study dealing with the problems of 35 patients and their families three months and six months after the former had been injured. The mean age of the group is 35 years, and all have a post-traumatic amnesia exceeding 24 hours.

At three months emotional problems were more common than

physical ones, and spouses commented that they were aware of feelings of tiredness in the injured person very often, and that they noticed poor memory, impatience, depression, and irritability only slightly less often. By six months irritability was declared the most frequent symptom, and tiredness and memory had become less common.

The frequency of symptoms does not appear to be a necessary correlate of the burden experienced by relatives. For example, whereas three months after injury patients' emotional symptoms showed a significant correlation with burden in relatives, this had been replaced by dependence of the head injured person on those around him three months later. As the frequency of emotional symptoms remains high these observations suggest that relatives may have developed means of coping with the emotional difficulties they encountered initially and that more general aspects of caring became a problem to them as time past.

These findings will be discussed in detail against the background of previous work leading to the study, and their significance for management planning will be examined.

Acta Neurochirurgica, Suppl. 28, 126—127 (1979)
© by Springer-Verlag 1979

Institute of Neurological Sciences,
Southern General Hospital and University of Glasgow, Scotland

The Nature of Physical, Mental and Social Deficits Contributing to the Categories of Good Recovery, Moderate and Severe Disability in the Glasgow Global Outcome Scale

M. R. Bond, W. B. Jennett, D. N. Brooks, and
W. McKinlay

In 1975 Jennett and Bond published an account of a Global Outcome Scale which they developed for use in the assessment of individuals who have had head injuries. The Scale has been used widely in several contries including Britain, Holland, and the United States, and familiarity with it has brought several criticisms. The main ones are, first, that it is a crude measure and not sensitive to subtle changes in patients' status and, second, that there is little background information about the nature and extent of physical and mental handicaps which make up the first three elements of the Scale. In other words, we wish to know what constitutes good recovery, moderate disability and severe disability. Jennett and others (1978) accept the first of these criticisms, and in a response to it have expanded the categories mentioned above from three to six thereby giving increased sensitivity. In order to deal with the second criticism a careful study of the mental and physical deficits of two groups of brain injured individuals has been carried out. Four kinds of disability have been examined. In a first sample of 150 patients physical, cognitive, and personality deficits have been graded as nil, mild, moderate, or severe, and related to outcome at six months after injury by which time most of these deficits are established. In a second sample, which is still under study, in addition to the deficits examined in the first group, the social consequences of disability are being examined in detail. Results from the first study show that some deficits, albeit mild, were detectable in 97 % of the patients examined. Two-thirds had personality change, two-thirds had cognitive change, and 93 % had one or other of both of these mental deficits. Physical handicaps were present in 75% of patients, but were less significant than mental handicaps which dominated recovery in just over half the patients in the survey. This pattern was repeated in each of the three outcome categories examined. In more detail, in 30% of patients the only detectable deficit was a change in personality, a figure which increased to 60% in patients without physical deficits or one of only a mild degree, and to a similar extent in those with nil or mild cognitive deficits.

The detailed nature of the physical, mental and social disabilities of patients in the two studies will be presented in terms of their respective contributions to the Global Outcome Scale. By this means it is hoped that even greater use will be made of the Scale in an area of medical science where agreed methods of assessment are required.

Acta Neurochirurgica, Suppl. 28, 128—133 (1979)
© by Springer-Verlag 1979

Neurosurgical Department, Addenbrooke's Hospital, Cambridge, England

Long-Term Prognosis After Severe Head Injury

W. Lewin and A. H. Roberts

Over the last thirty years we have had the opportunity of treating non-missile head injuries in the setting of a main general hospital with a neurosurgical unit where all head injuries admitted, both minor and major, came under the care of the neurosurgical unit. From 1948 to 1961 a consecutive series of 7,000 cases were admitted to the Radcliffe Infirmary, Oxford, and analysed by a punch card technique. We defined severe head injury as producing unconsciousness or post-traumatic amnesia (PTA) for one week or longer. Among the 7,000 cases in the Oxford series were 479 patients who had sustained a severe head injury under the present definition. All but 11 were traced in a follow-up ten to twenty-five years later. A hundred and seventy-eight patients had died, and the cause of death was established. The remaining 291 patients were examined by an independent team consisting of a neurologist, a clinical psychologist, and a psychiatric social worker. In more than 90% of these patients in the complete survey it was possible also to interview the relatives independently (Lewin, Marshall, and Roberts 1978).

Results

Physical Disability

Various post-traumatic syndromes could be identified, and these have been analysed in greater detail elsewhere (Roberts—in press). They varied from decerebrate dementia to complete recovery. The encouraging feature about this severe group was that 40% recovered with either minimal or no physical disability and this improvement was subsequently maintained over the years. The best results were to be found among the young patients and in those who had not sustained further complication, such as an intracranial haematoma or brain penetration, but even in this group, of which there was 77, the same pattern of recovery could be seen although the time taken to reach the final state might well be longer, provided that infarction did not take place.

The second important finding was that, after severe head injury, two-thirds of the survivors with severe disability showed deterioration of their neurological state after admission to hospital. It is being increasingly recognized that vascular infarction plays a major role in this deterioration. If such an event can be prevented, therefore, then the overall prognosis should improve. This observation is a justification therefore for the intensive management of head injuries as an emergency in the early hours. It could well be that the more recent introduction of intracranial pressure monitoring and controlled ventilation, both of which were developed after this first series was completed, might well prove to be preventive measures, but this remains to be seen.

Mental Disability

For the purpose of this analysis, physical and mental disability were analysed separately although they are essentially inter-depent, and the severer the injury the more likely it is that they occur together. The physical deficits have received a good deal of attention in the past, yet it is true that the adverse mental effects after severe head injury are not only as important but are indeed more often the determining factor as to whether there is a satisfactory social adjustment and possibility of return to work. The various syndromes have been fully described over the years under various names, but in summary are confirmed in this survey. In adolescence and young adults, frontolimbic dementia (50 cases) was associated with the severest physical disabilities. It consisted of frontal personality change together with profound memory impairment, irritability, and rage reactions. This latter symptom rather than the overall dementia or indeed the physical disability was often the crucial factor in making any adjustment in the social and occupational spheres. On the other hand mental disability after middle age was more often associated with anxiety/depression, or a neurotic reaction in which case this was usually in association with minimal physical disability. These features have been re-examined more recently by Bond (1975).

Predicting the Outcome

The well-established clinical predictive factors such as age at injury, the worst state of neurological responsiveness after injury, and the duration of PTA were once more confirmed in this survey and, put together, could give a reliable guide to the long-term outcome. Having said this, however, it should be stressed that it remains a guide only, and does not take account of individual variability. Nevertheless, more accurate knowledge of the final residual syndromes of mental and neurophysical disability enables one to recognize when progress is out of keeping with the normal pattern and suggest investigation of individual factors which may then help in more effective rehabilitation. Within these limitations, it is possible to make some observations.

Children (less than 15 years) whose injury has not caused decerebration will do well and be left with minimal or no disabilities. Those with decerebration may still make a good recovery although persistent decerebration longer than three months was not compatible, in this series, with recovery beyond total dependence. In general, children may recover over a much longer time than is the case with adults, and a poor prognosis should not be assumed within five years of injury.

Adolescents and young adults, if no more than confused, even for more than a week should recover without neurological disability. Those decerebrate for a day and with a PTA of less than two months will seldom be physically disabled although some memory impairment or personality change may be expected. However, those in whom post-traumatic amnesia after initial decerebration is greater than two months, will be severely disabled by their mental and physical disability.

In the middle-aged and older, initial coma with decerebration from the primary brain lesion carries a bad prognosis. Indeed in this series (excluding those complicated by a haematoma), no patient over 46 years of age made a practical recovery or indeed survived for a long period. Persisting mental symptoms were commoner at this age in those with a PTA of more than one week, but those initially confused only were unlikely to be severely disabled.

Some general statements can also be made about outcome in its relation to the rate of recovery.

1. No-one walking unassisted within $3^1/_2$ weeks of injury had any physical disability due to neural lesions in the long-term (excepting cranial nerve lesions).

2. Decerebration lasting longer than $2^1/_2$ weeks in children was compatible with little residual neuro-physical disability, but in adults was invariably followed by severe and permanent disability precluding a normal domestic, social, or occupational life, as did coma in adults lasting longer than a month and if walking unassisted was delayed six months.

3. If walking unassisted was delayed for three months this was seldom succeeded by worse than moderate physical disability even in adults.

4. Decerebration in adults and children persisting longer than three months never allowed recovery beyond vegetative or analogous states.

5. Spasticity and moderate difficulty in using a limb might persist for a year but still improve thereafter, so that there was finally negligible disability.

6. Recovery from mental disorder lagged behind the final residual physical disability and might continue for a further two years, causing moderate disability, yet thereafter resolve.

Progressive Deterioration

An earlier study of repeated minor head injuries in boxers revealed a progressive neuronal degeneration attributable to this cause and not associated with the histological characteristics of normal ageing. Roberts (1969) attention was paid to this point in the present survey. Progressive intellectual deterioration was not a rare occurrence in this group and was seen in 31 cases of the consecutive series, that is to say 11 %. However, there were no specific features of the head injury in those who did dement either immediately or after delays that distinguished them from the rest of the sample. At the present time it is likely that one is seeing the normal effects of ageing on a brain already depleted of its functional reserve by injury.

Prolonged Unconsciousness

Clinical observation for some years has recognized that a period of unconsciousness of over one month separated sharply the majority of patients in whom recovery might be expected from a much smaller group where the prognosis was very different. We have used the term prolonged unconsciousness to include the time the patient is in coma or only reacting to pain, proceeding to a stage where the patient is mute, often tetraparetic, and requiring artificial feeding (Lewin 1976). This description is similar to that of Giovanelli et al. (1975) in defining an incomplete apallic syndrome. It is among this group that so many of the present anxieties of management and the extent to which patients should be treated have arisen. In order to attempt a fuller picture of this condition we can now comment on 139 such patients alive and dead who have remained unconscious for more than one month after injury and who have been followed up. This is a selected group, for not only does it include the 73 cases in the Oxford series but 66 from a further series of patients treated in the Army Neurosurgical Unit, and at Addenbrooke's Hospital, Cambridge 1948-1970 by one of us (W.L.). Of the 134 patients traced, 70 are now dead. With five exceptions, where death was clearly due to other causes, it was decided that all the other fatalities should be assumed to have been related in some way to the head injury. The overall mortality after one month and within the first six months after injury of 33 % had risen by the end of two years to 43 %. This remained steady for some years—47 % at 5 years to reach the present mortality rate of 54 % in the group at periods of from 6 to 25 years later. The follow-up of the 64 survivors confirms that some patients can still make excellent recovery after this severe acute picture. Thus 19 of them, 30 %, have ended with only minimal physical disability, and a further 29 have improved to the extent that they are at home or at work, although with major disabilities, either mental or physical, or both. Put together, the two groups give a practical recovery rate of 75 %, and 16 remain totally dependent and unable to walk. The accent in these figures is on the physical disability, but as stated earlier the mental disability is as important, and when the two are put together it is found that although only in 16 (14 %) could the final disability be called minimal and recovery excellent, there was a further 40 % gainfully employed. In only 18, or 28 %, of the survivors was constant care still required.

The same factors already described in the unselected group concerning recovery, apply to this group. Age is particularly important and, provided there is no added complication, a good recovery can still be made. All the patients with a good recovery were under 25 at the time of injury and as age increases the prospect of a good recovery diminished. The second main predictor was not only the pattern during the first month but the rate of recovery during that period. Failure to make any improvement whatsoever during this period carried a bad prognosis as did fixity of the pupils (even though not dilated) for longer than the first 48 hours after injury. Similarly, persistent gross decerebration with tetraparesis after one month carried a bad prognosis. However, if definite improvement took place during the first month, even though the patient was still unconscious, there could be substantial improvement, particularly in the young.

Comment

It is hoped that this long-term study may be helpful in providing some predictive factors, based not only on the severity of the injury at outset but on the pattern of improvement in the succeeding weeks and months, and a close identification of the final disabilities that may be encountered. Even among the severest group, with prolonged unconsciousness, the percentage of survivors achieving a practical recovery although with some disability could be said to be encouraging. However, there is another side to the coin that has to be examined.

The team conducting the follow-up soon became aware of the fact that both in the patients and the relatives the experience of a severe head injury was at the best disturbing, often terrifying, and might be disastrous. For the patients who made a recovery, memory impairment, defects in concentration, anxiety over their amnesia, and the physical effects with imbalance and vertigo were major problems. As far as the relatives were concerned, although they could often deal with the physical effects, the distress caused by a major personality change could be intense. Rehabilitation programmes so far have concentrated very much on the physical disabilities, but it would appear that in the future more psychotherapeutic support should be arranged both for patients and relatives.

From an economic point of view the increasing number of patients totally disabled or severely disabled is serious. Thus if one considers England and Wales alone on the basis of this series (and we have reason to believe that the 7,000 cases of the unselected series from Oxford is reasonably representative), each year will leave 210 patients totally disabled, and 1,500 with profound disability one year later. In succeeding years those with total disability remain much the same although improvement from profound disability will reduce the 1,500 to about half. However, one has to realise that a new cohort of the same number is being added each year. The need for arrangements for their care is obvious as is the continued study of predictive factors at various stages after a head injury to guide us in the treatment and rehabilitation procedures that should be offered.

References

Lewin, W., Marshall, T. F. de C., Roberts, A. H., In press.

Roberts, A. H., Brain damage in boxers: London: Pitman Medical. 1969.

Bond, M. R., Ciba Foundation Symposium No. 34 new series. Amsterdam: Elsevier. 1975.

Lewin, W., Brit. med. J. 2 (1976), 1234.

Giovanelli, M., et al., Proc. Fifth Congress E.A.N.S., abstract 8, Oxford, 1975.

Acta Neurochirurgica, Suppl. 28, 134—136 (1979)
© by Springer-Verlag 1979

III. Factors Determining Prognosis

a) Prognosis and Series of Patients

Neurosurgical Clinic, University Medical School,
Ljubljana, Yugoslavia

Factors Determining Prognosis in Acute Subdural Haematoma

B. Klun and M. Fettich

The purpose of this paper is to present and analyse the clinical signs observed in a series of acute subdural haematomas and ascertain how they influence the outcome. A rating system was developed which allows a prognostic evaluation.

The series consists of 304 cases treated during the period 1963-1977. Cases of spontaneous subdural haematomas in infancy were excluded. Every space-occupying subdural blood collection which accumulated within the first five days after injury was included. Seventy-one per cent were combined lesions with contusions and lacerations. We also included cases with combined haematomas (epidural or intracerebral, or both), provided the subdural haematoma was the predominant one. Thirty-six per cent of the entire series had concomitant injuries, mostly to the chest or extremities or both.

Age factor showed the following influence:

Age in years	No. of cases	No. of deaths	%
Up to 10	14	5	35.7
11-20	20	12	60.0
21-30	36	20	55.5
31-40	46	26	56.5
41-50	68	41	60.2
51-60	48	34	70.8
61-70	45	32	71.1
71-80	26	21	80.7
above 81	1	1	100

Mortality/consciousness relationship:

State of consciousness at time of surgery	No. of cases	No. of deaths	%
Alert	14	3	21.4
Semicoma	72	22	30.5
Coma	213	168	78.8
No data	5		

Pupillary changes and the mortality rate:

	No. of cases	No. of deaths	%
Reacting pupils	92	35	38.0
One pupil non-reacting	95	66	69.5
Both pupils non-reacting	93	82	88.2
No or unreliable data	24		

Signs of brain stem damage (bilateral extensor responses, extensor spasms, vegetative disturbances):

	No. of cases	No. of deaths	%
Present	102	86	84.3
Absent	202	106	52.5

One of the most crucial prognostic factors seems to be the rapidity of the development of the blood collection and therefore the speed of brain compression.

Dynamics of development:

Time	No. of cases	No. of deaths	%
Up to 6 hours	209	160	76.5
Up to 12 hours	8	5	62.5
Up to 24 hours	32	9	37.5
Up to 2 days	18	7	38.8
Up to 5 days	18	6	33.3
No data	19		

Size of the subdural haematoma has only a limited prognostic value, because of the concomitant brain injuries, which may be moderate in a sizable haematoma, and vice versa.

	No. of cases	No. of deaths	%
Small	64	32	50.0
Sizeable	135	91	67.5
No data	105		

We have tried to analyse the clinical signs and their relation to final outcome, as observed in a fairly large series. The overall mortality was 63.1%, and the most important signs predicting the prognosis seem to be the following: the time from injury to clinical presentation of the haematoma, followed by signs of brain stem damage, pupillary changes, state of consciousness, and age. Little importance is attached to different methods of operative treatment.

In keeping with these data, a rating system was elaborated to determine the prognostic expectancy.

Acta Neurochirurgica, Suppl. 28, 137—139 (1979)
© by Springer-Verlag 1979

National Institute of Neurosurgery, Budapest, Hungary

Factors Influencing the Outcome of Coma in Severely Injured Patients

Éva Orosz

Material

Case histories of 160 patients, who were in coma for more than 5 days following admission to the Intensive Care Unit of the Institute of Neurosurgery of Budapest, are analysed in this paper. This group represents 33 per cent of the whole series of 479 severe cranio-cerebral traumatic cases treated in a five years period. Patients who died within 36 hours are not included in this series.

Fatal outcome occurred in 68 cases (43 per cent), and 30 out of the 92 survivors had severe sequelae at the time of discharge.

Eighty-four patients were operated on the basis of angiographically proven signs of space-occupying lesions, with a mortality rate of 54 per cent. Mortality of patients not operated on was 30 per cent.

Following the required circulatory and respiratory reanimation and the eventual surgical intervention patients were treated according to the same pattern of intensive care. Brain swelling was controlled by the administration of Dexamethasone (60 mg/day), Frusemide (40-60 mg/day), and Mannitol as required. Automatic ventilation was used only in cases, when respiration was not satisfactory, but not to fight cerebral oedema. Intracranial pressure was not monitored as a rule, only in cases, when intraventricular drainage was otherwise indicated.

Besides the monitoring of the routine vegetative parameters, blood-gases were analysed and EEG recorded regularly.

In the few cases, when also lumbar puncture was performed lactate, pyruvate content and acid-base parameters of the CSF were measured.

The following factors considered possible significant determinants in later prognosis, were analysed: age, level of coma, vegetative state, presence of decerebrate rigidity, blood-gas values and EEG.

Results

Table 1 demonstrates the breakdown of mortality rates with request to the mentioned factors, in the 160 patients studied.

Patients were separated in 4 age-groups (children were not included in this material). The rise in mortality proportional to age is conspicuous.

Table 1

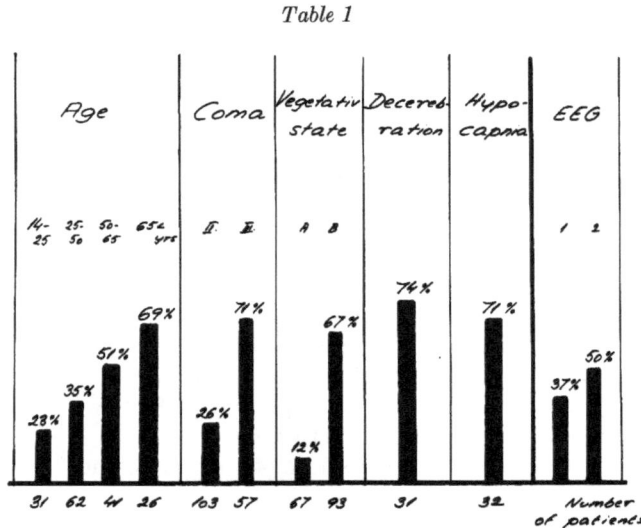

All of our patients were in a coma state of grade II and III according to Fischgold and Mathis. In coma II patients were unarousable but had at least (coordinate or incoordinate) motor responses. In coma III either total lack of motor responses was present or decerebration could be detected. High mortality in deeper coma is also obvious.

Most striking difference was encountered with respect to outcome of coma, when patients were separated according to their vegetative state. In state A, a patient's circulation and respiration was relatively stabilized and no hyperthermia was present. In state B, either systemic circulation or respiration, occasionally both, were seriously damaged with or without a tendency to hyperthermia.

The relation between high mortality and decerebration as well as arterial hypocapnia is also very impressive.

Analysis of early EEG recordings were far less predictive concerning the vital prognosis. In group 1 spontaneous or evoked periods of high amplitude slow waves, sleep patterns, and reactivity to various stimuli were characteristic, and considered as favourable prognostic signs. In group 2 tracings showed unorganized, polymorph slow activity which were non-reactive to any stimulus.

On the other hand, we emphasize the importance of long term EEG follow up. Pattern of time course in cortical electrical activity can give valuable information regarding the late prognosis and the state in which the patient will survive.

In the few cases where CSF acidity and lactate level were also measured we had the same experience as several authors, viz. high lactate level and low pH values proved to be very unfavourable prognostic signs.

Summary

From this analysis we may conclude that the most important factors influencing the outcome of coma due to injury are age, vegetative state, level of coma, decerebration, and hypocapnia. In all cases where a combination of four or more of any of the above-mentioned factors was present the patient died.

EEG seems less predictive in the early period, but may give some information for late prognosis.

Acta Neurochirurgica, Suppl. 28, 140—143 (1979)
© by Springer-Verlag 1979

Institute of Neurological Sciences, Glasgow, Scotland,
and Department of Mathematics, University of Nottingham, England

Age and Outcome of Severe Head Injury

G. Teasdale, A. Skene, L. Parker, and **B. Jennett**

With 2 Figures

Opinions about the importance of age as a prognostic factor after head injury have varied. For instance, Carlsson *et al.*[1] emphasized a close correlation between increasing age and a decreasing change of mental recovery; but others[2] report that age has little influence on the prospects for recovery.

Patients and Methods

Patients were studied in Scotland, the Netherlands, and the U.S.A., as described previously[3]. All were in coma for at least six hours after injury although in one third of cases prolonged coma developed only after a period of relative lucidity. Outcome in survivors was assessed six months after injury[4].

Results

When we inspected the data it was apparent that numbers were insufficient to support analysis based upon each individual year of age, but that the division into cohorts of successive 5 years epochs was practical.

The relationships between groups of variables were modelled using a log-linear analysis[5]. This may be regarded as the discrete analogue of the more familiar analysis of variance. The calculations were accomplished using the GLIM data analysis package[6].

Fig. 1 shows the age distribution of patients in the data bank and the distribution of those who died within six months of injury. The mean age in the series is 33 years, the mode 19 years. Children under five have been omitted from subsequent analyses because of the unusual selection of this group in the contributing centres and also because of the biological differences of head injury in the very young[7].

Fig. 2 shows the proportions at various ages who died. The pattern is of steadily increasing mortality with increasing age, with a possible

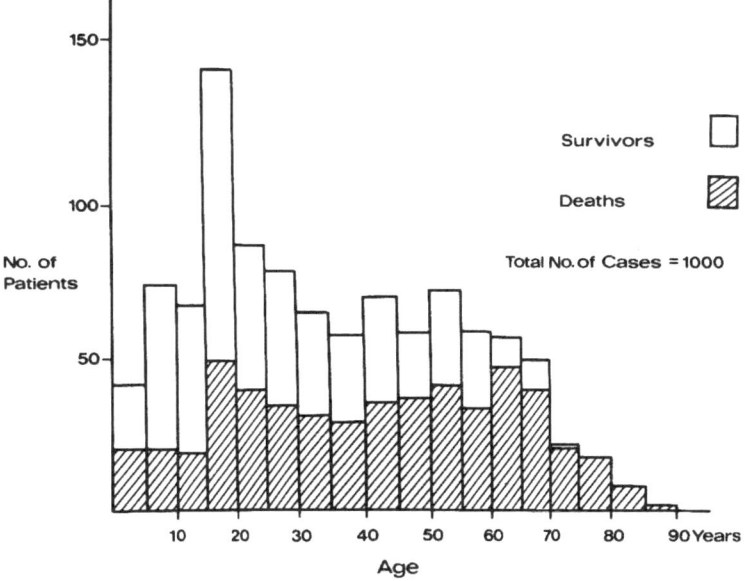

Fig. 1. Outcome following severe head injury

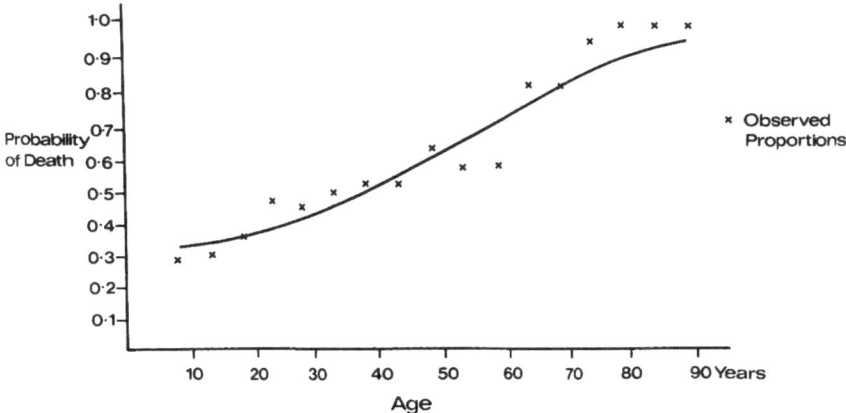

Fig. 2. Fitted curve giving probability of death as a function of age (excluding under 5's)

anomaly in the 50–59 year olds; no patient over 75 years of age survived, but this observation was based upon relatively few patients.

The fitted curve in Fig. 2 was obtained by observing how the ratio of the probability of death to the probability of survival varied with age. This ratio increased rapidly with age and could be described by an exponential curve where the exponent was a quadratic function of age, *i.e.*

$$\frac{\text{Probability of death}}{\text{Probability of survival}} = \exp\left(C_0 + C_1 \text{ age} + C_2 \text{ age}^2\right)$$

Disability

Severe disability among survivors was related to age, the proportion increasing from less than 15 % in patients under 20 years old, to more than 30 % in the over-60-year-olds.

Haematoma; Age; Outcome

Half of the patients in this study had an intracranial haematoma and their coma persisted after its removal. Haematoma occurred more frequently in patients who were older, and so did a bad outcome (Table 1).

Table 1. *Outcome From Severe Head Injury, Age, and Haematoma*

	% Occurrence of haematoma	% Dead/vegetative	
		haematoma	no haematoma
< 20	30	43	29
20–40	42	53	42
40–60	67	57	54
60–80	68	85	88
> 80	66	100	100

The worst outcome associated with an intracranial haematoma (in those severely affected patients) was significant at the 5 % level in the under 20 s, at only the 10 % in the 20–40 s, but there was no effect on outcome in patients over 40 years old.

Conclusion

Age has an important influence upon outcome after severe head injury, and this is not explained solely by the increased frequency of intracranial complications in older patients. In survivors increasing age is associated with an increasing rate of severe disability due to brain damage.

The relationship between haematoma, age and outcome is only one of many possible interactions. The results presented here were drawn from an extensive data analysis which showed that age remains an indicator of outcome, even when many other factors have been considered. It is therefore necessary to take age into account when considering the prognosis of an individual patient and also when comparing series of patients managed in different centres or treated in different ways.

References

1. Carlsson, C. A., von Essen, C., Lofgren, J., Factors affecting the clinical course of patients with severe head injuries. I. Influence of biological factors. II. Significance of post-traumatic coma. J. Neurosurg. *29* (1968), 242—248; 248—251.
2. Becker, D. P., Miller, J. D., Ward, J. D., *et al.*, The outcome from severe head injury with early diagnosis and intensive management. J. Neurosurg. *47* (1977), 491—502.
3. Jennett, B., Teasdale, G., Galbraith, S., *et al.*, Severe head injuries in three countries. J. Neurol. Neurosurg. Psychiat. *40* (1977), 291—298.
4. Jennett, B., Bond, M., Assessment of outcome after severe brain damage. Lancet *I* (1975), 480.
5. Bishop, Y. M. M., Fienberg, S. E., Holland, P. W., Discrete multivariate analysis in theory and practice. Cambridge: M.I.T. Press. 1975.
6. Nelder, J. A., General linear iterative modelling. Numerical Algorhithms Group. Oxford, 1975.
7. Bruce, D. A., Schut, L., Bruno, L. A., *et al.*, Outcome following severe head injuries in children. J. Neurosurg. *48* (1978), 679—688.

Acta Neurochirurgica, Suppl. 28, 144—147 (1979)

Department of Neurosurgery Agia Sophia Childrens Hospital,
Athens, Greece

Early Prognosis of Severe Head Injuries in Children

St. C. Comninos

This study is a retrospective analysis of the outcome of 120 severe head injuries in children, evaluating early findings which could be used for an early prognosis.

Material and Methods

Our material includes cases in coma, as defined by the Neurotraumatology Committee of the WFNS (Brihaye *et al.* 1978 and Frowein *et al.* 1976), either immediately after injury or after a lucid interval. In the study are considered cases in which unconsciousness had exceeded six hours, although the first estimation was performed on admission.

For the grading of coma in children of 18 months to 14 years old we applied the 15-point Glasgow coma scale (Jennett *et al.* 1975). Comatose infants from 1 to 18 months old were evaluated according to the two groups of clinical signs scale of the Neurotraumatology Committee of the WFNS.

Additional information on eye signs as well as blood pressure, heart rate, and respiration were included in the study.

The outcome was classified for both groups of cases (infants and children) according to the Glasgow coma scale (Bond *et al.* 1975).

The cause of the injury was in 36 cases (30%) road accidents, in 82 cases (68,3%) falls, and in 2 cases (1.7%) assault. Obstetric head injuries were not included in our survey.

Thirty (25%) were infants from 1 to 18 months old, and ninety (75%) children from 18 months to 14 years old.

The time of admission varied from one hour to thirty-six hours after the injury. Thirty cases (30%) had lucid intervals.

Of the 120 total cases 24 cases (20%) had other associated injuries such as long bone fractures and thoracic or abdominal injuries. Forty-two cases (35%) had one or more linear fractures of the vault of the skull, 12 cases (10%) a depressed fracture, and 18 cases (15%) a fracture of the base of the skull with otorrhoea and rhinorrhoea. Twenty-four cases (20%) presented with an intracranial mass. From these 24 cases 12 had an epidural haematoma, 8 a subdural haematoma, and 4 cases an intracerebral haematoma (2 hemispheric and 2 cerebellar).

Reexamination of the patients was performed at 3, 6, and 12 months after injury.

Early Signs and Symptoms and Outcome of Injury

Group I: Infants aged from 1 to 18 months old. Total cases 30.

Of the total 30 cases 3 died, giving a mortality rate of 10 %. All three cases were flaccid, with bilateral fixed pupils, absent oculovestibular response, hyperpyrexia, increased blood pressure, and tachycardia. The two groups of clinical signs coma score was classified as 4.

None of the cases remained in persistent vegetative state.

There was one case (3 %) with severe disability. This case showed decerebration, bilateral fixed pupils, impaired oculovestibular response, and a coma duration of six weeks. The coma score was classified as 4.

Another six cases (20 %) showed a moderate disability. Four of the six cases showed subdural haematoma, and the other two presented diffuse brain oedema proved by CT scan. The clinical signs presented by these six cases were decerebration, impaired oculovestibular response, and anisocoria. The coma duration in these cases was two weeks. The coma score was classified as 3.

Finally, 20 cases (67 %) had a good recovery. In these 20 cases 5 had an acute epidural haematoma, and 15 cases had diffuse brain oedema prooved by CT scan. Seven of these cases presented normal motility, nine incoordinated motility, four cases mono—or hemiparesis, and five cases anisocoria. The oculovestibular response was intact. The coma duration was 24 hours to 7 days. The coma score was classified between 1 and 2.

Group II: Children aged from 18 months to 14 years old. Total cases 90.

Of the total 90 cases 18 died, giving a mortality rate of 20 %. Of these 18 cases 10 were flaccid, 8 were decerebrate, 12 showed bilaterally fixed pupils, 12 had an absent oculovestibular response, 16 had hyperpyrexia, 10 had increased blood pressure, and 10 had bradycardia with cardiac arrhythmia. The Glasgow coma score in these 18 cases was classified between 1 and 3.

None of the cases remained in persistent vegetative state.

Of the remaining 72 cases, 5 were severely disabled. All were decerebrate with fixed pupils and impaired oculovestibural responses. The coma duration was more than two weeks. The Glasgow coma score was classified between 3 and 5.

Another 17 cases (23 %) were moderately disabled. Seventeen cases were decerebrate with intact oculovestibular responses. Ten of them had anisocoria. The verbal response in all cases was from none to incomprehensible words. The coma duration was more than one week. The Glasgow coma score was classified between 3 and 5.

The other 50 cases (55 %) recovered. The motor function in these 50 cases was slow and uncoordinated, with localizing or withdrawing movements. Twenty-five cases showed anisocoria. The verbal response was from none to incomprehensible words. The oculovestibular response was in all cases intact. The coma duration was less than three days. The Glasgow coma score was more than 5.

The incidence of early seizures was 6 % in infants (2 cases) and 20 % in children (18 cases). The incidence of late seizures was 10 % (12 cases) in infants and 7 % (6 cases) in children. The overall incidence of late seizures was 20 % (18 cases).

EEG examination with conventional equipment and evoked somatosensory potentials was not useful in the prediction of outcome.

Conclusions

As shown in Table 1 the overall mortality in our study was 17.5 %. This is higher than that reported by C.H.O. Ph (Bruce et al. 1978). The mortality in children (20 %) was twice as high as in infants (10 %). A significant difference in severe disability existed between infants and children (3 % and 5.5 %). There was no significant difference in moderate disability (23 % and 20 % respectively). Sixty-seven per cent of the infants and only 55 % of the children recovered completely.

Table 1. *Coma Level at First Assessment and Outcome of Injury*
Total cases 120—Overall mortality 17.5 %

Group A. Infants 30 Outcome		The two signs coma score	Group B. Children 90 Outcome		The Glasgow coma score
Died	3 (10 %)	4	Died	18 (20 %)	1-3
Severely disabled	1 (3 %)	4	Severely disabled	5 (5.5 %)	2-5
Mod. disabled	6 (20 %)	3	Mod. disabled	17 (23 %)	3-5
Recovered	20 (67 %)	1-2	Recovered	50 (55 %)	> 5

From our survey we can conclude that infants with open fontanelles and cranial sutures have a better prognosis than children.

Important factors in the prediction of the outcome were the time between the injury and the time of admission, and the time between injury and specific treatment (Overgaard 1973).

Motor functions and eye signs were the most important early symptoms affecting the prognosis in both age groups.

A decisive factor affecting the prognosis was the duration of coma. Recovery was almost complete in cases with coma of less than three days duration. Twenty per cent of infants and 23 % of children in coma for more than one week were moderately disabled. In patients (infants and children) with coma for more than two weeks the outcome was almost always unfavourable.

References

1. Bond, M. R., Outcome of severe damage to the central nervous system. Ciba Found. Symp. *34* (1975), 141—157. Amsterdam: Elsevier.
2. Brihaye, J., Frowein, R., Lindgren, S., Loew, F., Stroobandt, G., Report on the meeting of the W.F.N.S. Neuro-Traumatology Committee. Brussells 1976. Acta Neurochir. (Wien) *40* (1978), 181—186.
3. Bruce, D. A., Schut, L., Bruno, L., Wood, J. H., Sutton, L., Outcome following severe head injuries in children. J. Neurosurg. *48* (1978), 679—688.
4. Frowein, R. A., *et al.*, Classification of coma. Acta Neurochir. (Wien) *34* (1975), 5—10.
5. Jennett, B., Bond, M., Assessment of outcome after severe brain damage. A practical scale. Lancet *I* (1975), 480—484.
6. Overgaard, J., Christensen, S., Hvid-Hansen, O., Haase, J., Land, A. M., Hein, O., Pedersen, K. Y., Tweed, W. A., Prognosis after head injury based on early clinical examination. Lancet *II* (1973), 631—635.

Acta Neurochirurgica, Suppl. 28, 148 (1979)

Neurosurgical Clinics of Amiens, Bordeaux, Colmar, Genève, Grenoble, Liège,
Marseille, Montpellier, Nice, Paris-Creteil, Toulouse

Prognosis in Diffuse Injury

A Cooperative Study

J. Delcour, F. Cohadon, J. Baumgartner, A. Werner, J. Berney,
J. de Rougement, J. P. Bonnal, R. Vigouroux, C. Gros, J. Duplay,
J. P. Caron, J. Espagno, and G. Lazorthes

For prognostic evaluation of head injuries with diffuse lesions, twelve French-speaking neurosurgical units started a cooperative study on patients admitted to hospital within the twelve first hours following injury; the cases were strictly selected according to five criteria related to time before admission, the lack of any expanding lesion on the angiogram or the CT scan, good respiratory status at time of examination, lack of any anoxic hypoxic or ischaemic event, and the level of consciousness as evaluated according to the Teasdale and Jennett scale.

Only comatose patients were considered for study.

Thirty-six immediate and simple clinical parameters were used for the cooperative study: they are concerned with the background (5 items)—the noticeptive response (10 items), the state of eyes and pupils (10 items) the vegetative state (2 items), skull fracture (2 items), and associated lesions (7 items).

As a first step, these different parameters were correlated with survival and duration of the coma according to the multivariate factorial analysis. The statistical cloud of the data is referred to its principal axis which determines the main factors acting upon the prognosis—the cloud is projected on several planes containing various combinations of the main factors: the projected data on these planes can be separated in groups more strongly related to each of the main factors. The basic results of this cooperative study are exposed and discussed.

Acta Neurochirurgica, Suppl. 28, 149—152 (1979)
© by Springer-Verlag 1979

Universities of Glasgow, Groningen, Rotterdam, and Southern California

Prognosis in Patients With Severe Head Injury

B. Jennett, G. Teasdale, S. Galbraith, R. Braakman, C. Avezaat,
J. Minderhoud, J. Heiden, T. Kurze, G. Murray, and L. Parker

Data been collected prospectively on patients with severe head injury—studied in collaboration between Glasgow, Rotterdam, Groningen, and Los Angeles[1]. This data bank allows detailed analysis of the relationship between early features in the head-injured patient at various stages in the first week after injury, and ultimate outcome. All patients were in coma for at least six hours after injury, although in a third of cases this developed only after a period of relative lucidity. Coma was defined as "no eye-opening, no uttering of words, no obedience to commands", no matter how strong a stimulation was applied. This definition is comparable to that suggested by the Coma Committee of the WFNS—a state of "unrousable unresponsiveness"[2]. Severity in the early stages after injury has been assessed by clinical criteria: responsiveness on the Glasgow Coma Scale, abnormal motor patterns, pupillary responses, eye movements, and autonomic responses.

Results

The data bank now contains 1000 cases, and the additional data underline the similarities between severely head-injured patients in the different centres, both in early features (Table 1) and in outcome (Table 2).

Even after going into coma, the state of the patients was labile, in particular within the first 24 hours. Thus, at some time during this period almost half of the patients showed an absent or extensor motor response (coma sum 3/4), but in many patients this was only a transient phase, and in the majority of patients some better form of motor responsiveness was observed at some time within the first 24 hours. A similar phenomenon occurs with non-reacting pupils and disordered eye movements (Table 3). Because of this discrepancy, if patients were judged only upon their worst state, an over-pessimistic prognosis would

Table 1. *Features in Three Countries*

	Glasgow 593	Netherlands 239	Los Angeles 168
Mean age	35 yrs	32 yrs	35 yrs
Lucid interal	32%	25%	23%
Intracranial haematoma	54%	28%	56%
Extracranial injury	32%	51%	51%
Responsiveness (24 hours best)			
Coma sum 3/4	17%	20%	21%
Coma sum 5/6/7	52%	55%	66%
Pupils not reacting	19%	29%	31%
Eye movements: absent/impaired	45%	37%	40%

Table 2. *Outcome at 6 Months*

	Glasgow 593	Netherlands 239	Los Angeles 168
Dead	48%	50%	50%
Vegetative	2%	2%	5%
Severe disability	10%	7%	14%
Moderate disability	18%	15%	19%
Good recovery	23%	26%	12%

Table 3. *Frequency of Severe Dysfunction in the First 24 Hours*
(as % of patients for whom observations available)

	Best State		Worst State	
Coma scale score 3 or 4	176	19%	467	49%
Non-reacting pupils	226	23%	424	44%
Absent/bad eye movements	186	23%	268	34%

be obtained. Thus, 13% of all patients who had a coma sum of 3 or 4 at some period in the first 24 hours were able to make moderate or good recoveries; by contrast, only 7% of the patients who remained at this level, even at their best state, made a moderate or good recovery. The difference in prognostic significance of taking account of either pre- or

Table 4. *Outcomes Associated With Best Level of Responsiveness in First 24 Hours*

	n	Dead/ Vegetative	Moderate disability/ Good recovery
Coma Scale Score			
> 11	57	12 %	82 %
8/9/10	190	27 %	68 %
5/6/7	525	53 %	34 %
3/4	176	87 %	7 %
Pupils			
Reacting	748	39 %	50 %
Non-reacting	226	91 %	4 %
Eye Movements			
Intact	463	33 %	56 %
Impaired	143	62 %	25 %
Absent/bad	186	90 %	5 %

postoperative responsiveness, was even greater; 15 % of 120 patients with a coma sum of 3 or 4 preoperatively made moderate or good recoveries, but none of the 6 patients who survived out of 63 still in this state 6 hours after operation was better than severely disabled[5].

The need to avoid over-pessimistic predictions has led us to rely upon information about a patient's *best* state when reporting prognostic criteria. The relationship between various features and eventual outcome in this series are shown in Table 4.

Some factors had surprisingly little effect on outcome; these included the kind of event responsible for the injury, the location of damage in the right or left hemisphere, and the presence of major extracranial injury.

Conclusions

Clinical features in the first few days after injury have been shown to correlate with outcome at six months. It is, however, important to be very precise about the stage after injury at which patients are assessed, because of the variability in patients' responsiveness in the first week; the state on admission can be particularly deceptive.

The data bank may now be used in a variety of ways. Series of patients managed in different ways, whether in the original centres, or in new centres, using the same methods of assessment, can be compared in order to determine the efficacy of methods which aim to improve outcome, as described elsewhere[3].

The prognostic power of simple clinical parameters has proved to be considerable, but additional laboratory data may provide valuable additional information. With clinical data alone it is already possible to make reliable predictions of outcome in many individual patients, employing a variety of statistical techniques[4]. These methods may prove of considerable value in deciding whether or not a particular treatment is required or justified, and whether the results of a new method of treatment substantially affects expected outcome.

References

1. Jennett, B., Teasdale, G., Galbraith, S., Pickard, J., Grant, H., Braakman, R., Avezaat, C., Maas, A., Minderhoud, J., Vecht, C. J., Heiden, J., Small, R., Caton, W., Kurze, T., Severe head injuries in three countries. J. Neurol. Neurosurg. Psychiat. *40* (1977), 291—298.
2. Frowein, R. A., Classification of coma. Acta Neurochir. (Wien) *34* (1976), 5—10.
3. Teasdale, G., Parker, L., Murray, G., Jennett, B., Comparing series of head injured patients. Proceedings of the European Association of Neurosurgical Societies. Paris, July 1979.
4. Teasdale, G., Parker, L., Murray, G., Knill-Jones, R., Jennett, B., Predicting the outcome of individual patients in the first week after severe head injury. Proceedings of the European Association of Neurosurgical Societies. Paris, July 1979.
5. Teasdale, G., Galbraith, S., Acute traumatic intracranial haematomas. Progress in Neurological Surgery, Vol. 10. Basle: Karger. In Press.

Acta Neurochirurgica, Suppl. 28, 153—157 (1979)
© by Springer-Verlag 1979

Neurosurgical Clinic, University of Belgrade, Yugoslavia

Prognostic Factors in Acute Head Injuries— Brain Stem Contusion During the First Week

B. Babić, Ž. Djordjević, and M. Janićijević

Introduction

In deep unconsciousness the estimation of the intracranial state is based on the evaluation of intracranial pressure, dynamic neurological signs, and vital functions. In comatose patients showing general clinical signs of brain stem injury, neurological examination is directed towards brain stem reflexes which may indicate the anatomical level of the lesion. At the same time, brain stem reflexes, as the integral part of the total clinical picture immediately after injury, may be used as one of the factors for early prognosis. Generally speaking, the level of intracranial pressure, motor postural reflexes, and brain stem reflexes almost always provide a forecast of the results of severe craniocerebral injuries and particularly brain stem injuries (primary and secondary).

Material and Methods

In comatose patients showing decerebrate rigidity, brain stem reflexes (pupil reactions, corneal reflex, ciliospinal reflexes, oculocephalic reflex, and oculovestibular reflex are examined. We have analysed 48 such patients who have been treated at the Neurosurgical Clinic of the School of Medicine, Beograd University, Beograd during a period of 18 months (1977-1978). Clinical course and final result of the injury had been followed, and certain relevant factors analysed afterwards. Conclusions are made on the basis of the statistical analysis.

Results

Out of a total number of 48 patients who have been in a state of coma on admission to the clinic and have shown signs of decerebration, four survived, whereas 44 patients (92%) died.

Half of the surveyed number of patients were between 11 and 30 years of age. No survivor was older than 20. In all patients brain stem reflexes have been examined immediately upon admission to the clinic, vital functions have been recorded, and three syndromes of brain stem lesion, mesencephalic, mesencephalopontine and ponto-medullary, have been established on the basis of the results.

Table 1 shows the distribution of the patients and results of injuries in particular syndromes. Out of four survivors three have had a neurological picture of a lesion of the rostral part of the brain stem (mesencephalic syndrome), whereas out of 25 patients with low brain stem lesions (ponto-medullary level) 24 died. A large number of patients, 24 out of a total number of 48 patients (or 50%) have had

Table 1

Brain stem syndrome	Number of patients			
	Survived	Dead	Total	%
Mesencephalic	3	8	11	23
Mesencephalo-pontine	—	12	12	25
Ponto-medullary	1	24	25	52
	4	44	48	100%

mydriatic and paralytic pupils, as a sign of transtentorial herniation. In four survivors this sign was missing. Distribution of injured patients according to injuries is significant. In this light, two groups of injuries have been established based on the results of clinical and neuro-radiologic examination (Table 2).

It is evident that the patients in the series having brain stem contusion have had considerably greater chance of survival than the ones having impression fracture or intracranial haematoma besides contusion. Thirteen patients have had fractures of extremities and thorax bones, besides craniocerebral injuries, and only one of the patients from this group survived.

Time interval from the moment of injury to death varies very much, and ranges from one to sixty days. The average time of survival of the whole group is 9.5 days, and the majority (11 patients, or 25%) lived five days (Table 3). The greatest number of injured patients having ponto-medullary syndromes died during the first five days, while the length of existence of the patients having the other two syndromes varies very much in correlation with the type of craniocerebral injury.

The type of craniocerebral injury has been diagnosed by clinical examination, standard skull X-ray, and carotid angiography im-

Table 2

Group of injury	Number of patients			
	Survived	Dead	Total	%
I. Brain stem contusion with-without linear skull fracture	4	22	26	54
II. Brain stem contusion and other space-occupying compressive lesion (impression fracture, intracranial haematoma)	—	22	22	46

Table 3

Time interval from injury to lethal results, in days	Number of patients	%
First three days	12	27.2
4-7 days	21	41.7
8-14 days	4	9.0
Over 14 days	6	16.1
	44	100%

(Editor's note: Three are arithmetical errors in Table 3)

mediately on admission. In 25 patients (24%) tracheostomy has been effected within the first three days after injury. Gaseous analyses were carried out continuously, and water and electrolyte balance was followed two times a day, if necessary. Beside other break-downs of metabolic parameters, increased and high values of urea of extrarenal origin in blood have been registered in a great number of patients (50%) during the first days after injury.

Four of the survivors have certain common characteristics: all of them have been young persons (not older than 20). All had brain contusions as clinically diagnosed pathoanatomic substrates, without any other space-occupying compressive lesions; they were treated in hospital for 6-13 weeks. Subtemporal decompressive craniectomy was done in two patients (in one of them it was bilateral). Three cured patients had the same clinical course: from a comatose state with decerebration they passed into the apallic syndrome (in one of the patients it was complete and in the other it was a functional apallic syndrome) from which they progressed to complete psychological and physical restitution, and thus they are now completely socially independent individuals.

Discussion

In the majority of cases, the injured persons with the clinical signs of brain stem lesion have, as a rule, an unfavourable prognosis. Such a great degree of mortality in our series (92%) may be explained by the fact that the majority of patients (52%) had signs of transtentorial herniation of the caudal, ponto-medullary segment of the brain stem. On the other hand, a significant number of injured (48%) had clinical signs of unilateral transtentorial herniation caused by an additional compressive lesion (intracranial haematoma). All survivors showed signs of brain stem contusion without space-occupying compressive lesions. Tracheostomy at an early stage and correctly controlled balance of water and electrolytes affect prognosis favourably. We are inclined to believe that in two cases significant decompressive craniotomy had a considerable influence in restoring health. The height of intracranial pressure in some of our patients has been evaluated on the basis of clinical parameters (without measuring by instruments). Although intracranial pressure is one of the significant parameters for prognosis of craniocerebral injuries in general, we think that in the cases of such severe injuries as brain stem lesions, recording of postural reflexes and brain stem reflexes is sufficient for prognosis immediately after injury.

Summary

Based on our analysis of early prognostic factors in patients in a state of coma and with the signs of decerebration, it is possible to develop two clinical models:

I. With the greatest chance of survival are patients having brain stem contusions without additional compressive or destructive lesions and with preserved brain stem reflexes (signs of mesencephalic syndrome), and young people (children and persons not older than 20).

II. Unfavourable early features of brain stem injuries would be: presence of additional compressive lesions (intracranial haematomas in various locations), presence of the signs of transtentorial herniation, extinguished brain stem reflexes (ponto-medullary syndrome), and old age. Early diagnostic procedures should include carotid angiography or computerized axial tomography.

In therapy, besides hyperosmolar solutions and corticosteroids and appropriate surgical operation, continuous control (from the moment of injury) of gaseous values, and of water and electrolyte balance in blood and CSF is essential, as well as provision of an unobstructed passage within the respiratory system (endotracheal tube or tracheostomy).

References

1. Bruce, A. D., Langfitt, W. T., The prognostic value of ICP, CPP, CBF, and $CMRO_2$ in head injury. Head Injuries, Second Chicago Symposium on Neural Trauma, Chicago, 1975, pp. 23—35.
2. Becker, P. D., et al., Early prognosis in head injury based on motor posturing, oculocephalic reflexes and intracranial pressure. Head Injuries, Second Chicago Symposium on Neural Trauma, Chicago, 1975, pp. 27—30.
3. Shapiro, M. H., Intracranial hypertension. Anesthesiology 43, No. 4, Oct. 1975.
4. Espagno, J., Tremoulet, M., The prognosis of brain stem lesions in patients with recent head injuries. J. Neurosurg. Sci. 20 (1976), 33—38.
5. Rossanda, M., Intensive care of traumatic brain stem injuries. J. Neurosurg. Sci. 20 (1976), 43—48.
6. De Pascalis, C., Fernandez, E., Gentilomo, A., Considerations on clinical "brain stem" semiology in acute post-traumatic coma. J. Neurosurg. Sci. 20 (1976), 5—16.

Acta Neurochirurgica, Suppl. 28, 158—160 (1979)
© by Springer-Verlag 1979

b) Prediction of Outcome

Neurosurgical Clinic, Medical Faculty of the University of Rotterdam,
The Netherlands

Prognosis of the Individual Patient With Severe Head Injury

J. D. F. Habbema, R. Braakman, and C. J. J. Avezaat

With 3 Figures

Clinical prognosis in an individual patient always entails a certain amount of uncertainty. Categorical statements are seldom correct. Probability prognosis is preferable. Various chances are then given to one of a group of outcomes; *e.g.* this patient has a chance of 95% of being dead after one week and 5% of remaining alive. Such prediction is then based on the course so far and the expectations about the future course.

Early adequate and reliable prognosis of the individual patient with severe head injury is important, *e.g.* to inform the family early and correctly, to plan adequate rehabilitation programmes adjusted to the most probable outcome, or to evaluate alternative treatment regimes. If there are several treatment types it is easier to assemble groups of patients who are well-matched for severity if the factors which influence outcome are known. There have been many studies which have identified features observable soon after head injury which correlate with outcome. Most of them, however, provide information about the value of a certain feature for the prognosis of groups of patients, not for the individual patient. This report regards a study which is so far different from previous studies that

A: the population for which the prognostic rules apply has been defined sharply. All patients were in coma (*i.e.* did not open their eyes, did not obey commands, nor uttered any recognizable word) for at least six hours at some stage after injury, either immediately or after a delay.

B: a large number of features during the course of the illness were sharply defined, and scored within certain time periods in the same way in three countries (Fig. 1). Currently this data bank of patients

<pre>
                                        on admission
                                        within 24 hours
        70 features observed   day 2-3
        after start of coma   day 4-7
                                        day 8-14
                                        day 15-28
</pre>

Fig. 1

death
persistent vegetative state
severe disability
moderate disability
good recovery

Fig. 2

age
sum response score $(E + M + V)$
best motor response arms
motor pattern (hemiparesis etc.)
eye movements
pupils
change (improvement or deterioration)
apnoea

time to deterioration
respiratory frequency
blood pressure
tonic spasms
period accident—coma

best sum response score precoma
respiratory pattern

Fig. 3. Features with prognostic significance

contains all the details of more than 1000 comatose head-injured patients.

C: the outcome categories were sharply defined and limited in number (Glasgow outcome scale) (Fig. 2).

Most probably the rate of correct, accurate, and reliable individual prognostic probabilities for a certain outcome increases if many features at the same time can be taken into account. Those features are preferable which can be assessed simply and reliably by even junior nursing and medical staff, clinically and at the bedside. They may include investigations such as ICP, EEG, and CT scan. Features should be observations, not interpretations; terms such as purposeful, decorticate, diencephalic etc. are to be avoided.

There are various statistical models for this purpose. In one of them the assumption is that the prognostic significance of the various features are mutually independent. Among the various statistical models this model, which is partly incorrect, provides so far the best results. Through a stepwise method the feature which provides a maximum amount of information with a minimum number of incorrect scores is identified. In the next step subsequently the next ranking feature is included, and this goes on until no further improvement in information is obtained.

Summarizing our results so far it can be stated that

1. there is only a limited number of features (10-15-) which determine prognosis (Fig. 3). If these are included in a predictive exercise no further information is obtained by the scores of other data;

2. it is feasible in an unexpectedly large number of patients to make probability statements about outcome in the first few days after injury:

3. the features which are of prognostic significance in the first few days after injury are different from those observed in the next few weeks.

Acta Neurochirurgica, Suppl. 28, 161—164 (1979)

Institute of Neurological Sciences, Southern General Hospital,
and University of Glasgow, Scotland

Predicting the Outcome of Individual Patients in the First Week After Severe Head Injury

G. Teasdale, L. Parker, G. Murray,
R. Knill-Jones, and B. Jennett

Introduction

The establishment of a large collaborative data bank has allowed the relationship between early features and ultimate outcome after head injury to be identified. In turn this has permitted statisticians to predict the outcome of individual patients. We have already described the results of applying an "independence model" to the prediction of outcome of head—injured patients[1,2]; other methods in use include latent class models[3], linear discrimination[4], and kernel density methods[5]. In this paper we consider the use of the independence model to make predictions at different stages in the first week, using differing amounts of information and the purposes for which predictions might be used.

A Confident Prediction

Results

A "confident" prediction is made when one of the outcome categories is predicted with high probability. The level chosen to define "high probability" can be varied with consequent changes in the number of patients predicted confidently and the accuracy of these predictions. We have found a level of 0.97 to be a suitable threshold (Table 1).

Data from 344 "known" cases, used to predict outcomes of 165 "new" patients, from data at 2-3 days. Serious error = predicted dead but survived.

Table 1. *Level of Confidence and Predicted Yield*

Confident probability	% Patients predicted with confidence	% of those correct	Serious errors
.90	76	92	3
.95	67	96	1
.97	61	98	—
.99	49	99	—

Predictions at Different Stages in the First Week

Table 2 shows that more confident predictions are made at 2-3 days than in the first 24 hours, but the accuracy of these confident predictions is similar. There is less improvement in confidence after the first few days. The number of outcomes being predicted also affect the proportion of patients in whom a prognosis can be given. Prediction of only two outcomes (death as against survival) enables more confident predictions to be made than if an attempt is made to identify severely disabled survivors. This group seems particularly difficult to identify.

Table 2. *Prediction at Various Epochs After Onset of Coma*

Data Base	2 Outcomes Dead/Veg or Survive		3 Outcomes Dead/Veg or Sev or Mod/Good	
	% confident	% of those correct	% confident	% of them correct
24 hours	45	94	37	92
2–3 days	61	98	52	97
4–7 days	68	93	43	90

Confident = probability > 0.97

Predictions Using Different Numbers of Features

Although the computer initially had access to more than 25 items of data at any one epoch after injury, when a confident prediction was made, the probability reached 0.97 on the basis of a much smaller number of items.

We have chosen eight features which were useful predictors, were likely to be clinically reliable, were seldom missing, and did not contain data which were likely to be overly redundant. These were age, Glasgow Coma Score, best motor response score, motor abnormality pattern, pupillary responses, eye movements, whether or not apnoea had occurred, and whether or not the trend within an epoch was towards improvement or deterioration. With this number of items it is possible for clinicians to make predictions, using a set of tables and a programmable hand-held calculator, which compare well with those made by the computer, using the complete list. Until now predictions of a patient's outcome have not been transmitted to those caring for the patient while he or she was still under treatment. The provision of statistical information about a patient's probable outcome to the clinicians responsible for his care might have little effect upon management, but the rational response would be to focus resources on those most likely to benefit. In this context it is important to note that it is only a small proportion of even the severely injured patients in the data bank who are predicted confidently as having little or no prospect of recovery. In the remaining patients the implication would be that an acceptable recovery is either likely or at any rate still possible; this in turn could mean that all these patients should be regarded as potentially benefiting from continuing intensive management, even if not all to the same extent. Indeed, where a particular method of management involves prolonged expensive use of resources, or is associated with possible complications, the selection of patients for treatment might be based upon their not being confidently predicted to recover with more conventional therapy.

Predictions based solely upon clinical experience and judgement may vary markedly between different doctors, and such predictions are usually made with less confidence than the available data justify. Predictions made on the basis of the data bank make reliable use of data from 1000 previous cases; it is unlikely that a single doctor would ever accumulate experience of this number of cases, and even were he to do so his recall would certainly by imperfect.

One of the major uses of the data bank may be as a source of reference against which the results of other series can be judged; comparison between the expected outcomes of patients in a new series, as predicted on the basis of data from the bank, with their actual outcomes may be a powerful method of testing any differences[6].

References

1. Jennett, B., Teasdale, G., Braakman, R., Minderhoud, J., Knill-Jones, R., Predicting outcome in individual patients after severe head injury. Lancet *1* (1976), 1031—1034.
2. Knill-Jones, R., Clinical decision-making—diagnostic and prognostic inference. Health Bulletin *35* (1977), 213.

11*

3. Skene, A., Latent class models in medical diagnosis. Submitted for publication.
4. Habbema, J. D. F., Hermans, J., van den Broek, K., A stepwise discriminant analysis program using density estimation. Compstat 1974. Proceedings in Computational Statistics. Wien: Physica Verlag. 1974.
5. Titterington, M., Analysis of incomplete multivariate binary data by the kernel method. Biometrika *64* (1977), 455—460.
6. Teasdale, G., Jennett, B., Murray, G., Parker, L., Comparing series of head injured patients. Submitted to Neurosurgery.

Acta Neurochirurgica, Suppl. 28,165—170 (1979)
© by Springer-Verlag 1979

Neurosurgical and Psychometrie Units, Hospital General de Asturias, Oviedo,
Spain

Head Injury Prognosis: Calculations From Clinical Data

A. F. Serrats and S. A. Parker

With 2 Figures

In order to establish a more accurate clinical prognosis in head
injuries, a series of 600 consecutive cases without previous history or
associated lesions (secondary intracranial or general) were analysed.

Material and Method

All cases were seen within an hour of accident. Four hundred and
ninety-four cases had initial loss of consciousness, and 145 were in coma
at arrival, while 349 were in different levels of consciousness. A total of
156 were in coma at some time (109 caudo-cranial evolution; and 47
cranio-caudal).

Daily clinical assessment, complementary studies, and a three year
follow-up on survivors were done, as well as postmortem studies in
deceased patients.

The following parameters were used: a) *The brain stem specific reflex
activity.* b) *The patients basic general reactions* (motor, arousal, and
mimic), and c) *the degree of integrity of higher mental functions.* The
evolution of these cases could be displayed in graphic form and plotted
against time, the appearance and disappearance of clinical signs
compared in upwards and downwards evolving cases; signs appearing
always in the same relative order of succession could be taken as
evolutive landmarks. Thus, a clinical picture appearing constantly in a
similar position on the graph, associated with a given landmark, can be
taken also, as a *Functional Level of neurological integration* (FL) and
used to indicate evolutive stages of a dynamic process without
implying, a priori, any anatomical significance. Thus, neurological
grading as a necessary step for devising a Head Injury Prognostic Scale
could be done by using those levels.

In this way, we have been able to draw the following levels from our evolutive charts and compare them with postmortem and complementary studies:

I. Apnoea and total arreflexia, corresponding to a Medullary level.

II. Vegetative reflexes only (*Ponto-Medullary* level).

III. Extensor motor reaction (E); some deglutition (2. component); spontaneous respiration can be present. Irregularly dilated pupils (*Mid-Pontine* level).

All patients from these levels (more than one hour) died.

IV. Extensor response; corneal and deglutition reflex. Mid-dilated and fixed pupil. Spontaneous breathing (seems to correspond to *Upper-Pontine* level). Recovery was possible.

V. Extensor (E) or Flexor (F) response, mostly downwards corneomandibular reflexes. Fixed and mid-dilated or small pupils. Postmortem and radiological studies point to *Mesencephalic* level.

From here onwards, in upward (ascending) comas, the cases may follow one of three evolutive lines: a) Still presenting a extensor motor reaction at the end of the first week and remaining so in the following levels. We did not find recovery. b) Those showing a non-specific (flexor) reaction at the end of the first week and entering such condition in the next stages. On reaching arousal, they can proceed in one of two ways: either they regain menace or normal motor reaction during the second week (with good prognosis) or, failing to do so, the prognosis is poor (remaining demented in our series). c) Those showing normal (N) motor reaction within the first week made a good recovery.

VI. Positive vestibular reaction and oculo-cephalio reflexes, seem to correlate, in progressing comas, with recovery or integrity of Mesencephalic level.

VII. Reappearance of arousal and Blink reflex (2. component), seems to indicate recovery of Mesencephalic-Diencephalic reticular formation.

VIII. Reappearance of menace reflex (and the disappearance, shortly before, of the oculo-cephalic), seems to mark the beginning of corticalization.

IX. Full cortical level is represented by this level, comprising a series of transitional syndromes: obnubilation, confabulation, severe amnesia, mutism etc.

X. This level corresponds to normal condition.

I. Prognosis/Neurological Condition/Evolutive Time Relationship

We found in our series that probability of recovery, on the whole, increased with recovery of neurological function and the speed of its recovery (Fig. 1).

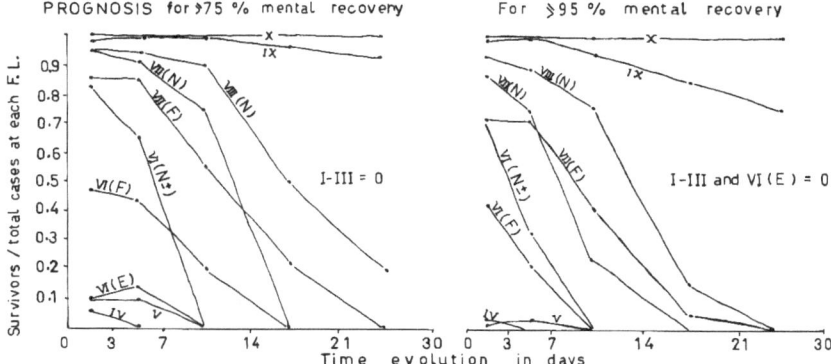

Fig. 1. Diagnosis, functional level and time of recovery relationship in our series of evolutive head injury cases. *I–X* neurological functional levels. (*E*), (*F*), (*N*±), (*N*) extensor, flexor, semi specific and normal motor reaction

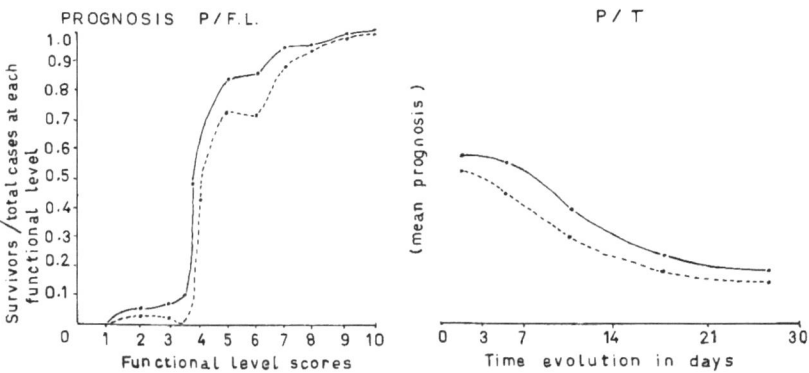

Fig. 2. Prognosis (*P*), functional level (*FL*) and time of recovery (*T*) relationship in evolutive head injuries as $P = f(FL/\Delta T) + C$. Prognosis for 75 % mental recovery (continuous line), prognosis for 95 % mental recovery (dotted line)

Taking the initial evolutive time (T_0) as the first 48 hours after head injury, and putting all *Initial Functional Levels* ($FL_{am} T_0$) and the *Times* ($T_0 — T_x$) on the X-axis, and the *Number of Successes/Total Cases* (P) at each level and time on the Y-axis, we obtained two semi-logarithmic inverse curves:

a) The probability of recovery of each "Functional level" at initial time and, b) the graphical expression of the patient's changing

prognosis as he remains on the same neurological level as time passes
(Fig. 2).

Thus we can say that. Prognosis is a direct function of the
Neurological level $(P = f(FL)$, and an inverse function of the time of
recovery $(P = f(l/T))$. Prognosis of evolutive head injuries at a given
time (Tx) of their evolution and at a given Neurological condition
(FL_m) could be expressed as *the theoretical prognosis that that particular
condition should have had at initial time* $(FL_{m \cdot To})$ *plus the increment in
prognosis as time increases from* T_0 *to* T_x. Thus, with $P_{n/t(o-x)}$ *the mean
prognostic* curve from the initial condition to the actual one, we have

$$P_{n/t (o-x)} = P_o + P_o = (\textstyle\int f' (\log FL_{a-m \cdot To}) + C) - (\int f' (\log T_{o-x}) + C')$$

$$Prognosis = (\log FL_{To}^2/2 + C)_a{}^m - (\log T^2/2 + C')_o{}^x \qquad (1)$$

Values for FL and T were drawn from Fig. 2 and were:

a) *For FL:* I. to III. = 1; IV. = 2; V. = 3; VI. (E) = 3.5; VI. (F) = 4;
VI. (N) = 5; VII. (F) = 5; VII. (N) = 7; VIII. (N) = 8; IX = 9; and
X = 10.

b) *For T:* 1 to 3 days = 1; 3 to 7 days = 2; second, third, and fourth
week = 3, 4, and 5 respectively.

The constants of integration C and C are arbitrary constants, and
their values and relations were found from the data by trial and error:

a) C was the logarithm of a biological variable, dependent on the
motor reaction in relation to two landmarks: alertness and the menace
reflex. The values of this variable were found to be: 1 for extensor
response; 2.75 for the flexor response, give or take 0.75 for the presence
or absence of alertness; 3.9 for semi-specific; and 3.75 for normal motor
response, give or take -0.25 for the presence or absence of menace.

b) C is also a variable related to Time and Neurological Function. It
has a positive sign, except at cortical levels (9 and 10), and for the first
and the first T and second ΔT on levels 6 and 8. Furthermore, provided
that we consider these results above 1 and below 0 as 1 and 0
respectively, we feel that we can safely propose as a general rule
$(\alpha \leq 0.01)$, that C be equal to 0.01 multiplied by the following values for
each ΔT:

Applying these values to formula (1) gives us the mean Prognostic
Curve $(P_{n/t})$ for Survival and $\geq 75\%$ mental recovery [with S.D. of
confidence intervals for the 95 % population $(S_{p(P95)}) \leq 8.5$]. Prognosis
for $\geq 95\%$ mental recovery obeys the same rules but follows a lower
(0.1 to 0.3) irregular curve (Figs. 1 and 2). At initial time it is equal to
$P \geq 75\%$ in fully conscious patients; 92-98 % of it in cortico-
subcortical; 89-83 % above mesencephalic level and only 50-20 % of
that below.

0

Time: (weeks)		T_0—1/2—1.—2.—3.—4.					
	(scores)	1	2	3	4	5	
Fl_{a-m}	motor response	scores					
I–III.	extensor	1	2	2	2	2	
IV.	extensor	2	$2^{1.5}$	2	2	2	(Example: C' for
V.	extensor	3	2	2	2	2	the ΔT from 2. to
VI.	extensor	3.5	2	2	2	2	3. week is:
VI.	flexor	4	2	2^3	2^3	2^3	$= 0.01 \times 2 \times 2 \times 2 = 0.16$)
VI.	inspecifio	5	2	2^3	2^3	2^3	
VII.	flexor	6	2^4	2^3	2^3	2^3	
VII.	normal	7	2	2^2	2^4	2^4	
VIII.	normal	8	2	2^2	$2^{1.7}$	2	
IX.	normal	9	2	$2^{2.6}$	2°	2°	
X.	normal	10	2^2	2^2	2^2	2^2	

More accurate calculations for $P \geq 95\%$ can be done by using a graph for each level (S.D. of $S_{p(P95)} \leq 6.79$).

II. Age Factor (f(a))

Age distribution in our series was a random one, as may be expected in any cross-section of population, with three age groupings: ≤ 25; $> 25 < 40$ and > 40, with mean age falling in the middle group, which shows a similar distribution of successes as $P_{n/t}$. Thus the whole series corresponded to a standard distribution curve with mean (middle group) standardized at $P_{n/t}$, S.D. of one, random variables ($Z_{\leq 25}$ and $Z_{\leq 40}$) with values of 0.2 and 0.32 and corresponding probabilities of $P_{<25} = +0.0792$ and $P_{<40} = -0.12552$ above and below the mean $P_{n/t}$ respectively. Thus, an age factor $(f(a)) = P_a(1 - P_{n/t})$ can and should be added to the main Prognosis ($P_{n/t}$) to get a correct probability (P_c).

$$\text{Thus: } P_o = P_a(1 - P_{n/t}) + P_{n/t} \qquad (2)$$

III. Added Factors: Complications

Up to now we have been considering patients with pure concussional syndromes with neither associated intracranial secondary lesions (Collections, contusion-oedema, etc.), nor intercurrent general problems (respiratory, metabolic, BP, etc.), such as may arise in any patient or in polytrauma cases. Prognosis should be expanded to include the possibility of such events. This can be done by subtracting from the main P_o in formula (2), the increment in mortality—morbidity (M), should such eventualities arise.

If F_r is the probability of one of these events occurring in head injury, and P_r its Prognosis in sucha case, the complete Prognosis P_T would be:

$$P_T = F_r P_r (1 - P_o) + P_o \qquad (3)$$

where P_o can be substituted from formulae (1) and (2).

Summary and Conclusions

As the original lesion causing the initial clinical picture in a head injury follows its natural evolution, one sees, in both horizontal and caudocranial direction, either an aggravation due to the existence of some associated dynamic factors (compression, ischaemia, metabolic factors, etc.), or a functional recovery of some non-permanently damaged structures.

As recovery advances and new clinical pictures emerge, one realises the existence usually of an irregular upward extension of the lesion, the importance and extent of which cannot be properly assessed initially and which is frequently ignored.

In order to attempt an assessment and grading of such clinical states one must avoid the general tendency to consider them as separate clinical syndromes, as they are not static entities but, most often, part of an evolutive-involutive process, following an irregular and apparently unpredictable lesion-path, in which each step shows a combination of lesions of different structures and anatomical levels. The emerging picture is really the functional level of cerebral integration, at any given time of the evolution from the beginning, expressed by the whole remaining function shown by the patient at that time.

Theoretically, one can admit the possibility of a great number of combinations of damaged structures but, in practice, such a random distribution does not occur to such an extent as to make it impossible to pick out the most significant combinations and to group them clinically into a certain number of functional levels. This would be of an academic importance only if one was unable to correlate these functions with a particular localization or with the patient's evolution and use them as evolutive stages with a practical meaning in the diagnosis of the case.

Through analysis of our series we came to the conclusion that prognosis is a direct function of the neurological level and an inverse time-function and that, by integration of both functions and considering together with the age- and complicationfactor, we could reach a prognosis by the use of a simple pocket calculator. Also the formula can give us the degree of neurological affectation from added complications or can be used, as coded formulae, to store information.

Acta Neurochirurgica, Suppl. 28, 171—173 (1979)
© by Springer-Verlag 1979

Neurosurgical University Clinic Graz
(Head: Prof. Dr. F. Heppner) and
Neurosurgical Department Salzburg
(Head: Prof. Dr. H. E. Diemath), Austria

Predicting Outcome After Severe Head Injury— A Computer-Assisted Analysis of Neurological Symptoms and Laboratory Values

L. Auer, G. Gell, B. Richling, and R. Oberbauer

The prognosis of outcome in the acute stage after severe head injury is of outstanding interest for both the patient's doctor and relatives. The course of neurological symptoms and biochemical data during the first days after injury has been evaluated by several authors to find out parameters that correlate with the clinical course and the outcome of the patient (Jennett and coworkers, Heller and Oldenkott, Brodersen and Jorgensen).

Our plan was to find a pattern of routine laboratory values and neurological symptoms that indicates no survival chance for the injured. By other means we wanted to find out if there is a possibility of drawing the absolute no survival chance conclusion for such patients in the early stage after injury. It was clear that such a system could only cover the immediate consequences of primary lesions, but no secondary complications.

To date our study covers 130 patients treated in one of the two neurosurgical units cited above. All data were put together in a joint study, and evaluated by means of a computer programme. All patients were comatose for at least three days. Seventy-five per cent had an isolated head injury, 25% had polytrauma. The same therapeutic schedule was used in both intensive care units. In the first 96 patients 80 operative interventions were performed, and 38% did not survive. The other patients were scaled using the Glasgow-outcome scale: 11% remained in a persistent vegetative state, 14% came out with severe deficit, 12% had mild deficit; 30% recovered well.

During the first seven days after injury, the following data were evaluated daily for computer analysis:

1. Laboratory values: Serum-osmolality, electrolytes, urea, uric acid, creatinine, coagulation factors, proteins, pH, bicarbonate, blood cells, blood sugar, lactate, pyruvate; CSF-haemoglobin and total protein.

2. Neurological symptoms: An evaluation schedule according to the Glasgow coma scale was used, which includes eye opening, verbal response, and motor response (A-V-M). Evaluation was performed by calculating a mean score of the hourly investigated signs. 1 was the worst score for every sign, a mean score of 1 thus representing the worst situation possible for the patient. In addition, pupil reaction was evaluated qualitatively in four groups: fixed maximally dilated, anisocoria, pinpoint pupils, and normal. Oculocephalic reflex and vestibulo-ocular reflex were also qualitatively evaluated.

3. Vegetative parameters: blood pressure, body temperature, pulse frequency, respiration, evaluated with a scoring-schedule. All parameters were evaluated in respect of their exclusive existence in non-survivers.

Therefore, as a first step, we checked the parameters that significantly differed between survivors and non-survivors; these data are listed below; they are mean values over the whole week or the survival time:

Serum-osmolality	$p < 0.001$	platelets	$p < 0.01$
Serum-sodium	$p < 0.001$	part. Thr. time	$p < 0.001$
Serum-chloride	$p < 0.005$	blood sugar	$p < 0.005$
Serum-calcium	$p < 0.01$	platelet aggr.	$p < 0.005$
Serum-urea	$p < 0.001$	CSF-total prot.	$p < 0.005$
Serum-uric acid	$p < 0.001$	A-V-M.	$p < 0.001$
Serum-creatinine	$p < 0.001$	SAP	$p < 0.005$
Serum-total bilirubin	$p < 0.001$	body temp.	$p < 0.001$

As a next step these significant parameters were checked for their statistical variance, those overlapping too widely being eliminated from further evaluation. Thereafter, the following parameters could be used for further calculations: serum osmolality, urea, total bilirubin; pupil reaction; AVM-system; vegetative parameters. The prognostic significance of parameters, chosen for our prognosis-schedule, fits with earlier investigations (Auer *et al.*).

A score for every parameter was found that occurred in certain non-survivors but in none of the survivors, at least for two days or until early death. The percentage of non-survivors with parameters beyond the survivor-limit was then evaluated. A no-chance-score in patients with at least one positive parameter was found in 80%. Evaluation of laboratory values alone covered 42 % of non-survivors. Neurological signs + vegetative parameters alone covered 80%. Maximally dilated and fixed pupils, once diagnosed, were followed by lethal outcome in all but one patient, the latter surviving with severe deficit. Therefore, we combined all parameter groups, and gave a no chance-score only to those patients that had at least two positive parameters, thus covering 50 % of all non-survivors.

The no-survival-chance prediction cannot be made before the third day after head injury.

Undoubtedly a larger series of patients is needed to test this predicting system and adapt it to different age groups since different patterns might be valuable for different ages. Nevertheless it does not seem to be possible to cover all non-survivors with such a prognostic schedule nor to say anything about positive survival chances. Investigation of laboratory values does not increase the percentage of non-survivors to be detected with the no chance-system, but it increases the probability of a true prediction.

Acta Neurochirurgica, Suppl. 28, 174—178 (1979)

Neurosurgical Clinic (Director: Prof. Dr. W. Grote)*
and Institute of Neuropathology (Director: Prof. Dr. L. Gerhard)**,
Essen University, Federal Republic of Germany

Risk Factors in Severe Head Injury

H.-E. Nau*, V. Reinhard, E. B. Bongartz*,
and R. Floßdorf****

The evaluation of prognostic and risk factors has been one of the most important topics in neurotraumatology. These factors would enable the neurosurgeon to modify therapeutic procedures according to prognosis. Different authors have tried to determine the outcome of injured patients by analysis of clinical data: age[9], ICP[15,16], CBF and cerebral metabolic rate for oxygen[4], motor posturing and oculocephalic reflexes[1,2], and EEG patterns[3,12]. Studies based on neurological findings and their relations to patients' outcome were given by different authors[5,6,8,10,11,13,14].

Patients and Method

One hundred patients with severe head injury were studied. One group consisted of 50 patients who died and in whom autopsy was done. The other group had 50 patients with favourable outcome.

We differentiated three types of factors: 1. pretraumatic, 2. traumatic, and 3. posttraumatic factors (Table 1).

Results

Pretraumatic Factors

In each group we found 35 males and 15 females. The average age of the non-survivors was 41 years, that of the survivors 22 years. Additional diseases were present in six patients in the group with a favourable outcome and in 27 in the other group. In eight patients only were these pretraumatic factors known from the history. In the 50 patients who died, autopsy revealed the following risk factors: atherosclerosis of the Willisian circle (16 patients) and of aorta (12 patients), coronary sclerosis (9 patients), myocardial diseases (11 patients), pulmonary sclerosis (8 patients), emphysema (4 patients),

Table 1. *Investigated Factors in Severe Head Injury*

Pretraumatic Factors

Age   Sex

pre-existing diseases (clinical and morphological findings)

Traumatic factors

Kind of accident	Time between accident and admission
Unconsciousness	Shock
Assisted ventilation	Pupils/light reaction
Pain reaction	Reflexes/motor disturbances
Extension rigidity	Kind of skull fracture
Additional injuries	Intracranial space-occupying lesions
Morphological findings	

Post-traumatic Factors

Operations	Unconsciousness
Extension mechanisms	Seizures
Infections	Intracranial pressure
Blood pressure	Blood chemistry
EEG	Therapeutic managements
Morphological findings	

fatty liver (5 patients), and renal atherosclerosis (4 patients). The average age of the patients with risk factors was 57.5 in the non-survivors' group, contrasting with 36.5 years in the survivors' group. In both groups the ages of patients without risk factors were nearly equal (21.3 and 20.4 years).

Traumatic Factors

The causes of admission were always accidents, mainly traffic accidents (52 to 56 per cent), followed by falls (30 to 20 per cent). The time between accident and clinical neurosurgical admission was 8.3 hours in the fatal group and 11.8 hours in the other. Forty-one patients arrived within an hour of intury (21 in one group, 20 in the other).

The cause for admission to our clinic was primary unconsciousness in 88 per cent in the fatal group and 72 per cent in the survivors' group, and secondary unconsciousness in 12 per cent and 18 per cent respectively in the two groups.

Among the non-survivors 18 had signs of shock, whereas 9 patients of the group with a favourable outcome had shock. In the fatal group 36 patients arrived with assisted ventilation compared to 38 in the other group. In both groups all patients had to be intubated.

An abnormal reaction to light stimulus was found in 60 per cent of the non-survivors and 36 per cent of the survivors. In the latter group

reaction to pain stimuli was inadequate in 40 per cent contrasting with
74.5 per cent in the group with a fatal outcome. Among these patients
81 per cent showed motor disturbances, whereas in the other group we
found motor disturbances in 52 per cent. In the survivors' group no
open skull brain fracture could be found, compared with 23 per cent in
the fatal group. In summary we found 48 skull fractures in the fatal
group and 22 among the survivors. Twenty-two had additional
concomitant injuries (most of them bone injuries), and so had 18
patients in the other group. Radiological investigations (CT, angiography) revealed space-occupying lesions in 81 per cent of the fatal
group and 20 per cent in the other. In the patients with fatal outcome
autopsy demonstrated renal shock in four cases and suprarenal necrosis
in two.

Post-traumatic Factors

In the non-survivors 53 operations were done, and in the survivors
48 operations. In the fatal group most of the operations wer done
because of space-occupying lesions, in the other group for continuous
ICP monitoring. Raised ICP was found in 30 per cent in the non-
survivors' group, in the other in 4 per cent only. In the fatal group 11
patients showed a temporary clinical improvement. Extension rigidity
and mechanisms were observed in 37.5 per cent, in the other group in 16
per cent. Post-traumatic seizures were nearly equally frequent (17.5
and 14 per cent). Blood pressure difficulties developed in 55 per cent of
the patients with fatal outcome, in the others in 10 per cent. The blood
sugar level was raised in the fatal group in 55 per cent, in the other
group in half of the patients. Serum electrolytes were normal without
correction in 5 per cent of the non-survivors, in the survivors in 30 per
cent. Urea and creatinine levels were pathologically changed in 12 per
cent of the non-surviving patients and in 4 per cent in the others.
Temperature disorders were observed in both groups in about 80 per
cent. EEG derivations showed severe general slowing in all patients in
the two groups.

In the survivors' group unconscionsness lasted for five days on an
average. Most of the patients with an unfavourable outcome died in the
first post-traumatic days: 19 on the first day, 9 on the second and third,
only one on the 6th day, and all other patients after the seventh day.

In these patients autopsy revealed pulmonary fat embolism in two
cases, thrombembolism of the pulmonary artery in five cases,
thrombosis of femoral and pelvic veins in seven cases. Seventy per cent
of these patients had signs of raised ICP. Alterations of the
diencephalon were found in 32 per cent, in the caudal brain stem in 24
per cent, and in the internal capsule and basal ganglia in 32 per cent.

Discussion

Our results in both groups and their comparison demonstrate that none of the conditions is absolutely fatal[7]. Therefore one should speak of risk factors and not of prognostic factors. These risk factors should be differentiated according to their importance.

Age in itself appears to be no risk factor, but since at a higher age the probability of patients having one or more diseases of vital organs increases. Age is an indirect risk factor, which is in accordance with the clinical observations of Jennett[10]. The fatal outcome in young patients, with the exception of one downs-syndrome, revealed no diseases of internal organs, but included generally very extensive fractures or special post-traumatic complications.

Among the most important traumatic factors are open skull fractures, fractures of the base of the skull and the posterior fossa, space-occupying lesions, wide pupils, inadequate reaction to light and pain stimuli, and shock[8, 9]. Among the post-traumatic factors in both groups, disorders of intracranial pressure[13], blood pressure, and temperature seem to be the most important ones. These disorders reflected the neuropathological findings of diencephalic and brain stem lesions.

In accordance with internal medicine the combination of more than one risk factor can be correlated with prognosis.

References

1. Becker, D. P., Miller, J. D., Ward, J. D., Greenberg, R. P., Young, J. F., Sakalas, R., The outcome from severe head injury with early diagnosis and intensive management. J. Neurosurg. *47* (1977), 491—502.
2. Becker, D. P., Vries, J. K., Sakalas, R., Young, H. F., Ward, J., Early prognosis in head injury based on motor posturing, oculocephalic reflexes, and intracranial pressure. In: R. L. McLaurin: Head Injuries, pp. 27—30. New York-San Francisco-London: Grune&Stratton. 1976.
3. Brenner, R. P., Schwartzman, R. J., Richey, E. T., Prognostic significance of episodic low amplitude or relatively isoelectric EEG patterns. Dis. Nerv. Syst. *36* (10), (1975), 582—587.
4. Bruce, D. A., Langfitt, Th. W., The prognostic value of ICP, CPP, CBF, and $CMRO_2$ in head injury. In: R. L. McLaurin: Head Injuries, pp. 23—25. New York-San Francisco-London: Grune&Stratton. 1976.
5. Bues, E., Stöwsand, D., 104b. Prognose der schweren gedeckten Hirntraumen im akuten Stadium nach dem klinischen Syndrom. Langenbecks Arch. Klin. Chir. *319* (1967), 627—630.
6. Busch, E. A., Brain stem contusions: differential diagnosis, therapy, and prognosis. Clin. Neurosurg. (Baltimore) *9* (1963), 18—33.
7. Caronna, J. H., Plum, F., Prognosis and medical coma. In: R. L. McLaurin: Head Injuries, pp. 3—9. New York-San Francisco-London: Grune&Stratton. 1976.

8. Frowein, R. A., Steinmann, H. W., Auf der Haar, K., Terhaag, D., Karimi-Nejad, A., Limits to classification and prognosis of severe head injury. Advances in Neurosurgery *5* (1978), 16—26.
9. Heiskanen, O., Sipponen, P., Prognosis of severe brain injury. Acta Neurol. Scandinav. *46* (1970), 343—348.
10. Jennett, B., Prognosis of severe head injury. In: R. L. McLaurin: Head Injuries, pp. 45—47. New York-San Francisco-London: Grune & Stratton. 1976.
11. Jennett, B., Teasdale, G., Galbraith, S., Pickard, J., Grant, H., Braakman, R., Avezaat, C., Maas, A., Minderhoud, J., Vecht, C. J., Heiden, J., Small, R., Caton, W., Kurze, T., Severe head injuries in three countries. J. Neurol. Neurosurg. Psych. *40* (3) (1977), 291—298.
12. Nau, H.-E., Bock, W. J., Electroencephalographie (EEG) differentiation of the apallic syndrome in severe craniocerebral injuries. Advances in Neurosurgery *5* (1978), 44—51.
13. Overgaard, J., Reflections on prognostic determinants in acute severe head injuries. In: R. L. McLaurin: Head Injuries, pp. 11—21. New York-San Francisco-London: Grune & Stratton. 1976.
14. Overgaard, J., Hvid-Hansen, O., Land, A.-M., Petersen, K. K., Christensen, St., Haase, J., Hein, O., Tweed, W. A., Prognosis after head injury based on early clinical examination. Lancet (1973), **631—635**.
15. Tindall, G. T., Fleischer, A. S., Intracranial pressure (ICP) monitoring and prognosis in closed head injury. In: R. L. McLaurin: Head Injuries, pp. 31—34. New York-San Francisco-London: Grune & Stratton. 1976.
16. Vapalahti, M., Troupp, H., Prognosis for patients with severe brain injuries. Brit. Med. J. *3* (1971), 404—407.

Acta Neurochirurgica, Suppl. 28, 179—182 (1979)
© by Springer-Verlag 1979

Department of Neurosurgery, Pinderfields Hospital, Wakefield, England

The Prediction of Outcome of Patients Admitted Following Head Injury in Coma With Bilateral Fixed Pupils

D. J. Price and R. Knill-Jones

With 2 Figures

The decision to transfer a patient in coma and often with multiple injuries to a Neurosurgical Department some distance away is usually difficult. If the patient has been in coma since impact it might be presumed that he is not developing a treatable intracranial hae-matoma, and if both pupils are also unreactive to light we could well presume that he has sustained an overwhelming brain injury for which energetic and expensive treatment is not indicated. Such presumptions can, however, easily lead to unnecessary morbidity and mortality, and for this reason prediction of outcome is of some value provided a forecast with virtually 100 % certainty can be made within the first few critical hours of injury when intensive management in a Neurosurgical Department is being considered.

The aim of the study is to identify the three most powerful predictive indicants for good survival and to establish a simple system of recognizing whether a particular patient can be included in any of the following three groups:

1. 100 % certainty of survival with return to work.
2. 100 % certainty of death or survival with severe disabilities.
3. 100 % certainty of death.

We chose a clearly defined group of patients expected to have a low incidence of survival. It consisted of a consecutive series of patients admitted after head injury to an intensive care unit in coma with bilateral medium or dilated unreactive pupils. The only patients excluded from the series were those already moribund who died during the first half hour of resuscitation. One hundred and fifty patients were included in this partly retrospective and partly prospective study over a 10 year period. One hundred and twenty-two were admitted within the first half hour after injury and 142 within the first hour, and the autopsy rate was 81 %.

12*

Bilateral unreactive pupils in patients in coma within half an hour of head injury may well denote impending brain stem death but in this series 21 survived, and of these 14 were able to return to work.

A very simple coma scale (1 to 8) was used, as this study was mainly retrospective, and more detailed information was not available. The preliminary analysis showed that on admission 10 % did not obey commands but responded to pain purposefully (level 4), 23 % did not obey commands but responded to pain without purpose (level 3), 56 % were unrousable by any means but retained a cough reflex (level 2), and 9 % were unrousable with no cough reflex and had inadequate respiration (level 1).

Eighty per cent of the patients had sustained road traffic accidents, and the chances of survival of a car occupant was half that of a pedestrian. Although 5 out of 19 patients with decerebrate rigidity survived, none returned to his or her original employment. Of the 19 patients who had high blood pressure immediately after injury, none survived. The survival rate was halved in those 72 patients over 30 years of age as compared with that of the remainder under the age of 30.

The data-base comprised 40 parameters for each patient, and included details of clinical, operative, and autopsy findings. A large mainframe computer was used to form the cross correlation analysis with the aim of identifying the three parameters with highest significance. These three proved to be conscious level, pupil signs, and time from injury.

Before embarking on a predictive analysis, it was necessary to exclude three groups of patients.

1. 13 patients who died as a result of missed operable extradural or subdural haematomas.

2. 11 patients who died as a result of other injuries.

3. 9 patients who lived but in whom as time progressed it became evident that their pupil signs had been due to extra-cerebral causes such as oculomotor or optic nerve damage or hypoxia.

Within 24 hours of injury most of these patients were identified by their continuing improvement in their conscious level despite persistent unreacting pupils. They were progressively excluded from the time series analysis.

Results

It is not surprising that the probability of returning to work rises with improving neurological signs and time from injury. If at 24 hours conscious level remains at levels 1 or 2 and pupils are still unreactive, there is only a 10 % chance of returning to work. Such statistical information is in practice meaningless as clinical decisions can only be

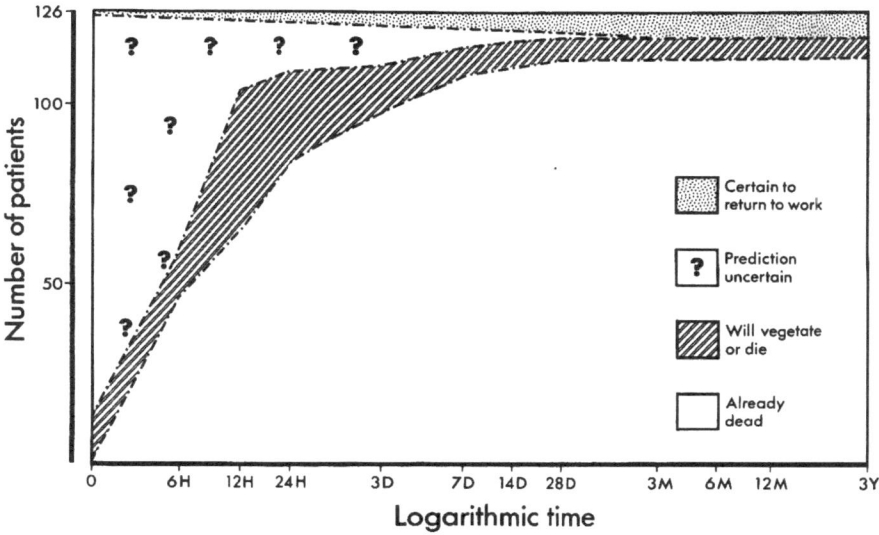

Fig. 1. Certainty of returning to work

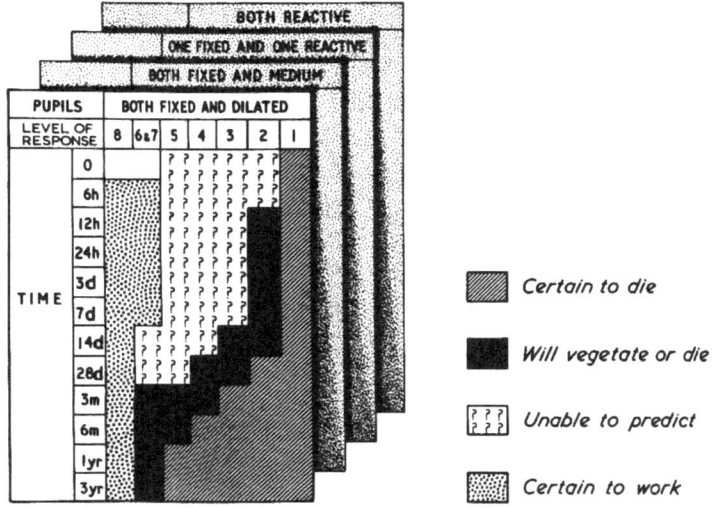

Fig. 2. Prediction of outcome. Data base: 150 patients admitted with fixed pupils

made when the certainty is virtually 100%. We therefore used multi-dimensional analysis to identify those patients in the three possible outcome grades and we found, as expected, that as time progressed the total number of fatalities increased and the number of patients with 100% certainty of dying increased. The number with 100% certainty of returning to some form of employment also increased, and the number with uncertain outcome gradually diminished (Fig. 1).

To facilitate access to our data-base we used a simple card system (Fig. 2). For example, a patient with continuing fixed dilated pupils six hours after injury with a very low conscious level (1) will die. Another patient at level 2 with continuing fixed dilated pupils 12 hours after injury would vegetate or die. It thus seems possible to make an accurate prediction for a small group of severe head injuries within a few hours of injury based on simple assessment of conscious level and pupil signs. We realise that the inclusion of brain stem function tests as additional predictive indicants could increase the percentage of patients for whom we have a 100% certainty of their eventual outcome within the first few hours after injury, but these tests have only been in routine use in recent years.

This predictive system has been applied to a further 115 patients admitted in coma with unreactive pupils to the same hospital during a further 7 year period. There had been no significant changes in management and we found the system entirely free of error for this very clearly defined group of severe head injuries.

This data-base may not be safely applied for prediction of outcome of a similar group of patients treated very aggressively with elective ventilation and intracranial pressure stabilization und we await the results of a continuing study.

Acta Neurochirurgica, Suppl. 28, 183—187 (1979)
© by Springer-Verlag 1979

Forecasting Peculiarities of Intracerebral Pressure and Local Cerebral Blood Flow Data and Methods of Outcome Forecasting in the Early Postoperative Period

V. V. Lebedev, L. G. Simonov, and J. K. Bayun

With 3 Figures

Mechanisms of cerebral blood flow disturbance in pathological conditions (such as cranio-cerebral trauma, acute disturbance of cerebral circulation etc.) differ. All cerebral blood flow changes are first of all based on intracerebral pressure (ICP) changes, caused by different factors. The problem of local cerebral blood flow (LCBF) changes in different degrees of intracerebral hypertension is also of great importance.

Comparison of ICP and LCBF correlations can serve as a test to forecast outcomes of brain diseases and injuries in the early postoperative period.

To carry out simultanecus dynamic study of ICP and LCBF, there was created a combined sensor (L. G. Simenov 1975), sunk into the medullary substance during operation. ICP was defined by capacity method LCBF—by the method of hydrogen clearance. The test was performed every 24 hours. On the 7th-13th postoperative day the sensor was removed without additional operation.

Seventy-two patients were reviewed: 50 with severe cranio-cerebral trauma, and 22 with acute disturbance of cerebral circulation. All patients were divided into two groups: I—favourable outcome (patients making satisfactory recovery), II—fatal outcome (dead patients).

Fig. 1 illustrates ICP, LCBF, and AP (arterial pressure) dinamics in patients with severe cranio-cerebral trauma. It shows progressive ICP reduction in the postoperative period in group I with further normalization on the 7th-9th days, whereas ICP in group II by that period of time is still increased. So, these data show reliable difference (P < 0,05) in ICP quantity between these two groups after the first postoperative day.

In the first two days LCBF in group I is certainly lower compared with group II blood flow. During the following day oscillation of LCBF in both groups is observed, preserving a high enough LCBF.

Investigation of LCBF and ICP made it possible to determine their critical levels. So, ICP above 1700 mm wg (water gauge) and LCBF

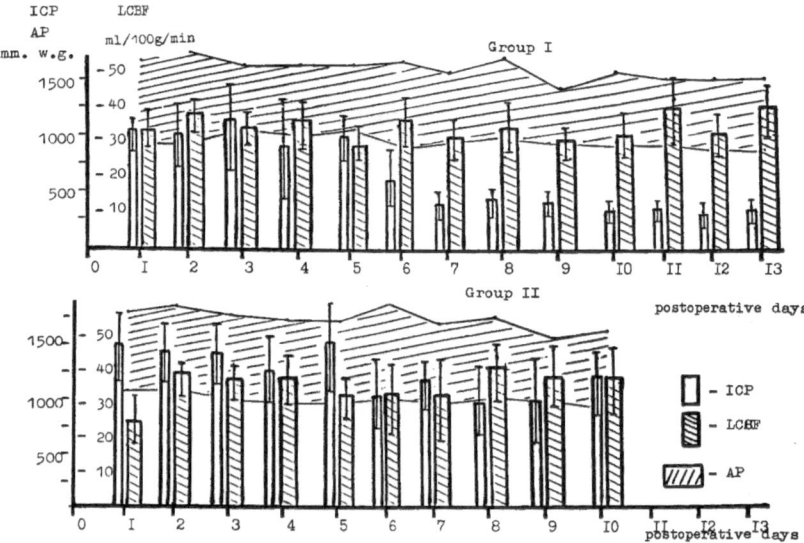

Fig. 1. The dynamics of intracerebral pressure (ICP), local cerebral blood flow ($LCBF$) and arterial pressure (AP) in patients with severe cranio-cerebral trauma

below 16 ml/100 g/min were observed only in fatal cases ($P < 0.05$). Both groups showed moderate rate of back dependence, thus, probably, showing only partial disturbance of autoregulation.

To achieve the possibility of outcome forecasting by means of observing ICP and LCBF in the early postoperative period the methods of mathematical statistics were used. Two logarithms were worked out to forecast brain injuries outcomes with the help of ICP and LCBF data.

Using logarithm 1 it is possible on the basis of ICP and LCBF data to set up daily control over a patient's condition in the postoperative period. As a result of the logarithm 1 usage one of the following solutions can be achieved:

1. favourable outcome is forecast (field A);

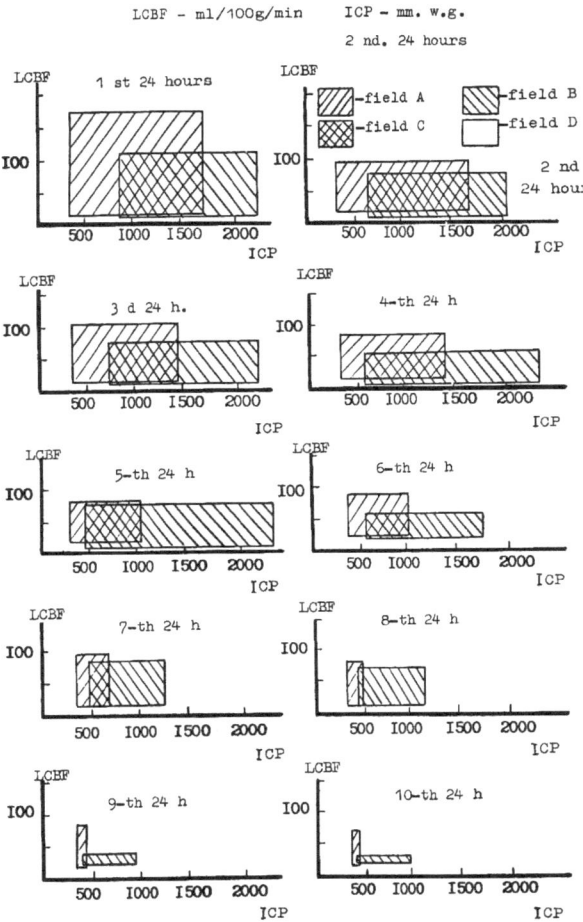

Fig. 2. Forecasting fields (A, B, C, D) obtained from ICP and LCBF in groups I and II (explanations in the text)

2. unfavourable outcome is forecast (field B);

3. forecasting is difficult because outcome is not differentiated (field C).

Fig. 2 is used to forecast outcomes according to logarithm 1. The results of daily postoperative ICP and LCBF qualities can be represented in a corresponding graph as dots.

Forecasting unfavourable outcome logarithm 1 does not point out

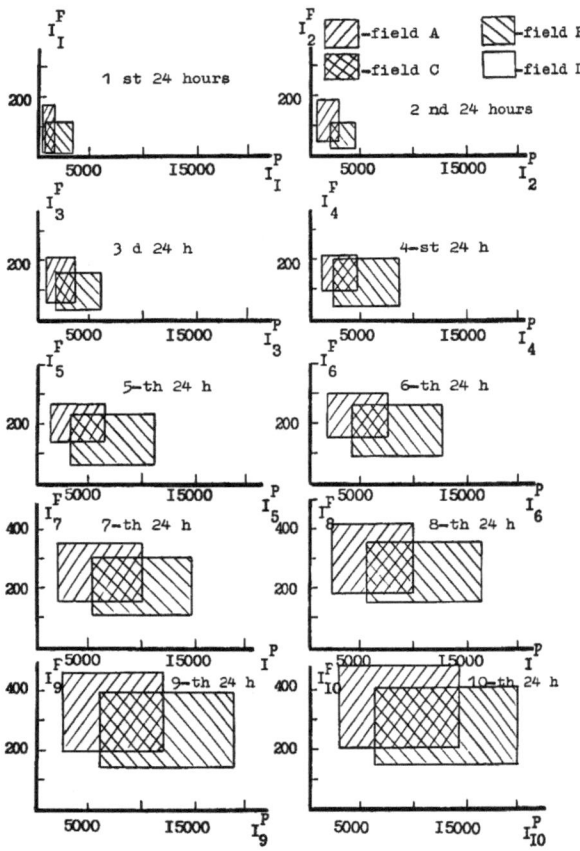

Fig. 3. Forecasting fields (A, B, C, D) for I_N^P and I_N^F meanings on the 1-10th postoperative days (explanations in the text)

the day of the fatal outcome, whereas logarithm 2 indicates possibility of fatal outcome during 24 hours after the last ICP and LCBF measurements.

To forecast possibly unfavourable outcome by logarithm 2, it is necessary (at the Nth postoperative day) to calculate the sum of the daily ICP data (including ICP data on the Nth day) marked as I_N^P and the sum of the daily LCBF data marked as I_N^F. Then the dot with I_N^P and I_N^F coordinates is put on a corresponding graph of Fig. 3. This dot can get into one of the following fields:

A field, where favourable outcome during the day is forecast;

B field, where unfavourable outcome during the day is forecast;

C field, where forecasting is difficult because here group I and group II dot data are found;

D field, where I_N^P and I_N^F meanings are not found.

The efficiency of these forecasting methods can be judged from the Table 1 data. This table represents percentage case correlations of concrete solutions based on initial statistical data (dot getting into field A or B).

Table 1. *Per Cent of Cases With Concrete Solation*
(dot getting into field A or B)

Postoperative days	1	2	3	4	5	6	7	8	9	10
Logarithm 1, % of dots getting into field C and B	48	57	66	74	66	52	47	92	87	92
Logarithm 2, % of dots getting into field A and B	52	82	78	85	82	76	63	81	62	65

The results of this investigation can be used to forecast brain affection outcomes, with the aim of carrying out optimum resuscitational neasures and to motivate rational postoperative therapy.

Acta Neurochirurgica, Suppl. 28, 188—192 (1979)

Division of Neurosurgery (Head: Prof. A. Benedetti),
City Hospital, Vicenza, Italy

Sleep Alterations During Post-Traumatic Coma as a Possible Predictor of Cognitive Defects

A. Alexandre, L. Rubini, P. Nertempi, and C. Farinello

Introduction

Enphasis has been recently laid on the problem of quantifying and treating neuropsychological deficits following severe head injuries[2, 10, 19, 20, 27]. Correlations have been sought with the entity of injury, expressed by parameters such as the duration of unconsciousness[20], of PTA[10, 19], or the presence of skull fractures and neurological deficits[10, 27]. In previous papers we[2] demonstrated a significant correlation with the neurological syndrome of level of lesion in the acute phase. Since in acute coma semiology the important and characteristic EEG alterations have a clearly demonstrated prognostic significance[5, 9, 30], our aim is that of studying the possible correlation between sleep and cognitive abnormalities.

Patients and Methods

This paper concerns a group of 20 severe head injuries admitted and operated on for intracerebral or extracerebral expanding lesions; in 12 the lesion was on the left, in 8 on the right. At admission the neurological situation was evaluated using the classification of Plum and Posner[24] and of Bricolo et al.[8, 9]: six patients showed the picture of a hemispheric, eight of a diencephalic, and six of a mesencephalic syndrome. EEG and electropolygraphic nocturnal recordings were performed in the acute phase, during PTA, and every two months thereafter, together with the application of neuropsychological testing by means of Wais, Raven, Corsi, Kimura, and Token tests.

Results

In the first week after injury abolition or severe reduction of REM sleep was observed in the six patients with mesencephalic syndrome and in four out of those with diencephalic syndrome. In the other four patients with diencephalic syndrome sleep was altered for prolonged phase 1 and 2 and for reduced REM sleep which was observed once or twice per night and lasted no more than twelve minutes. The table disregards the six patients with hemispheric syndrome, among whom only three showed reduction in REM sleep duration, who were all out of PTA at the third day, and who showed no cognitive defects. In all the other 14 patients there was a progressive restoration of the various sleep phases, paradoxical sleep always reappearing after complete restructuration of slow-EEG sleep. Only in three patients, more then one year after injury, did REM sleep remain poor.

Cognitive deficit evaluation was performed in each patient when out of PTA, that is one week after injury in three cases, four weeks in seven, seven weeks in eight. Twelve weeks after injury all the patients were out of PTA. In our table Mild deficits collects the subjects whose performance is up to 20% below the control group; those with lower performances are defined as Severe Deficits.

None of the 10 patients with initial severe REM alterations has a normal performance 14 months later, and the five patients with severe cognitive deficits had had acutely an abolition of REM sleep. The four patients who in the fourth week after injury, although not out of PTA, showed normal REM sleep, will completely recover their cognitive faculties; the sooner the EEG restoration, the earlier is cognitive normalization. Fourteen months after injury the five patients with severe neuropsychological defects show severe or mild REM sleep abnormalities, while a mild cognitive disfunction is present in three cases out of five with REM alterations. REM is normal in all patients free from cognitive deficits.

Comment and Conclusions

Temporal basal and medial structures, and particularly the hippocampus, assume a specialized function during REM sleep: there is evidence of a particular EEG activity[6, 17] that parallels an increase in CBF[15] in these structures having direct connections with the locus caeruleus[26], which is fundamental for inducing and maintaining REM sleep. Furthermore, hippocampectomy influences sleep activity, reducing fast sleep and increasing slow sleep[16, 22]. Clinical observations indicate in head injuries a reduction in REM sleep together with an increase of sleep phase 2[5, 21].

On the other hand the same encephalic structures bear a significant role in memory functions: specific electrical activity persists in

pyramidal hippocampal cells long after the end of elaboration of a
stimulus in the specific cortical areas[29]; there are several clinical[3]
observations of amnesia following occlusion of the posterior cerebral
artery which supplies medial temporal structures, among them the
hippocampus, and following surgical ablation of these structures[23, 25].
Bickford[4] could cause memory loss by stimulating the hippocampal
region, and in a case of Transient Global Amnesia electrical discharges
in the mesial temporal lobe were recorded[19]. Memory alterations in
head injuries have been frequently reported[2, 10, 19-21].

Table 1

Time after injury	REM sleep			No. pats out of PTA	Cognitive deficits		
	Severely reduced	Reduced	Normal		Severe	Mild	None
3 Days	10	4	0	0	0	0	0
1 Week	8	5	1	3	1	2	0
4 Weeks	5	5	4	7	3	4	0
12 Weeks	5	5	4	14	7	6	1
6 Months	4	6	4	14	6	6	2
14 Months	3	5	6	14	5	5	4

Furthermore, in normal subjects, REM sleep deprivation affects
mnesic processes[11, 28], and rats deprived of REM sleep have a reduced
learning ability[18].

In our series of patients sleep EEG alterations significantly
correlate with cognitive dysfunctions. Certainly traumatic cerebral
lesions are polytopistic[1, 7], and affect several neuronal systems, but
mesial temporal lobe involvement is frequent because of transtentorial
herniation, with compression of the posterior cerebral artery, or
because of direct traumatic contusion of underlying bony structures.

This damage involves both hippocampal cortex and the so-called
temporal stem, a structure which acquires nowadays a particular
importance in mnesic functions[14].

The validity of our proposed correlation between sleep and
cognitive alterations deserves evaluation in a larger number of patients,
since it may offer a further element in the individual prognosis of head
injured patients during the acute phase and PTA, when cognitive
assessment by means of the classical tests is not possible.

References

1. Adams, J. H., Graham, D. I., The pathology of blunt head injuries. In: Critchley, M., O'Leary, J. D., Bennett, B., Scientific foundations of neurology, p. 478. London: Heinemann. 1972.
2. Alexandre, A., Nertempi, P., Farinello, C., et al., Risultati preliminari dell'applicazione del test di Kimura nei traumatizzati cranici. Europa Med. Phys. 14 (1978), 85—90.
3. Benson, D. F., Marsden, C. D., Meadows, J. C., The amnesic syndrome of posterior cerebral artery occlusion. Acta Neurol. Scandinav. 50 (1974), 133—145.
4. Bickford, R. G., Mulder, D. W., Dodge, H. W., et al., Changes in memory function produced by electrical stimulation of the temporal lobe in man. Res. Publ. Ass. Nerv. Ment. Dis. 36 (1958), 227—243.
5. Bricolo, A., Prolonged post-traumatic coma. In: Handbook of clinical neurology. Linken, P. J., Bruyn, G. W. (eds.), pp. 699—755. North-Holland Publ. Co. 1976.
6. Bricolo, A., Neurosurgical exploration and neurological pathology as a means for investigating human sleep semiology and mechanisms. In: Experimental study of human sleep: Methodological problems. Lairy, G. C., Salzarulo, P. (eds.). Amsterdam: Elsevier Scientific Publ. Co. 1975.
7. Bricolo, A., Turazzi, S., Alexandre, A., et al., Decerebrate rigidity in acute head injury. J. Neurosurg. 47 (1977), 680—698.
8. Bricolo, A., Battistini, N., Bergamini, L., et al., A proposal for the classification of acute coma due to organic cerebral lesions. J. Neurosurg. Sci. 19 (1975), 113.
9. Bricolo, A., Signorini, G. C., Mazza, C., et al., Clinical criteria for the prognosis of acute cerebral traumatic coma. In: Present limits of neurosurgery. Fusek, I., Kunc, Z. (eds.). Prague: Avicenum. 1972.
10. Brooks, D. N., Wechsler memory scale performance and its relationship to brain damage after severe closed head injury. J. Neurol. Neurosurg. Psychiat. 39 (1976), 593—600.
11. Cambier, J., Personal comunication, 1978.
12. Greene, H. H., Bennett, D. R., Transient global amnesia with a previously unreported EEG abnormality. Electroenceph. Clin. Neurophys. 36 (1974), 409—413.
13. Held, J. P., Personal comunication, 1978.
14. Horel, J. A., The neuroanatomy of amnesia: a critique of the hippocampal memory hypothesis. Brain 101 (1978), 403—445.
15. Ingvar, D. H., Cerebral metabolism and circulation in wakefulness, sleep and coma. Astronautica Acta 17 (1972), 171—178.
16. Kim, C., Choi, H., Kim, C. C., et al., Effect of hippocampectomy on sleep patterns in cats. Electroenceph. Clin. Neurophys. 38 (1975), 235—243.
17. Lena, C., Parmeggiani, P., Hippocampal theta rhythm and activated sleep. Helv. Physiol. Acta 22 (1964), 120—135.
18. Linden, E. R., Bern, D., Fishbein, W., Retrograde amnesia: prolonging the fixation phase of memory consolidation paradoxical sleep deprivation. Physiol. Behav. 14 (1975), 409—412.
19. Mandleberg, I. A., Cognitive recovery after severe head injury. 3. Wais verbal and performance IQs as a function of post-traumatic amnesia duration and time from injury. J. Neurol. Neurosurg. Psychiat. 39 (1976), 1001—1007.

20. Mazeau, M., Ducarne, B., Held, J. P., Le devenir neuropsychologiques des traumatisés craniens sévères. 3rd World Congress of the IRMA, Basel, 2-8 July, 1978.
21. Najenson, T., Groswasser, Z., Mendelson, L., *et al.*, Rehabilitation of the severely brain injured. 3rd World Congress of the IRMA, Basel, 2-8 July, 1978.
22. Parmeggiani, P., Zanocco, G., A study of the bioelectrical rhythms of cortical and subcortical structures during activated sleep. Arch. Ital. Biol. *101* (1963), 385—412.
23. Penfield, W., Mathieson, G., Memory. Autopsy findings and comments on the role of hippocampus in experiential recall. Arch. Neurol. *31* (1974), 145—154.
24. Plum, F., Posner, J. B., The diagnosis of stupor and coma, ed. 2. Philadelphia: F. A. Davis. 1972.
25. Scoville, W., Milner, B., Loss of recent memory after bilateral hippocampal lesions. J. Neurol. Neurosurg. Psychiat. *20* (1957), 11—21.
26. Segal, M., Bloom, F. E., The action of Norepinephrine in the rat hippocampus: II. Activation in imput pathway. Brain Res. *72* (1974), 99—114.
27. Smith, E., Influence of site of impact on cognitive impairment persisting long after severe closed head injury. J. Neurol. Neurosurg. Psychiat. *37* (1974), 719—726.
28. Spinnler, H. B., Sterzi, R., Vallar, G., Le amnesie. F. Angeli Publ. Milano, 1977.
29. Vinogradova, O., Registration of information and the limbic system. In: Horn, G., Hinde, R. A. (eds.): Short-term changes in neural activity and behaviour. Cambridge: Univ. Press. 1970.
30. Williams, R. L., Karaca, I., EEG of human sleep. Amsterdam: Elsevier Scientific Publ. Co. 1975.

Acta Neurochirurgica, Suppl. 28, 193—194 (1979)
© by Springer-Verlag 1979

IV. How May Prognosis be Influenced by Therapy?

a) Surgical Treatment

Department of Neurological Surgery, Chiba University,
School of Medicine, Inohana-cho, Chiba-shi, Japan

Assessment of Outcome Following Large Decompressive Craniectomy in Management of Serious Cerebral Contusion

A Review of 207 Cases

H. Makino and A. Yamaura

Since 1966 unilateral or bilateral large decompressive craniectomy has been performed in acute serious cerebral contusion with or without concomitant intracranial haematomas. At the present moment, a total of 207 cases have accumulated, and short-term and long-term follow-up studies have been conducted in relation to the preoperative neurological scale, in a search for factors determining prognosis.

Material and Method

Surgical technique has been uniform in that a large bone flap over the cerebral contusion was removed and dura mater was widely incised to give a full decompressive effect. If this unilateral opening did not seem to be sufficient in its decompressive effect, a contralateral craniectomy was added. A bilateral procedure was required in 24% of patients.

This analysis is based on 2 series of a total of 207 cases; series 1 is composed of 154 patients (118 adults and 36 children), operated on between 1966 and 1974; a further 53 patients (40 adults and 13 children) were operated on between 1975 and 1976, and are summarized as series 2. Prognostic value of preoperative scale, obtained in series 1, was tested in series 2.

The outcome of the patients was analysed in relation with the three key-signs of "pupillary changes", "decerebration", and "respiratory disturbance", as the preoperative scale. The presence of such key-signs was recognized by any medical and co-medical staff, and could be recorded as "present" or "absent" without any possible mistakes. Grading of the preoperative neurological status was defined as follows: Grade I—There were no key-signs. Grade II—There was any one of the key-signs. Grade III—There were any two of the key-signs. Grade IV—All the key-signs were present. This grading is also a simple and practical method of classifying patients preoperatively.

In an analysis of a long-term follow-up study over a mean 50 months period, the patients were classified into five categories of social recovery: (A) full recovery, (B) returned to less activity, (C) confined to home, (V) vegetative, and (D) dead.

Results

General statistics. In 154 patients in series 1, there were 45 deaths (29%). Eighthy-three per cent of the survivors were in the state of functional recovery A or B and only three were in vegetative state for 2 to 10 years.

Age. The age is the most important "non-cerebral" factor in the outcome of serious head injury. Adults possess significantly less chance of survival (77%) and functional recovery (73%), compared with children, who have survival rates of 83% and 100% functional recovery. Break-point of age was 30 years. There were no deaths among eight children who were operated on within 24 months of birth. All of four patients in their seventies eventually died from complications.

Key-Signs. In adults, the presence of any key-sign resulted in a significantly high mortality (P < 0.01) and less chance of functional recovery (P < 0.01).

Grading of preoperative status. In adults, 90% survived, and 83% returned to a useful life in grade I, and survival rate and functional recovery steadily regressed with progress down the gradings. In grade III 9 out 27 patients survived, and only 3 returned to a useful life. In grade IV only 1 survived in a vegetative state and all other patients died within 48 hours of surgery. Even in children there was a very poor survival rate in grade IV.

Testing of prognostic value (mortality) of preoperative grading. The probability in each grading, obtained in series 1, was tested in series 2; 22 and 6 were expected to result in death in adult and children, and the actual deaths were 23 and 7, showing excellent reliability of the probability from series 1.

Influence of preoperative hemiparesis, concomitant intracranial haematoma, time from injury to surgery, and acute brain swelling need to be discussed.

Acta Neurochirurgica, Suppl. 28, 195—198 (1979)
© by Springer-Verlag 1979

Department of Neurosurgery, Kurume University School of Medicine,
67-Asahimachi, Kurume City Fukuoka, Japan

Outcome of Acute Subdural Haematoma Following Decompressive Hemicraniectomy

M. Shigemori, K. Syojima, K. Nakayama, T. Kojima, M. Watanabe,
and S. Kuramoto

With 2 Figures

Introduction

The survival rate for acute subdural haematoma and the functional recovery of the patients are still unsatisfactory although decompressive hemicraniectomy in addition to clot removal has been used over the last five years in our clinic. We have retrospectively reviewed and analysed the last 15 cases with hemicraniectomies performed for unilateral acute subdural haematomas for assessment of the outcome following this operative procedure.

Case Materials and Method of Evaluation

The patients in this series included nine males and six females with an age range of 5 to 82 years, all with rapid neurological deterioration when brought into hospital. The standard neurosurgical management consisted of adequate airway, steroids, and intravenous mannitol in all cases, and the majority of patients were operated upon within 10 hours of injury. At the time of admission quantitative evaluation based on the preoperative neurological examination of the patients, and recording of vital signs were carried out. Both an emergency computerized tomographic (CT) scan and carotid angiography were performed in all patients immediately after initial management. Intracranial pressure (ICP) was monitored in all patients using the fibre optic monitor system (manufactured by Ladd Research Industries, Inc. Burlington, Vermont) placed in the extradural space for 24 to 48 hours after operation. In some cases ICP during operation was also recorded. The changes of ICP and postoperative CT scans performed periodically were analysed in all patients.

Results

At the time of evaluation, 10 cases were comatose, four cases were semicomatose, and one case was lethargic. Decerebrate posturing was present in eight patients. Eight cases had anisocoria, and in seven cases

bilateral dilated pupils were noted. Ten patients had respiratory
abnormalities, and apnoeic respiration was found in four cases. Marked
systemic hypotension was present in five patients. Ten cases in this
series (64.3%) died within nine days after operation. Three of these died
of systemic complications. Four patients (26.7%) returned to normal
activity. The total survival rate was 35.7%. Poor filling of the cerebral

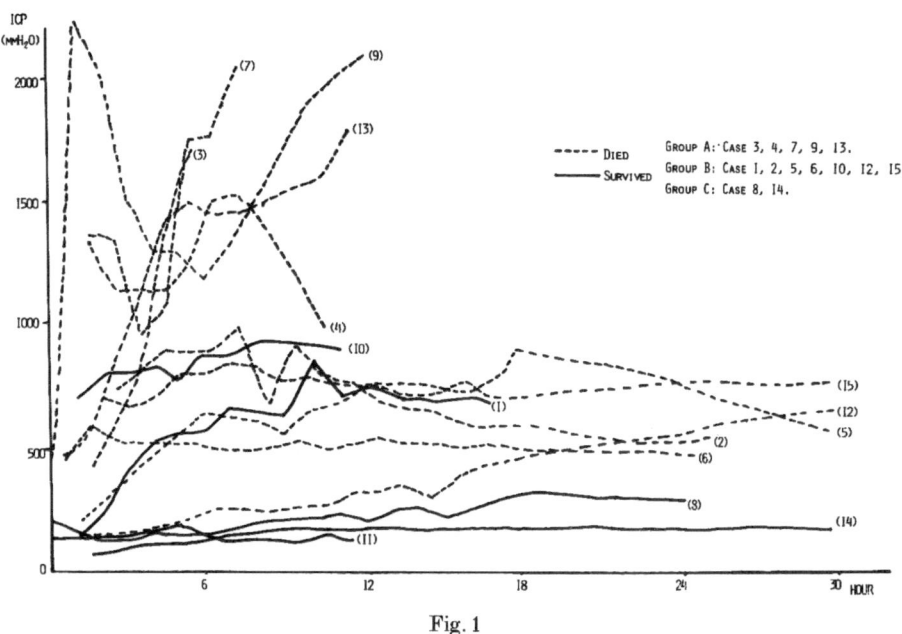

Fig. 1

circulation on preoperative angiography was demonstrated in eight
patients. Common findings on preoperative CT scan showing marked
shift of the midline structure and collapsed lateral ventricle on the side
of a haematoma. Non-visualization of the third ventricle and major
basal cisterns was noted in all cases.

Three different types of the course of ICP within six to eight hours
after operation were recorded, so that the patients in this series were
divided into three groups (A, B, and C) according to postoperative ICP
(Fig. 1). Five patients in A group with ICP over 1000 mm H_2O and
rising rapidly all died within a short time after operation. B group with
ICP between 500 and 1000 mm H_2O maintained constant for 24 to 48
hours included seven patients of whom two survived. In C group with

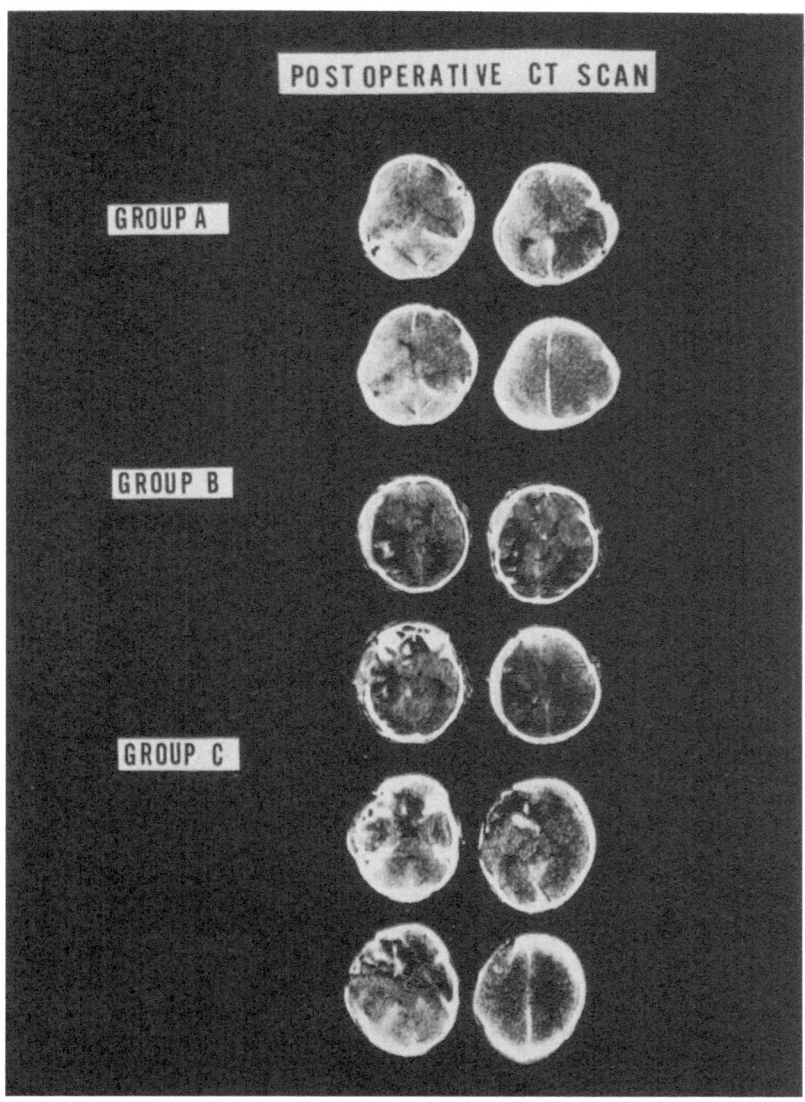

Fig. 2

ICP under 500 mm H_2O after operation, all three patients returned to normal activity. Preoperative neurological status, angiographic findings, and postoperative changes of ICP in the three groups were all correlated with the outcome following surgery. However, preoperative findings on CT scans were not always correlated with the outcome.

Fig. 2 indicates the postoperative CT scans performed within 24 hours in the cases of each group.

Complete collapse of the lateral ventricles on both sides and diffuse low density areas over the whole brain suggesting acute brain swelling were demonstrated in all cases of A group. In the cases in B group, the same degree of midline shift and unilateral collapsed ventricle as in the preoperative CT scan, and a low density area mixed with spotted high density over the hemisphere on the operated side were shown. The shift of the midline structures was still seen on the CT scan performed two weeks later in this group. Mild degree of midline shift without diffuse low density areas was present in all cases of C group; it disappeared within a few days after operation.

Conclusion

Retrospective analysis of fifteen cases with unilateral acute subdural haematoma treated by decompressive hemicraniectomy in addition to clot removal was carried out. The patients in this series were divided into three groups according to postoperative ICP. Decompressive hemicraniectomy was effective in all cases of C group compared to the cases of A group in which there were no survivals. Treatments additional to decompression were considered to be necessary for the cases of B group in order to increase the survival rate. The total survival rate was 35.7%. Preoperative neurological status, angiographic findings, and postoperative ICP within 24 to 48 hours were well correlated with survival. It seemed to be difficult to predict the outcome following surgery from the findings of preoperative CT scan. It may be concluded from the present results that an analysis of findings on CT scan and ICP during the early period after operation are important for assessment of outcome following surgery of acute subdural haematoma and for consideration of further additional postoperative managements.

Acta Neurochirurgica, Suppl. 28, 199—200 (1979)
© by Springer-Verlag 1979

A. L. Polenov Neurosurgical Institute, Leningrad, U.S.S.R.

Early Surgical Treatment of Traumatic Intracranial Haematomas and Laceration Foci as the Main Factor for Favourable Prognosis

V. M. Ugrumov, Yu. V. Zotov, and V. V. Shchedryonok

During last twenty years in all advanced countries an increase in trauma, mainly due to vehicle accidents, has been observed. It changes the character of craniocerebral trauma with an increase in severe cerebral contusions, subdural haematomas, and laceration foci.

In spite of considerable progress in the treatment of severe craniocerebral trauma the mortality in this group of patients is still high (70–85 per cent), and the long-term results in survivals are not satisfactory in terms of mental and intellectual recovery.

Nowadays the main prospect of achieving better results in treatment of severe craniocerebral trauma and prevention of disability lies in the improvement of surgery. Rehabilitation in patients with traumatic intracranial haematomas depends on operation timing. The importance of urgent diagnosis and surgical treatment of intracranial haematomas is stated enthusiastically by all neurosurgeons, yet the urgent surgical treatment of intracranial haematomas has not yet been widely introduced. One of the hindrances is the predominant view of slow and gradual haematoma formation. We have worked out a largely new thesis of traumatic intracranial haematoma formation during the first minutes and hours after trauma which greatly changes the examination, diagnosis, and surgical treatment of intracranial haematomas.

A system of diagnosis and surgical treatment of haematoma in the early period, mainly in the first three hours, has been elaborated. Three tactical variants of urgent examination are used: full, reduced, and minimal. Thirteen-year results in 400 patients show that early diagnosis and surgical treatment of traumatic intracranial haematoma, carried out in 90 per cent of patients in the first 3 hours after trauma, caused a decrease of mortality in the given category of patients by

22-25 per cent. For the urgent diagnosis of intracranial haematoma computer-assisted diagnosis has been effective.

In order to achieve better results of treatment of severe cranio-cerebral trauma the problem of treatment of contusion foci was reviewed.

A ten-year study of this problem allowed us to work out a system of early diagnosis and treatment of brain laceration foci. Surgical experience in 260 patients with severe craniocerebral trauma showed that the removal of brain laceration foci favourably affected the results of treatment in this category of patients. Postoperative mortality was 41 per cent. The most favourable results were obtained with brain laceration foci when the patients were operated on early. Seventy per cent were operated on in the first six hours after trauma.

Long-term results showed full social adaptation in 90 per cent of patients, in whom 50 per cent returned to their usual occupations.

The results of treatment, together with efficacy and degree of rehabilitation in patients with severe craniocerebral trauma depend to a great extent on surgical treatment of intracranial haematomas and brain laceration foci.

Acta Neurochirurgica, Suppl. 28, 201—202 (1979)
© by Springer-Verlag 1979

A. L. Polenov Neurosurgical Institute, Leningrad, U.S.S.R.

Local CBF in the Laceration Focus in Patients With Craniocerebral Trauma

E. N. Kondakov

The important role of CBF and metabolic changes in pathogenesis of craniocerebral trauma makes the objectivize assessment of these changes and their control during treatment necessary.

CBF measurements with Xe^{133} clearance before operation showed a decrease of blood flow in the laceration area (33.2 ± 2.0 ml/100 g/min). CBF values in the distant brain areas were 41.2 ± 3.3. Mean CBF in the more damaged hemisphere was also lowered (38.5 ± 1.6 ml/100 g/min).

CBF and pO_2 fluctuation polarographic studies in patients during and after operation demonstrated important peculiarities of developing changes. A certain topography of local CBF and pO_2 changes was seen, and three zones were determined: destruction zone with absence of blood flow, transitory zone with reduced CBF, and marginal zone with increased CBF.

Areas of tissue laceration with absent local blood flow and pO_2 were called destruction zone with CBF absence. In the postoperative period no return of local CBF and pO_2 was observed in laceration areas. As a rule there was no border-line between the damaged tissue and neighbouring areas. In brain tissue directly adjacent to a destruction zone (0.5-1.5 cm) the decrease of local CBF, increase of hypoxia (absence of pO_2 fluctuations), and CBF arrest on the fourth to sixth postoperative day was observed. Progressive local CBF decrease in these patients was observed on the background of gradual increase of systemic arterial pressure.

The area adjacent to the destruction zone, with low and gradually decreasing local CBF and with disappearance of pO_2 fluctuations was called the transitory zone (zone of reduced blood flow). The size of this zone was 0.5-1.5 cm around the perimeter of the non-ablated laceration foci. It underwent later necrosis.

Brain tissue area lying 3-5 cm from the destruction zone was called the marginal zone, with increased blood flow. Its width varied, but we stress that closer to the transitory zone the oscillation of CBF reactions was observed, while in distant parts of it CBF increased. With increase of systemic arterial pressure a gradual increase of local CBF in the marginal zone was observed, whereas in the transitory zone the arrest of CBF was seen.

Thus, in patients with cerebral contusion the local CBF changes in hemispheric laceration foci seen before operation became more obvious after it. The destruction zone expanded on the fourth to sixth day after trauma, gradually spreading to the transitory zone. As a result of brain oedema local CBF decreased round the focus, with increase of tissue hypoxia and lessening and disappearance of pO_2 fluctuations. The developing ischaemia resulted in enlargement of the necrotic area.

After total removal of lacerated and haemorrhagic tissue the prolapse of brain into the trephine hole decreased rapidly, and pulsation appeared. In tissue directly adjacent to the resection area gradual improvement of local CBF and pO_2 took place. In the marginal zone two phases of local CBF increase were observed, on the 1-2nd and 9-10th days after the operation. After that, CBF and pO_2 in this area were within normal limits.

Thus, in the postoperative period in patients with laceration foci resection including destruction and transitory zones the gradual CBF increase in adjacent tissue and normalization of CBF in the marginal zone were observed. After laceration focus resection the further growth of the necrotic zone in the operation area was not seen.

From this study we consider that local CBF and pO_2 changes round the laceration foci lead to hypoxia and then to ischaemia of the surrounding tissue (transitory zone) thus increasing the necrotic zone. The most effective surgical treatment in patients with severe craniocerebral trauma with laceration foci seems to be resection within the limits of the destruction and transitory zones.

Acta Neurochirurgica, Suppl. 28, 203—204 (1979)
© by Springer-Verlag 1979

Neurosurgical University Clinic, Belgrade, Yugoslavia

Brain Injuries—Causes of Death, and Life Expectancy

N. Sekulović and A. Ćeramilac

This work assesses the relationship between cerebral injuries and causes of death.

Material and Method

Autopsy protocols of 507 cases of cerebral injuries were analysed. Complex injuries where the cause of death was injury of some other organ or system were excluded.

Sections of brain tissue and meninges, as well as all other organs, were histologically examined.

Results

The frequency of some lethal brain injuries as well as life expectancy are shown in the table. The majority of those injured died shortly after trauma, due to brain stem lesions with blood vessel rupture, haemorrhage, and local ischaemic necrosis. Pneumonia as a complication of brain injury, usually caused by unconsciousness with consecutive circulatory and respiratory disturbances, is in second place as a cause of death. About the same number die of brain oedema in the area of the lesion and spreading to other parts or to the whole brain causing brain stem compresion. Oedema usually develops after 12 hours, and reaches its culmination in 7 days. The incidence of other causes of death is considerably lower, and among them the most important are brain contusions with intracerebral or extracerebral haemorrhage causing death most frequently 12 to 24 hours after injury. Next is aspiration of blood from skull base fracture with mortality over 85% within the first hour after injury. Later complications such as leptomeningitis and sepsis are represented by a low percentage, and appear after the seventh day following injury. Other causes of death were pulmonary thromboembolism, brain abscess, late traumatic apoplexy, and two cases of asphyxia due to blood aspiration from tracheostomies.

Cause of death	Life expectancy								Totals
	within 1 hour	within 12 hours	within 24 hours	within 48 hours	within 7 days	within 14 days	within 30 days	over 30 days	
Injury brain stem	of 256 85%	20 6.7%	21 7%	4 1.3%	— —	— —	— —	— —	301 59.4%
Brain oedema	— —	8 13.3%	18 30%	11 18.3%	19 31.7%	3 5%	1 1.7%	— —	60 11.8%
Brain compression	— —	5 14.7%	16 47%	7 20.6%	6 17.7%	— —	— —	— —	34 6.7%
Aspiration of blood	18 85.7%	2 9.5%	1 4.8%	— —	— —	— —	— —	— —	21 4.1%
Pneumonia	— —	— —	4 6.6%	11 18.0%	24 39.3%	17 27.9%	4 6.6%	1 1.6%	61 12.0%
Leptomeningitis	— —	— —	— —	— —	1 14.3%	4 57.1%	2 28.6%	— —	7 1.4%
Sepsis	— —	— —	— —	— —	— —	5 45.4%	4 36.4%	2 18.2%	11 2.2%
Other causes	— —	— —	— —	— —	— —	2 16.6%	5 41.7%	5 41.7%	12 2.4%
Totals	274 54.0%	35 6.9%	60 11.8%	33 6.5%	50 9.9%	31 6.1%	16 3.2%	8 1.6%	507 100%

Conclusion

Our material is based on 507 autopsies of head and brain injury cases, without injuries of other organs or systems.

The majority of injured died due to direct lesions of brain stem within the first hour after trauma. A large number died within the period from 12 hours to 7 days, due to developing brain oedema, brain compression, and pneumonia.

Brain oedema reaches its culmination as a cause of death on the 7th day after injury, brain compression has its climax between the 12 and 24th hours, and over 85 % of deaths were caused within the first hour after injury by blood aspiration.

Acta Neurochirurgica, Suppl. 28, 205—208 (1979)
© by Springer-Verlag 1979

b) Evaluation of Therapeutic Procedures

Institute of Neurological Sciences, Southern General Hospital,
Glasgow, Scotland

On Comparing Series of Head Injured Patients

G. Teasdale, L. Parker, G. Murray, and B. Jennett

The data bank that developed as a result of collaboration between centres in Scotland, the Netherlands, and America, currently contains information about the early features and ultimate outcome of more than 1000 patients who sustained severe head injuries—defined as those that are followed by coma for at least 6 hours[1].

One of the applications of this bank is as a source which can be compared with other series of patients managed in different centres or in different ways. When making these comparisons, certain methodological considerations need to be taken into account, and these are reviewed in this paper.

Reliability

It is necessary to ensure that assessment of early severity and ultimate outcome has been made in the same way and at the same stage after injury. The observer variability of the methods used in the collaborative study has been reported[2,3], and the labile state of patients in the first week has been noted[1].

Sample Size

A major limitation in making comparisons is the high degree of variability in small samples. Table 1 shows that the smaller the sample the larger the range over which an observed frequency may vary without differing significantly from the frequency observed in the data bank.

Table 1. *Ranges of Observed Frequencies in a New Sample Which Would not Differ Significantly (at 5 % on a χ^2 Test) From Observed Frequencies in the 1000 Data Bank*

Size of sample from new centre	Data bank frequency	
	20% Range of variation	50% Range of variation
20	5–35%	30–70%
50	10–30%	36–64%
100	12–28%	40–60%
200	14–26%	42–58%
1,000	17–23%	46–54%

Matching Distribution of Features

Factors important in determining prognosis include age, responsiveness as assessed by the Glasgow Coma Scale, motor abnormalities, and signs of brain stem dysfunction. Direct comparisons between series can be made only if the distribution of features within each series is similar. It would thus not be appropriate to compare a group of children directly with the data bank. Table 2 gives an admittedly contrived example which shows that it would not even be sufficient to demonstrate that the two series had similar mean ages, because the overall distribution of age could differ with a consequent difference in expected outcome.

Table 2. *Effect of Age Distribution on Expected Mortality in Series of Severely Head Injured Patients*

Age Group	Mortality*	Proportion of patients		
		Series I	Series II**	Series III
10–29 years	35%	62.5%	50%	25%
30–49 years	40%	0%	25%	75%
50–69 years	80%	37.5%	25%	0%
Mean age for series		35 years	35 years	35 years
Expected mortality for series		52%	48%	38%

* Estimated from data bank.
** Approximates to 1,000 cases in data bank.

Even when matched for more than one individual factor, two series may still differ when combinations of factors are considered. Moreover, so many are the factors that influence outcome, that it is unrealistic to expect two series to be perfectly matched for all features, an important limitation when making direct comparisons between unselected series.

Outcome for Similar Severity—Individual Features in Multiple Patients

Even though the rate of occurrence of a feature may vary within two series, the outcome of patients showing that feature may still be the same. Thus, although there were differences in the frequency with which motor abnormalities were recorded in two of the centres, these centres showed no difference in outcome between patients who showed similar abnormalities (Table 3).

Table 3. *Motor Response Pattern (Best in First 24 Hours) in Two Centres*

a) Frequency of occurrence of motor pattern *worse than* hemiparesis (*e.g.* hemiplegia, bilateral abnormal response)

Glasgow	$298_{/571}$	52%
Los Angeles	$128_{/168}$	76%

$\chi^2 = 30.6$ Significant at 0.1%

b) Outcome distribution for patients with motor pattern *worse than* hemiparesis

	n	Dead/PVS	Severe	Moderate	Good
Glasgow	298	203 (68%)	31 (10%)	33 (11%)	31 (10%)
Los Angeles	128	82 (64%)	18 (14%)	20 (16%)	8 (6%)

$\chi^2 = 4.44$ (3 d.f.)   Not significant

Such a simple, direct comparison has advantages but does not take into account the many other factors that may affect prognosis; comparisons based upon groups matched for several factors are not feasible because of inadequate numbers.

Multiple Factors Predicting Individual Patients

It is possible to calculate the probable outcome of an individual new patient on the basis of his presenting features[4]. This method can be used to detect differences in the relationship between initial severity and outcome in two different series, data from one source being used to predict the outcome of each individual in the other. Table 4 shows the results of a comparison between cases in Glasgow and the Netherlands. Information from one group of Glasgow cases was used to predict the outcome of (I) a further 125 cases in Glasgow, and (II) 129 patients from the Netherlands. Similar proportions of predictions were made with "confidence", and amongst these similar proportions were correct.

Table 4. *Comparsion of Predicted Outcomes With Actual Outcomes*

Prediction of 125 Glasgow cases (I) and 191 Dutch cases (II), each based on 447 other Glasgow cases.

I. Glasgow-Glasgow Prediction			II. Glasgow-Dutch Prediction		
64 % Confident**; of these 96 % correct			59 % Confident**; of these 93 % correct		
	Predicted to die n = 31	Predicted to survive n = 49		Predicted to die n = 31	Predicted to survive n = 81
Died	31	3	Died	30	7
Survived	0	46	Survived	1	74

** A confident prediction is made when one of the outcome categories is predicted with probability > 0.97.

Conclusion

Some of the methodological pitfalls in comparing series of head injured patients have been considered in this paper; a powerful way of detecting differences due to alternative management in two series of patients analysed retrospectively is to predict each series from the other, and then to compare the predicted outcomes with the actual outcomes. The value of this method would depend upon the reliability of the predictive technique. The aim would be to determine if patients predicted to die or survive only with disability actually made good recoveries.

References

1. Jennett, B., Teasdale, G., Braakman, R., Minderhoud, J., Heiden, J., Kurze, T., Murray, G., Parker, L., Prognosis in series of patients with severe head injury. Submitted to Neurosurgery.
2. Teasdale, G., Knill-Jones, R., Van der Sande, J., Observer variability in assessing impaired consciousness and coma. J. Neurol. Neurosurg. Psychiat. *41* (1978), 603—610.
3. Braakman, R., Avezaat, C., Maas, A., Roel, M., Schouten, H., Inter-observer agreement in the assessment of the motor response of the Glasgow "Coma" Scale. Clin. Neurol. Neurosurg. In press.
4. Jennett, B., Teasdale, G., Braakman, R., Minderhoud, J., Knill-Jones, R., Predicting outcome in individual patients after severe head injury. Lancet *I* (1976), 1031—1034.

Acta Neurochirurgica, Suppl. 28, 209 (1979)

Hôpital de la Conception Neurochirurgicale, Marseille, France

Effect of Therapy on Prognosis of Cerebral Contusions

R. P. Vigouroux and P. Guillermain

Our study is based on the analysis of 544 observations of isolated hemispheric contusions—attritions without associated lesions, all of them surgically checked, or diagnosed by angiography or computerized tomography. In all these cases, trauma was recent and closed.

The general prognosis of these lesions has greatly benefited from recent attainments in the field of medical therapeutic and monitoring common to all brain trauma we concentrated on checking respiratory functions and on correction of hypoxia by the use of controlled respiration, and also on prevention of neurovegetative disorders and of cerebral oedema. Treatment may be directed or corrected according to results of intracranial pressure registered in a systematic way.

Surgical treatment has greatly improved as a result of operative indications from CT. In our opinion this is the only investigation which enables us to distinguish between the part played by oedema from that due to haemorrhage or tissue destruction. Surgery is more often required in the case of haemorrhage than with other lesions.

Many factors interfere with surgical prognosis.

Operative timing. As we have often encountered bad results from emergency surgery we no longer perform it, and prefer to act a few days after trauma (our best results were achieved when surgery was performed between the fifth and eighth days after trauma).

Direct surgical approach to lesions. Under emergency conditions, when intracranial pressure is very high, we perform a large decompressive craniotomy without touching the cerebral lesion. In cases where we do perform surgery on a cerebral lesion, a large skull flap appears to be preferable to a small one.

Treatment of lesions. We prefer simple lavage with careful evacuation of distroyed tissues and clots to conventional lobectomy, the results of which appear mediocre to us.

Since 1970 our results have greatly improved, as our general death-rate for all these lesions both medically and surgically treated, fell from 50% to 38%.

Acta Neurochirurgica, Suppl. 28, 210—212 (1979)
© by Springer-Verlag 1979

Departments of Neurosurgery, University of Glasgow*, of Rotterdam**,
of Groningen***, and of Southern California****

The Assessment of the Efficacy of Different Therapies for Severe Head Injuries

B. Jennett*, G. Teasdale*, J. Frey*, R. Braakman**,
J. Minderhoud***, and J. Heiden****

Reviewing mortality over recent decades, Langfitt (1978) concluded that there had been little improvement in spite of the application of several measures designed to control the secondary events that threaten life after injury. Three explanations are possible. One is that therapy is ineffective. Another is that more efficient resuscitation and transportation enable more hopelessly injured patients to reach special centres, where they soon die; this maintains a high mortality rate—even though other patients are doing better than previously. The third is that methods of assessment vary so much from place to place,

Table 1. *Frequency of Treatments*

n	Glasgow 507	Los Angeles 224	Netherlands 302
Steroids	24 %	99 %	34 %
Tracheostomy	10 %	66 %	15 %
Intubation/ tracheostomy			
— 3 D	38 %	70 %	61 %
Assisted ventilation	18 %	62 %	28 %
Bone flap removed (% of craniotomies)	28 %	93 %	92 %
Osmotics	86 %	78 %	69 %
Dead or vegetative			
6 months after injury	49 %	54 %	50 %

Table 2. % Dead/Vegetative With and Without Various Therapies
(all centres combined)

	Glasgow coma score (24 hours best)	Without	With
Steroids	3/5	82 %	77 %
	6/7	48 %	47 %
	> 8	23 %	20 %
	Total	50 %	50 %
Osmotics	3/5	81 %	79 %
	6/7	41 %	58 %
	> 8	16 %	39 %
	Total	43 %	61 %
Intubation tracheostomy	3/5	68 %	83 %
	6/7	34 %	53 %
	> 8	14 %	40 %
	Total	30 %	62 %
Tracheostomy	3/5	83 %	72 %
	6/7	47 %	45 %
	> 8	22 %	39 %
	Total	48 %	53 %
Ventilation	3/5	75 %	85 %
	6/7	38 %	61 %
	> 8	18 %	54 %
	Total	40 %	70 %
Bone flap removal	3/5	68 %	88 %
	6/7	46 %	69 %
	> 8	26 %	29 %
	Total	44 %	67 %

or from time to time, that like is not compared with like, and the value of effective treatment is thereby obscured.

The last is the most readily dealt with, by the use of standardized systems for assessing initial severities, subsequent progress, and ultimate outcome. This has already been done for over 1000 patients prospectively collected as part of a collaborative study based on Glasgow, Netherlands, and Los Angeles[1]. Although methods of clinical assessment were rigorously controlled in this study, no attempt was made to standardize treatment—but the therapies used were recorded. There were marked differences between the three countries in the frequencies with which some treatments were used (Table 1). In some centres some methods of therapy were more often used in the more severely injured patients (those with low coma scores, poor motor responses, or non-reacting pupils). Even when these factors, the age of patient and the presence or absence of haematoma, were allowed for, statistical analysis showed that there was no difference in outcome when steroids were administered. Tracheostomy, intubation, controlled or triggered ventilation, use of osmotics, or removal of the bone flap (after evacuation of an IC haematoma) were each associated with a *higher* mortality than in patients of similar severity and age who were not so treated. This effect was independent of the presence of a major chest injury, although this was the reason for some patients having tracheostomy with assisted ventilation. These apparently adverse effects of certain treatment methods were often more marked in the *less severely affected patients* (Table 2) (as indicated by the best coma score in the first 24 hours). We could find no evidence that series of patients treated with each of these therapies had better outcomes than was predicted on the basis of patients not so treated.

The uniformity of the outcomes for series of patients well matched for severity and age, but treated by different techniques, does not prove that these various methods may not be effective for some patients in some circumstances. It does, however, suggest that, provided that all patients receive a high standard of care, outcome is mainly determined by age and severity. New therapeutic techniques, not considered in this study, may prove effective—and the assessment methods of the data bank could facilitate such evaluation.

Reference

1. Jennett, B., Teasdale, G., Galbraith, S., Pickard, J., Grant, H., Braakman, R., Avezaat, C., Maas, A., Minderhoud, J., Vecht, C. J., Heiden, J., Small, R., Caton, W., Kurze, T., Severe head injuries in three countries. J. Neurol. Neurosurg. Psychiat. *40* (1977), 291—298.

Forum B

Physiological and Clinical Basis of Cerebral Reconstructive Vascular Surgery

Acta Neurochirurgica, Suppl. 28. 215 —217 (1979)

I. Physiological Aspects

Phenomena Associated With Focal Ischaemia in the Central Nervous System

L. Symon* and J. Astrup

Occlusive vascular disease is the occasion of focal brain ischaemia. Whatever the primary nature of the vascular obstruction, the effect is the same, blood supply to the area supplied by the vessel in question is reduced, and a number of pathophysiological phenomena are set in train both in the area of ischaemia and in the surrounding regions where an attempt is made to replace the lost blood flow from collateral vessels. It is an everyday clinical experience that a dense neurological deficit soon after a cerebral ischaemic episode may gradually resolve and finally even disappear. It seems likely that cells may survive in a state of structural integrity yet with paralysis of function. Possible explanations for subsequent recovery may either be improvement in the residual circulation with expansion of collateral vessels from neighbouring cerebro-vascular beds, or modification of the neuronal metabolism itself so that function may be resumed at a lower basal level of blood flow.

With experimental middle cerebral occlusion in primates (Symon 1975) there is a contour of reduction of blood flow, the ischaemia being densest in the region of the Sylvian opercula and in the basal ganglia where flow is reduced to about 20 % of the basal control of around 55 ml per 100 gm per minute, i.e., to 10–12 ml per 100 gm per minute. There is a graduated reduction in the flow, decreasing in intensity as the midline and parasagittal areas are approached.

The relation between reduced blood flow determined in this way, and the electrical function of cortical neurones can be assessed by the reaction of a somato-sensory evoked response recorded by a plate electrode on the post-Rolandic Cortex. We have demonstrated (1974) a

* L. Symon, TD, FRCS, Professor of Neurological Surgery, The National Hospital Queen Square, London WC1N3B9, England.

threshold relationship between regional blood flow and the somato-sensory evoked response, the response being maintained to levels of blood flow of 20 ml per 100 gm per minute, while at levels below 12 ml per 100 gm per minute the response is absent. In the area of 14-16 ml per 100 gm per minute there is a very sharp decline in the evoked response, the 50% reduction of response being at 16 ml per 100 gm per minute. Similar findings have been reported by Boysen *et al.* (1973) in Scandinavia, looking at the relationship between EEG frequency and carotid perfusion during endarterectomy. Heiss (1976) and his colleagues have also found a similar relationship between rCBF and neuronal activity in the cat.

The Relationship Between Blood Flow and Structural Integrity

Detailed pathological studies after perfusion fixation (Brierley, Symon 1977) indicate that the ultimate area of infarction is confined to areas where blood flow reduction in the acute stage of the stroke is certainly below values of 10 ml per 100 gm per minute, indicating that in the acute stage of infarction loss of function will affect neurones in a much wider distribution than the ultimate structural loss. In accordance with this view, Morawetz *et al.* (1978) found that histopathological signs of structural infarction following a 2-3 hour period of focal ischaemia in the monkey were only obtained at sites where local blood flow was below 10-12 ml per 100 gm per minute.

From these observations, we have developed a concept that an area of structural loss in stroke was probably surrounded for some time in the acute phase, by an area of functional neuronal suppression, in which the structural integrity of the neurones was immediately, and even permanently, preserved. This we termed the ischaemic penumbra.

We now have some evidence that in the penumbral areas certain basic physiological mechanisms of the neurone remain intact, particularly concerned with ionic homeostasis at the cell membrane level. Potassium has long been known to accumulate in the extracellular space during hypoxia but in our experiments (Astrup *et al.* 1977) control levels of extracellular potassium ranging from 3-9 millimoles (mean 5.7 ± 1.5) were maintained with only minor changes at about the level of the threshold for electrical function, significant and massive movements of potassium ion into the extracellular space occurring only when flow fell to between 7 and 11 ml per 100 gm per minute, a level significantly lower than the levels for failure of electrical function. The assumption must be, therefore, that there is a differential failure of neuronal metabolic poroceses so that in the penumbral area synaptic transmission is impaired but the energy state and the ionic balance are maintained at normal levels.

The Development of Oedema

Recent work from our own laboratory (Symon *et al.*—in press) and from Hossmann and Schuier (1978) has indicated a definite relationship between the development of cerebral swelling and the intensity of brain ischaemia.

We find that significant ischaemia is associated at $1^1/_2$ hours with an increase in water content in the most densely ischaemic zones and in the area of the penumbra; a significant relationship between the increase in water content and blood flow is evident. Movement of water occurs when flow falls below 20 ml per 100 gm per minute, and it appears to be the initial depth of ischaemia that acts as a trigger mechanism releasing water which thereafter advances through the hemisphere as described for cold oedema fronts. Experiments in which ischaemic areas have been reperfused indicate that after $1^1/_2$ hours of ischaemia reperfusion is associated with an increase rather than a decrease in ischaemic oedema. Restoration of blood flow after a significant period of ischaemia may thus compound the problem of brain swelling.

References

Astrup, J., Symon, L., Branston, N. M., Lassen, N., Cortical evoked potential and extracellular K^+ and H^+ at critical levels of brain ischaemia. Stroke *8* (1977), 51—57.

Boysen, G., Engell, H. C., Trojaborg, W., Effect of mechanical rCBF reduction on EEG in man. In: Cerebral Circulation and Metabolism (Langfitt, T. W., McHenry, L. C., Jr., Reivich, M., Wollman, H., eds.), pp. 378—379. Berlin-Heidelberg-New York: Springer. 1975.

Branston, N. M., Symon, L., Crockard, H. A., Pasztor, E., Relationship between the cortical evoked potential blood flow and local cortical flow following acute middle cerebral artery occlusion in the baboon. Experimental Neurology *45* (1974), 195—208.

Brierley, J. B., Symon, L., The extent of infarcts in baboon brains three years after division of the middle cerebral artery. J. Neuropath. and Appl. Neurobiol. *3* (1977), 217—218.

Heiss, W. D., Hayakawa, T., Waltz, A. G., Cortical neuronal function during ischaemia. Effects of occlusion of one middle cerebral artery on single unit activity in cats. Arch. Neurol. *33* (1976), 813—820.

Hossmann, K. A., Schuier, F. J., The metabolic (cytotoxic) type of brain oedema following middle cerebral artery occlusion in cats. Proc. of the Princeton Conference, 1978. (In press.)

Morawetz, R. B., de Girolami, Ojemann, R. G., Marcoux, F. W., Crowell, R. M., Cerebral blood flow determined by hydrogen clearance during middle artery occlusion in unanaesthetised monkeys. Stroke *9* (1978), 143—149.

Symon, L., Experimental model of stroke in the baboon. Advances in Neurology *10* (1975), 199—212.

Acta Neurochirurgica, Suppl. 28, 218—221 (1979)
© by Springer-Verlag 1979

National Institute of Neurosurgery and Semmelweis
Medical University Department of Anatomy

Experimental Cerebral Hypoxia and Ischaemia in Cats

A. Pásztor, E. Pásztor, Cs. Léránt, and J. Hámori

With 2 Figures

The purpose of this study was to produce standard hypoxic and ischaemic insults and to study the pathological changes in brain caused by hypoxic and ischaemic processes. We thought that the pathological brain changes caused by hypoxia differ from the changes created by ischaemic processes.

EEG, systemic arterial blood pressure (SAP), systemic venous pressure (SVP), and ECG were measured during the hypoxia and ischaemia. The hypoxia was caused by stopping of ventilation, and ischaemia was brought about by elevating intracranial pressure (ICP) above the level of SAP.

Material and Methods

Twenty adult cats weighing 2.5-3.5 kg were anaesthetized with pentobarbitone sodiuni (Nembutal) 30 mg/kg. A tracheostomy was performed, and the animals were ventilated with a Harvard animal respirator. The animals were paralysed with Flaxedyl (gallamine triethiodide) 4 mg/kg and placed in a sterotaxic head holder. Femoral arterial and venous catheters were inserted, and a needle was introduced into the cisterna magna for measurement of ICP and infusion of mock cerebrospinal fluid (CSF). The SAP, SVP, ICP, ECG, and EEG were recorded on an eight-channel Elema-Schönander polygraph. Ischaemia was produced by rapidly increasing ICP to the level of SAP in five animals. Hypoxia was created in five other animals by stopping artificial ventilation for a period. Ten animals formed a control group. When the SAP fell below 60 mm/Hg the procedure was halted to allow recovery from hypoxia and high ICP. The insult was repeated many times. The animals were then killed, and the brains were perfused with Hayat solution. Material from the brain was removed from frontal cortex, thalamus n ventromedialis, and calamus scriptorius. Analysis of the material was done with the Jeol 10 MB electron microscope.

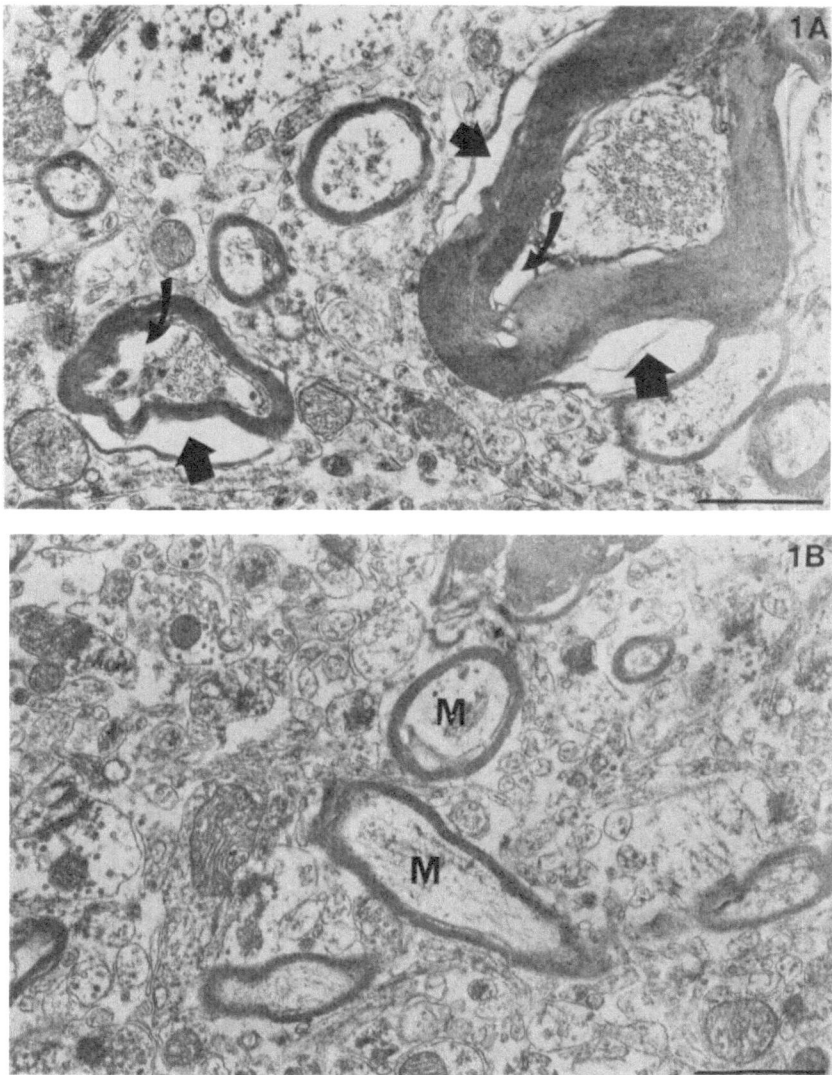

Fig. 1

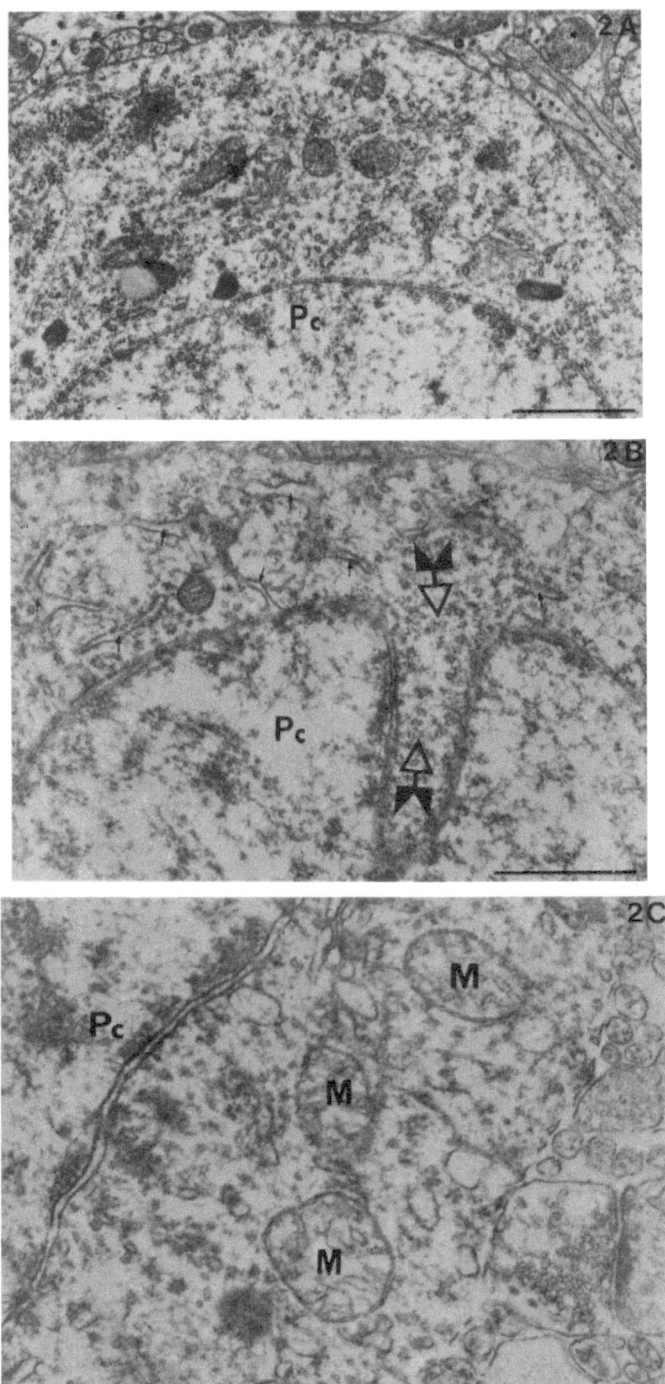

Fig. 2

Results

1. *Myelinated axons:* in the course of high ICP and hypoxia, axoplasms of thick (3.5-4 μm) myelinated axons become detached from the internal layers of the myelin sheath in ascending systems of the medulla oblongata as well as in the fibrae arcuatae internae. Less marked changes were found in the myelinated fibres of the same regions.

In deeper areas of the brain (nucl. ventromedialis thalami) a similar detachment can be seen in the thinner myelinated axons. Also, external lamellae of the myelin sheath are seen to be detached (Fig. 1A). In the case of acute hypoxia, such alterations cannot be seen in myelinated fibres of similar sizes within the same nucleus (Fig. 1B).

2. *Cells.* Glial cells and Golgi II (Gc) type interneurons are most vulnerable to hypoxia and raised ICP. Within Golgi II type cells large vacuoles appear, probably representing dilated endoplasmic cisterns.

The most severe alterations were observed after elevated ICP and acute hypoxia in glial cells. While the nucleus (N) is more or less intact, the perykaryon appears to be entirely empty, mitochondrial cristae disappear, and a homogeneous dense substance remains.

Pyramidal cells (Pc) in the fifth layer of the cortex are more resistent to increased ICP than to acute hypoxia. After high ICP, alterations are confined to the endoplasmic cisterns which are slightly more dilated than in control samples (Figs. 2A, B). Moreover, after hypoxia and raised ICP the quantities of free ribosomas are enhanced.

In addition to the above alterations, after acute hypoxia mitochondria are impaired. They are swollen, the numbers of cristae are decreased, and the ground substance is lighter than normal. The nucleus envelope is intact (Fig. 2C).

3. *Neuropil.* Alterations of neurophil are identical after high ICP with those seen in acute hypoxia. Synaptic vesicles are clustered both in terminals and in non-synaptic areas of the axons. Mitochondria are usually rounded with wellpreserved cristae. Here and there vesicles can be seen in the darkened matrix substance.

Acta Neurochirurgica, Suppl. 28, 222—225 (1979)
© by Springer-Verlag 1979

Department of Neurosurgery* and Department of Biochemistry**,
Hiroshima University School of Medicine, Hiroshima, Japan

Experimental Middle Cerebral Artery Embolization and Embolectomy

Y. Okada*, T. Shima*, M. Yamamoto*,
T. Uozumi*, and T. Kawasaki**

With 2 Figures

This experiment was performed to study clinicopathophysiology and cerebral metabolism of regional cerebral ischaemia produced by embolization of the trunk of the middle cerebral artery (MCA) of the dog, in contrast with that produced by trapping of the trunk of MCA. Embolectomy as a treatment for cerebral embolism is a contraversial subject. The effect of embolectomy within three hours after embolization is evaluated in this model.

Material and Method

Forty-five dogs, weighing 8 to 15 kg, were anaesthesized by intravenous injection of sodium pentobarbital (10-15 mg/kg) and relaxed by pancronium bromide (0.1 mg/kg). After endotracheal intubation, respiration was controlled mechanically and adjusted to ensure normocapnia and normoxia.

A silicone rubber cylinder 1.1 mm in diameter and 8 mm in length was placed in the cervical internal carotid artery, and segmental occlusion of MCA was performed. In eight animals embolectomy was completed microsurgically within three hours after embolization. To facilitate embolectomy, 4-0 nylon thread was embedded in the cylinder, and a tip of thread was left protruding from the distal end of the embolus. In a separate group, MCA trunk was exposed through a subtemporal approach and Scoville clips were applied to its proximal and distal ends.

The regional cerebral blood flow (rCBF) was measured by the hydrogen clearance method in the temporal cortex on the occluded side. The clearance curve was recorded during inhalation of 10% hydrogen gas for one to two minutes, and a calculation of rCBF was made by the initial slope method.

The cortical evoked potential on the occluded side in response to contralateral median nerve stimulation was recorded for six hours after MCA occlusion (Fig. 2 A).

In 20 animals the regional cerebral metabolism were observed at 1, 3, and 5 hours after embolization. The brain samples taken from both temporal lobes, parietal lobes, and deep parts of the hemispheres were frozen in liquid nitrogen. The ATP and lactate concentrations were analysed in each sample.

The animals in each group were kept alive for four to seven days, and neurological deficits were evaluated after recovery from anaesthesia by Smith's neurological evaluation score. After death, the brain was removed and explored grossly, and then fixed in 10% formalin solution. Coronal sections 5 mm in thickness were cut, and the infarct volume was calculated by the average end area method.

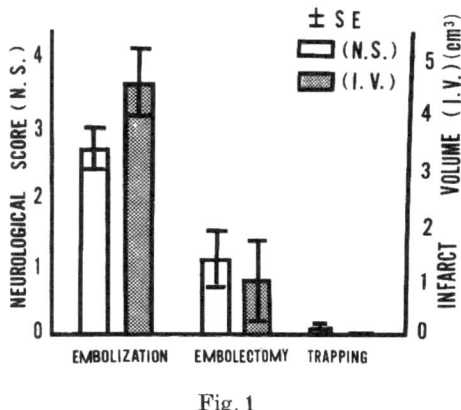

Fig. 1

Results

1. Embolization Group

The embolized animals exhibited remarkable neurological deficits, and the infarcts involved the lobus pyriformis, caudate nucleus, and thalamus. The mean neurological evaluation score was 2.7 ± 0.34 (mean $\pm$ SE), and the mean infarct volume was 4.6 ± 0.5 cm³ (Fig. 1).

Segmental occlusion of MCA trunk produced a decrease in rCBF from the original mean value of 53.0 ± 8.1 ml/100 g/min (mean $\pm$ SD) to 39.3 ± 10.7 at one hour after embolism. The rCBF remained almost unchanged during a period of 6 hours (Fig. 2 C).

The amplitude of EP decreased progressively from a resting value of 100% to $83.7 \pm 15\%$ one hour after embolism, $68.9 \pm 12.1\%$ at two hours, and $57.0 \pm 11.7\%$ at three hours (Fig. 2 B).

The changes in regional cerebral energy metabolism as ATP depletion and lactate accumulation were most prominent in the deep cerebrum of the embolized hemisphere. The changes became significant at three to five hours after embolization.

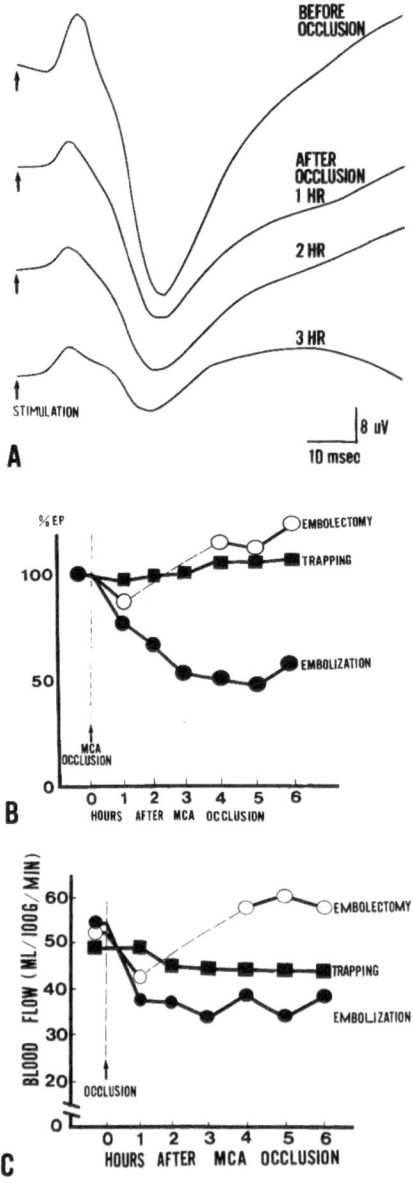

Fig. 2

2. Trapping Group

In this group no significant changes were found in rCBF and EP amplitude over a period of six hours (Figs. 2 B, C).

After recovery from anaesthesia all five animals were able to walk, but one animal showed forced circling movement. No infarction was found in any (Fig. 1).

3. Embolectomy in Embolization Group

After embolectomy rCBF increased from 42.3 ml/100 g/min over the preocclusional level (Fig. 2 C).

The amplitude of EP also increased to $115.4 \pm 26.8\%$ one hour after embolectomy (Fig. 2 B).

One animal died of brain swelling, and two showed motor weakness, but the other five exhibited no neurological deficits. The mean neurological evaluation score was 1.1 ± 0.45, which was significantly less than that of embolization group (P 0.01) (Fig. 1). The mean infarct volume was 1.1 ± 0.47 cm^3. A subacute intracerebral haematoma of 4 cm^3 was found in the temporal lobe in one animal, which was probably caused by retraction of the brain during embolectomy. In two animals small haemorrhagic infarctions were found around the caudate nucleus. The other five animals had no infarction, but shift of the midline structures to the opposite side was observed a week later.

Conclusion

The perforating afteries of the MCA play an extremely important role in the development of infarct in dog.

The decline of EP amplitude is probably due to functional disturbance of the second sensory neurone and thalamic nuclei, and seems to correspond well with the degree of neurological deficit.

Microsurgical embolectomy within three hours after embolization may prevent or alleviate ischaemic brain damage in the dog.

Acta Neurochirurgica, Suppl. 28, 226—230 (1979)
© by Springer-Verlag 1979

Department of Neurological Surgery, School of Medicine,
University of Pittsburgh, The Veterans' Administration Medical Centre,
and the Montefiore Hospital

Pentothal Protection for Delay Cerebral Revascularization *

H. Yonas, M. Dujovny, R. Segal, and D. Nelson

With 3 Figures

Summary

Thiopentone (20 mg/kg/bolus and 20 mg/kg/three hours) was effective in preventing infarction in five dogs with six hours of middle cerebral occlusion. Nine control animals sustained massive to large infarctions. Utilizing this regime therapeutic blood levels were rapidly attained for over 12 hours without side effects.

From the experimental and human experience with focal cerebral ischaemia, there appears to be a finite grace period in which cerebral revascularization can be undertaken. In canine and primate models this time has been about five hours, following which the infarction process may not be reversible (Sundt et al. 1977, Laha et al. 1978). Seeking to prolong this grace period, thiopentone was selected as an ideal drug for this purpose, and its effect on the revascularized canine middle cerebral distribution was evaluated at six hours following embolectomy.

Key words: focal cerebral ischaemia, thiopentone, cerebral embolism, cerebral revascularization.

Method

Fourteen mongrel dogs weighing between 15 and 22 kilograms were divided into two groups: nine controls and five thiopentone-treated. All animals underwent silastic cylinder embolization of the middle cerebral artery via the cervical internal carotid artery (Dujovny et al. 1976). Thiopentone (20 mg/kg/bolus and 20 mg/kg/hours for three hours) was begun 15 minutes after embolization. All vital functions were monitored, blood gases were maintained

* Supported in part by Grant-in-Aid, Western Pennsylvania Heart Association, 1977—1978.

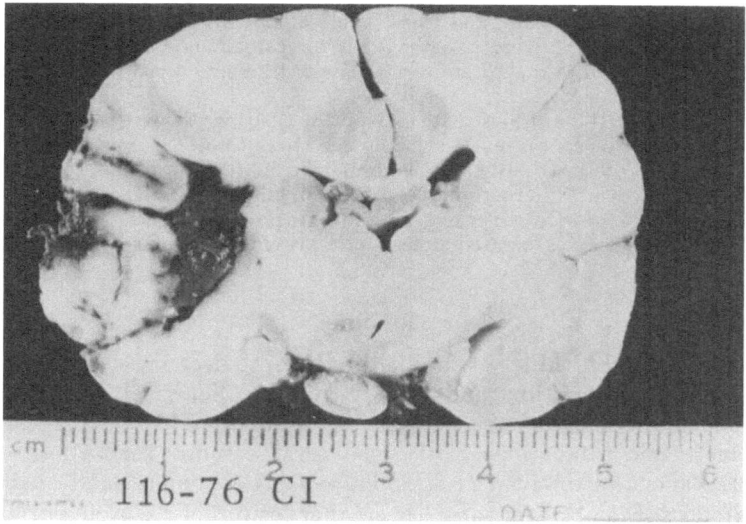

Fig. 1. Control animal developed a haemorrhagic infarction of the right middle cerebral distribution following unprotected emobolectomy at six hours

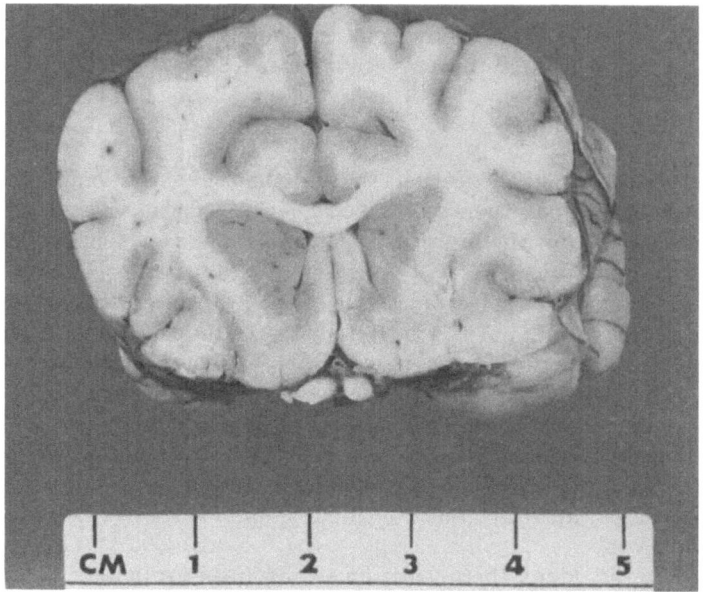

Fig. 2. Normal thiopentone-treated animal embolectomized at six hours

15*

within normal parameters, and blood levels of barbiturate were obtained at intervals. The emboli were removed with microtechnique and flow was re-established by six hours. All animals received intensive supportive care until self-sufficent.

The brains of the animals that survived for three weeks were perfused with 10% formalin. For all animals, including the three that died prematurely, the brains were studied grossly and then immersed in 10% formalin. The middle cerebral artery was microscopically patent in all animals. The brains were coronally sectioned after fixation, and photographic enlargements were made. The infarct size was calculated as described previously (Dujovny et al. 1976).

Results

Three of the nine control animals embolectomized six hours following embolization and died within 48 hours. These animals remained unconscious, and at autopsy were found to have massive haemorrhagic infarctions of the ipsilateral cerebral hemisphere. Six control animals survived 21 days. Three of these animals had massive infarctions (Fig. 1), and three had smaller lesions of the pyriform lobe.

The thiopentone groups usually required two to three days of respiratory assistance, but dit not require cardiovascular support. They woke very slowly, but by four days were observed to be neurologically intact. Coronal sections of these brains were grossly normal, except for a very small lacunar area of caudate softening in one animal and a small area of external capsular softenig in another (Fig. 2).

Blood levels of barbiturates were obtained as noted in Fig. 3.

Discussion

The present experimental data suggest that the early administration and maintenance of therapeutic blood levels of thiopentone protect cerebral tissue from the injurious effect of ischaemia and delayed post-ischaemia reperfusion.

A barbiturate was selected because of the known cerebral protective effects of this family of drugs (Hoff 1978). Thiopentone is the most lipid-soluble barbiturate (10 fold-that of pentobarbitone, Mark et al. 1958) whose property should permit maximal delivery of the drug within the ischaemic area. In order to sustain blood levels over at least the period of vessel occlusion, a bolus, followed by constant perfusion of the drug, was given. This technique allows saturation of all body depots (muscle, viscus, and fat), and a predictable and relatively slow decline of blood levels.

To date, no ideal therapeutic level has been established for focal cerebral ischaemia, and the range of 2-4 mg% was chosen from the literature (Marshall et al. 1977). These dosages and blood levels, while protecting from ischaemia, are below those that may induce cardiac toxicity and hypotension.

We believe that controlled introduction of thiopentone has a place especially in the treatment of acute focal cerebral ischaemia that may occur in the hospital environment during angiography, aneurysm surgery, or accidental embolization of the middle cerebral artery, with

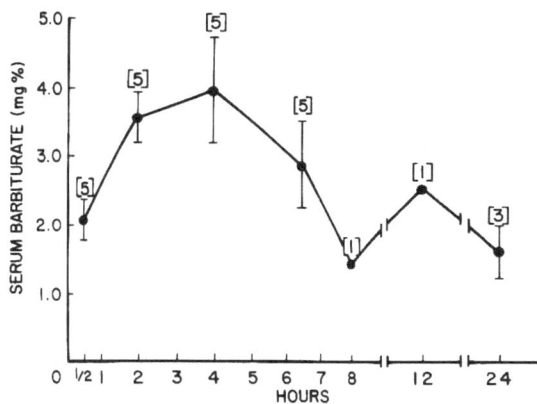

Fig. 3. Thiopentone blood levels over 24 hour period

muscle or gelfoam in the treatment of a carotid cavernous fistula or hemispheric arterio-venous malformation. Whether such significant cerebral protection as we have observed will be found with longer periods of delay before initiating therapy or re-establishing flow has not yet been determined.

The recent demonstration of the protective effects of both dimethylsulfoxide (DMSO) and low dose methyl prednisolone (Laha et al. 1978) are also encouraging. One would be hopeful that future combinations of these drugs with thiopentone may not be additive but synergistic in their ability to prolong the grace period for cerebral revascularization.

References

1. Dujovny, M., Osgood, C. P., Barrinuevo, P. J., et al., Middle cerebral artery microneurosurgical embolectomy. Surg. 80 (1976), 336—339.
2. Hoff, Julian, T., Resuscitations in focal brain ischaemia: Critical Care Med. 6 (1978), 245—253.

3. Laha, R. K., Dujovny, M., Barrionuevo, P. J., et al., Protective effects of methyl prednisolone and dimethylsulfoxide in experimental middle cerebral artery embolectomy. J. Neurosurg. 49 (1978), 508—516.
4. Mark, L. C., Burns, J. J., Brand, L., The passage of thiobarbiturates and their oxygen analogs into the brain. J. Pharmacol. Exp. Ther. 123 (1958), 70—75.
5. Marshall, L. F., Smith, R. W., Rouscher, L. A., Acute and chronic barbiturate administration and management of severe head injury. Presented American Association Neurological Surgeons Meeting, New Orleans, 1977.
6. Sundt, T. M., Houser, O. W., Sharbrough, F. W., et al., Carotid endarterectomy: Results, complications, and monitoring techniques. Advances in Neurology, Vol. 16, edited by R. A. Thompson and J. R. Green, pp. 97—119. New York: Raven Press. 1977.

Acta Neurochirurgica, Suppl. 28, 231—235 (1979)

II. Technical Aspects

Department of Neurosurgery (Head: Prof. W. Grote), University of Essen,
Federal Republic of Germany

Techniques of End-To-Side Anastomosis— Experimental Evaluation and Clinical Findings

H. M. Mehdorn, W. J. Bock, D. Rhode, and E. W. Strahl

With 2 Figures

The degree of improvement of cerebral function after the extra-cranial-intracranial (EC/IC) bypass procedure depends on many factors: preoperative cerebral function, cerebral perfusion as indicated by angiography and CBF measurements, and quality of available extra- and intracranial vessels. Besides these given factors which influence the indication for an EC/IC bypass, another major factor is the surgical technique used to perform the EC/IC anastomosis. Yaşargil[3] developed a technique that has been applied—with minor changes—in more than 4000 patients over the past 10 years. A major objection to this technique has been the fact that the recipient cerebral artery must be occluded with temporary clips over some 20-30 minutes.

For this reason, a new technique was suggested[2], that would reduce the critical occlusion time for the cortical vessel to 7-10 minutes. The donor artery is sutured to the posterior wall of the recipient cortical artery; next, this vessel is occluded using temporary clips, and an incision is made into it. Finally, the anterior wall is sutured, and all clips are released.

Experimental Model and Clinical Series

Using as experimental model the end-to-side anastomosis (ESA) between the femoral artery and the femoral vein in the rat, we performed 50 ESAs according to standard technique (Group A) and 30 ESAs according to the new technique (Group B). At intervals ranging from some hours to five months after the operation, the animals were sacrificed by transaortic *in vivo* perfusion fixation with 3% glutaraldehyde-phosphate buffer at physiological pressure, and specimens were prepared for light and scanning electron microscopy (SEM) according to standard techniques.

Furthermore, one of us (WJB) has previously used the new technique in certain patients of his series. These patients had suffered a moderate to severe stroke due to a high grade stenosis or occlusion of the internal carotid artery and underwent the EC/IC bypass 5 to 28 weeks after they had experienced the stroke. They were followed up postoperatively by angiography and clinical examination.

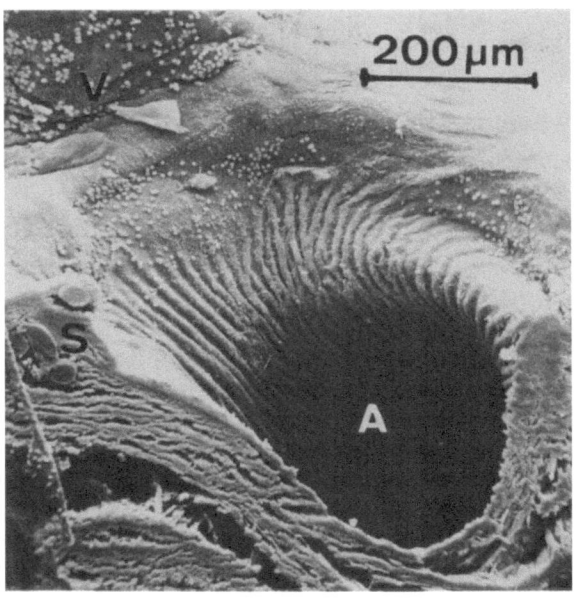

Fig. 1. End-to-side anastomosis, 4 weeks after operation, Group A. Note: Smooth junction between the artery (*A*) and the vein (*V*). *S* Suture material

Experimental Findings

All 80 ESAs remained patent. SEM observation of the specimens in Group A showed that most of the endothelium in both artery and vein was torn off immediately after the anastomosis had been completed and the blood flow had been restored. In the next 24–48 hours, the damaged endothelium, exposed subendothelium, and suture materials were covered by a layer of flattened platelets. The thickness of this non-thrombogenic layer varied depending on whether the blood flow was laminar or turbulent. Subsequently, the platelets were replaced by flat cells that had functional qualities of endothelial cells.

At 10–14 days after the operation, these cells have formed a complete layer of new endothelial lining. In specimens removed four weeks after the operation (Fig. 1) the transitional zone between artery and vein was covered with endothelium, and it was difficult to distinguish the border. Occasionally, one could see thickened endothelium and calcium deposits in areas where the blood stream hits the vein wall. These

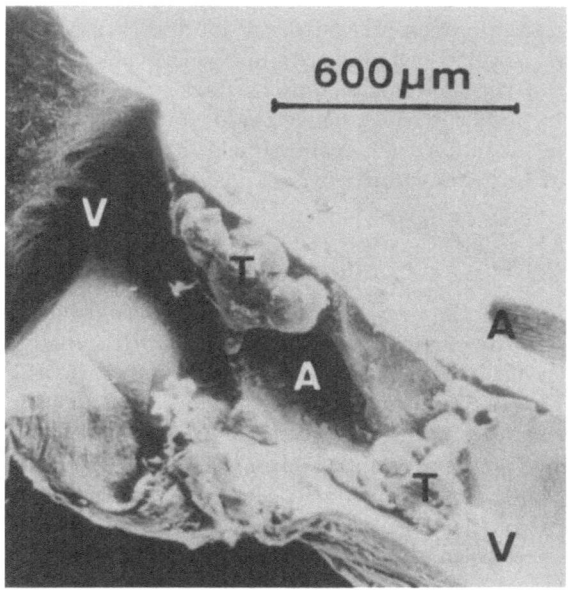

Fig. 2. End-to-side anastomosis, 4 weeks after operation, Group B. Note: Thrombus formation around the anastomosis and turbulences-indicating endothelial lining pattern on the venous side. (*A* Artery; *V* Vein; *T* Thrombus)

deposits became more frequent and increased in size over the next months. Eventually, they led to a labyrinth-like appearance of a cross-section through the vein, at light microscopic examination.

In Group B, the endothelium was denuded similarly and a new endothelial lining established. However, when compared to Group A, reendothelialization occurred at a much slower speed. After 4-5 weeks after operation, the endothelial lining was not yet complete (Fig. 2). The transitional zone between artery and vein was still covered with platelets adhering to a fibrin layer. Also, besides the deposits observed in Group A, another type of thrombi could be observed at the site of the

anastomosis that led to a severe stenosis of the anastomosis. Distally
from these thrombi, the endothelial cell pattern indicated a markedly
turbulent flow.

Clinical Findings

Follow-up examination of the patients operated on with the new
technique showed that all anastomoses had remained patent. However,
it was difficult to evaluate whether or not the extracranial artery had to
the same extent increased in size as it does when the standard
techniques are applied. Clinical examination revealed that there was
improvement of the neurological deficit, particularly of speech deficit,
after EC/IC bypass. However, our average follow-up interval was too
short to allow more accurate evaluation and comparison of the long
term effects of both techniques.

Discussion

The rationale for the new technique of ESA is to reduce the critical
occlusion time of the cortical vessel during the EC/IC bypass procedure.
This can indeed by achieved. However, as shown by the patients
operated on world-wide over the last ten years, even an occlusion time
of 40–50 minutes does not necessarily lead to a permanent neurological
deficit nor to histologically verified damage in the irrigated brain area[1].
On the other hand, SEM evaluation of the ESA performed with the new
technique indicated that platelets adhering to the inverted media and
adventitia of the vein may lead to a marked degree of thrombus
formation at the arterio-venous junction. This caused excessive stenosis
of the anastomosis and increased turbulences at the venous side of the
ESA. The shear stress which is exerted on the vein wall increased more
markedly than can be safely tolerated by the venous endothelium. This
probably will lead, over a longer period of time, to excessive new
thrombus formation and to some sort of atherosclerotic deposits on the
venous side of the recipient vessel which might seriously influence the
long-term patency rates after EC/IC bypass. The thrombi narrow the
anastomosis relatively more severely in small diameter vessels than in
larger vessels. Therefore, we suggest that there may be only a limited
use for the new technique of ESA. This would be the case when an
extracranial vessel would be anastomosed to a very proximal part of
the middle cerebral artery (MCA). Here, the short occlusion time of the
trunk of the MCA might be of benefit to the outcome after operation.

Further research is needed to evaluate the influence of anticoagulants and other platelet-affecting drugs on the formation of plugs

at the site of the anastomosis. Careful clinical evaluation of larger comparable series of patients might be usefull to elucidate further any possible use for this new technique.

References

1. Mehdorn, H. M., Chater, N. L., Townsend, J. J., Weinstein, P. R., Meyermann, R., Vessel wall response to microsurgical end-to-side anastomosis: Comparison of clinical findings with a laboratory model. Ann. Meet. Congr. of Neurol. Surg., 24.-29. 9. 1978, Washington, D.C., U.S.A.
2. Tulleken, C. A. F., A new technique for the end to side anastomosis between arteries of small calibre. Fourth Intern. Symp. on Microsurgical Anastomosis for Cerebral Ischemia, 6.-8. 9. 1978, London, Canada.
3. Yaşargil, M. G., Microsurgery applied to neurosurgery. Stuttgart-New York-London 1969.

Acta Neurochirurgica, Suppl. 28, 236—240 (1979)
© by Springer-Verlag 1979

Ursula Clinic, Wassenaar, Holland

A New Technique for End-To-Side Anastomosis Between Small Arteries

C. A. F. Tulleken, P. Hoogland, and J. Slooff

With 7 Figures

Introduction

The construction of an end-to-side anastomosis between arteries of small calibre, as in the extra-intracranial bypass procedure, will take, in experienced hands, about 25-40 minutes. During this period the receiving cortical artery is occluded. Since this artery is part of the leptomeningeal collateral circulation system, normally no local ischaemia develops. For an end-to-side anastomosis in the more proximal portion of one of the three main cerebral arteries (anterior, middle and posterior cerebral artery) this occlusion period is much too long, since collateral flow at this level is insufficient.

The use of an intraluminar shunt, as in carotid endarterectomy, is technically difficult in vessels of this calibre, and a sufficient flow can seldom be established. We experimented in our laboratory with a new technique for an end-to-side anastomosis between small arteries (in our experiments, the carotid arteries of the rat-diameter 0.8-1 mm). This new technique has the advantage of a very short time of occlusion of the receiving artery.

Technique (Figs. 1-6)

The artery which receives the end-to-side anastomosis is dissected free, but care is taken to leave the adventitia intact. The distal portion of the artery used for the anastomosis is prepared as is shown in Figs. 1-6. The distal opening of this artery is enlarged by a longitudinal cut with straight microscissors. With about ten interrupted sutures, using 10.0 Ethylon (R), which passes through all the layers of the donor artery, but only through the adventitia of the receiving artery, the end-to-side anastomosis is constructed for threequarters of its circumference. During this part of the procedure the lumen of the receiving

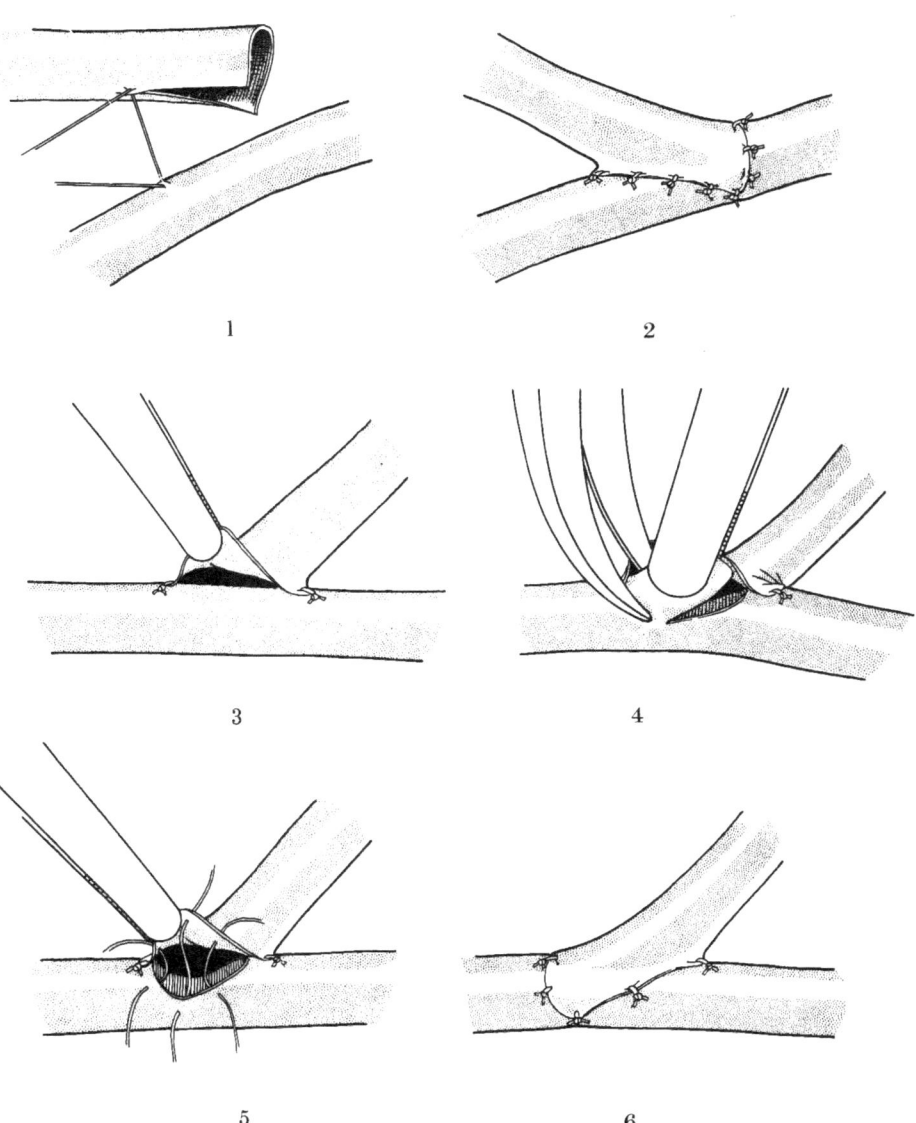

1

2

3

4

5

6

Figs. 1-6. Different stages of the new end-to-side anastomosis

artery remains patent, and the flow in this artery is, therefore, undisturbed.

If the needle is inadvertently introduced into the lumen of the receiving artery, brisk bleeding, that can be easily controlled by gentle tamponade with Surgical (R), occurs.

After completion of the end-to-side anastomosis for threequarters of its circumference, the receiving artery is then occluded by two microclips on both sides of the anastomosis.

With microforceps the wall of the receiving artery is grasped inside the anastomosis and with curved microscissors a hole is cut, which just fits the anastomosis. The site of the anastomosis is now flushed with a heparin in saline solution (0.25 ml heparine in 10 ml saline) and the end-to-side anastomosis is completed with three sutures, using 10.0 Ethylon, which pass through all the layers of the receiving and the donor arteries. The clips are removed, and gentle tamponade with surgical is exerted for 3-5 minutes at the site of the constructed anastomosis. When some experience is gained, the occlusion time necessary to complete the anastomosis is 5-7 minutes.

Methods

In a group of 15 rats chronic experiments were performed to check the patency of this new type of end-to-side anastomosis.

A. In a group of five rats the left CCA was proximally ligated and cut, and end-to-side connected to the right CCA.

B. In a group of six rats the left CCA was partially removed and put as a bypass on the right CCA using the new technique for one end-to-side anastomosis and the routine technique for the other.

C. In another group of four rats the left CCA was put as a bypass on the right CCA, using for both end-to-side anastomoses the new technique.

The animals were sacrified between 24 hours and 3 months after operation. The anastomosis was studied in three different ways:

inspection when the animal was still alive (pulsations, direction of flow) (all animals);

angiography (nine animals);

inspection of the anastomosis site, at autopsy after opening of the arteries, with the aid of the operating microscope (all animals);

histologically (three animals).

Results

a) Inspection when the animal was still alive showed good pulsations and a normal direction of flow in 14 animals. In one rat (left CCA put as a bypass on the right CCA using the new technique for both end-to-side anastomoses) the distal end-to-side anastomosis was occluded after 48 hours, and the proximal anastomosis was patent.

b) Angiography (nine animals: 48 hours, 72 hours, 8 days, 23 days, 5 weeks, 10 weeks, 3 months, 3 months) patent anastomoses in every case (Fig. 2).

c) Inspection at autopsy with the aid of the microscope disclosed patent anastomoses, without any thrombus formation, in 14 rats. In one rat (see a) the distal anastomosis was occluded by thrombus.

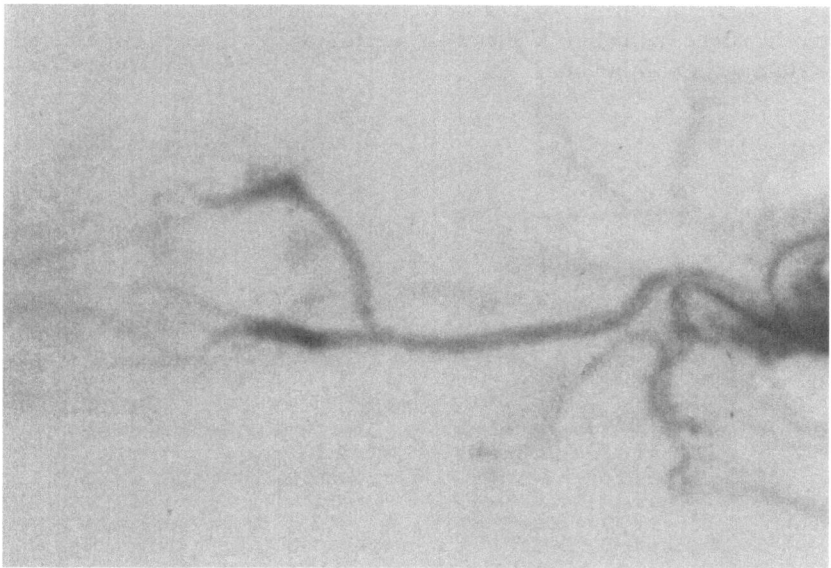

Fig. 7. Angiography (23 days after operation). The carotid artery is ligated between the two end-to-side anastomoses

d) Histological examination was performed in three rats (5 weeks, 10 weeks, 3 months). No thrombus formation was found.

N.B. In 4 rats, which were operated upon for a chronic experiment, the anastomosis was occluded in the immediate postoperative phase because of a technical error, and the animals were sacrificed.

Discussion

The new technique for an end-to-side anastomosis between arteries of small calibre, described in this communication, has the advantage of a very short occlusion period of the receiving artery: 5-7 minutes. As a consequence, this type of end-to-side anastomosis can possibly be performed on the more proximal portion of the cerebral arteries, where collateral flow is insufficient and therefore occlusion for a longer period of time is contra-indicated.

The experiments were started purely as a technical exercise, and without much hope of a patent anastomosis, since at the site of the anastomosis the three layers of the receiving artery are exposed to the blood stream. A thrombogenic influence by adventitia and media was expected, but, to our surprise, when the operation was correctly performed, no thrombus developed and the anastomosis remained nicely patent, as could be shown by angiography, at autopsy, and by histological examination.

Acta Neurochirurgica, Suppl. 28, 241—249 (1979)

Sophia Hospital, Zwolle,The Netherlands

A Scanning Electron Microscopic (SEM) Study of the Re-Endothelialization of the Carotid End-To-Side Anastomosis in the Rat

P. W. Gelderman

With 3 Figures

Summary

A carotid end-to-side anastomosis was made on 25 male Wistar rats (mean weight 197.8 g). At different time intervals, from 0 to 21 days after the operation, the animals were sacrified. The anastomosis was exposed, the aorta was cannulated, and the animals were perfused at a constant pressure of 80 mm Hg with a $2^{1}/_{2}\%$ glutaraldehyde solution. The anastomoses were taken out for further SEM and light microscopic (LM) study. The SEM results indicate that after the acute platelet-fibrin reaction in the first 48 hours the suture line itself becomes re-endothelialized after 4 days. On the stitches, however (Ethilon[R] 11 × 0, 2871 G, BV 7 needle) after two days a cellular population was seen, consisting of leucocytes transforming into flattened cells. The morphology of these cells and their role in the regeneration of endothelium is discussed. This study gives evidence to the possibility of a blood-borne genesis of endothelial cells *in vivo*.

Introduction

Much research has been done on the reaction of the vascular wall to trauma. Most of these investigations were inspired by the question of the pathophysiology of the development of atherosclerotic lesions. A greatly varying number of mechanical and chemical experimental models have been used, and a comparison is not easy.

This work has received a new impulse in recent years from the development of microsurgical vascular techniques.

SEM is very useful for the study of cellular changes that happen at the surface of the vessel wall in cases of trauma and repair of the

endothelium. This technique was introduced by the pioneers Shimamoto, Yamashita, and Sunaga in 1969 for the study of endothelium[25].
It is of the utmost importance to have standard methods in the
preparation and fixation of the specimens in order to get uniform and
reliable results and to avoid artifacts[6, 12].

Gregorius and Rand[14] described the most intense reaction to trauma
in microvascular anastomosis that takes place at some distance from
the suture line and at places where vascular clamps were applied.
Rosenbaum and Sundt[24] examined microvascular anastomoses in the
rat, and studied the acute thrombotic reaction at the site of the
anastomosis. Both papers pay attention only to the reaction of the
vascular wall in the first hours after surgical trauma. The aim of this
study was to pay attention to the process of re-endothelialization itself.

Materials and Methods

25 male Wistar rats (mean weight 197.8 g) were anaesthetized with
Nembutal[R] intraperitoneally. Under a Zeiss diploscope a horizontal incision
was made just above the manubrium sterni. The trachea and both carotid
arteries were exposed. A tracheostomy was made at the lower border of the
thyroid gland, and the animal was intubated. The left carotid artery was tied
off, cut tangentially just below the bifurcation, and washed out with heparin-
saline. A Scoville clamp was applied to the vessel as proximal as possible. On
the right common carotid artery two Scoville clamps were put at a distance of
1 cm from each other. An end-to-side anastomosis was made with interrupted
stitches of 11 × 0 Ethilon[R] (2871 G, BV 7 needle). At different time intervals,
from 0 to 21 days after the operation, the animals were sacrified. The
anastomosis was exposed, the aorta was cannulated, and the animals were
perfused at a constant pressure of 80 mm Hg (8) with a $2^1/_2\%$ glutaraldehyde
solution. The ends of the anastomosis were tied off, and the specimen was taken
out for further study. After four hours the specimen was opened and fixed on a
piece of cork for 24 hours in a $2^1/_2\%$ buffered glutaraldehyde solution, rinsed in
0.1 M phosphate buffer, and dehydrated in rising concentrations of acetone.
The tissue was dried by the critical point drying method. The specimens were
examined with a Cambridge Stereoscan S 4.

Results

In the first two days after the operation a platelet-fibrin reaction is
observed. Suture line and stitches are covered with a thin layer of
coagulum consisting of flocky threads of fibrin, that caught cellular
elements. This reaction markedly increases after 24 hours and stabilises
within two days. The fibrin threads and the long offshoots of the
platelets are mainly arranged in the direction of the blood flow.

Some stitches are not covered by thrombus. On them the first signs
of population appear after two days: platelets without offshoots and
leucocytes. Some of these cells lost their spherical appearance and

seemed to flatten out. Their coarse microvilli were refined and limited to the central part of the cell.

Three days after the operation the population of the stitches has increased and is more varied. Transient forms from leucocytes that stick

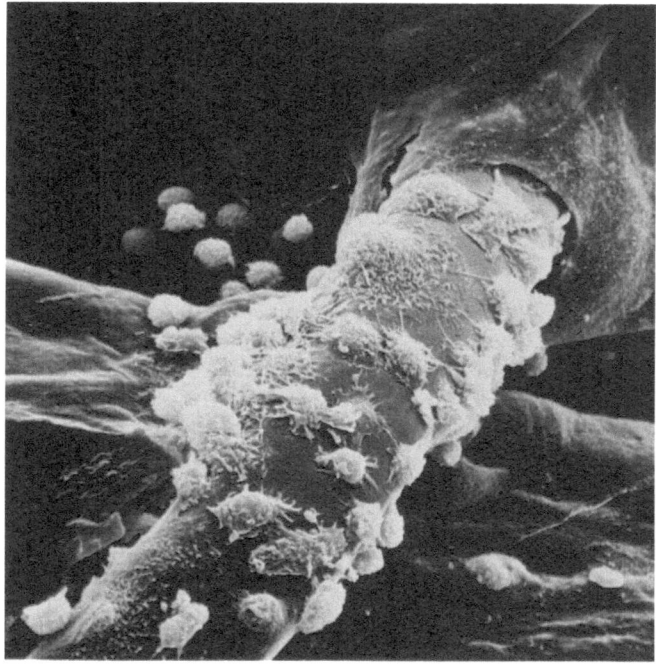

Fig. 1. Enlargement × 1,300. Stitch three days after the operation. Population of the thread. Leucocytes are flattening and flow centripetal over the surface. Top left: ant hill cell

with small pseudopodia on the sutures to flattened covering cells can be seen. The pseudopodia increase in number, spread out and flatten as the cytoplasm flows centripetal over the surface of the thread. The aspect of the microvilli has changed from coarse lobules into delicate dots. At the base of some stitches one sees an advancing re-endothelialization from the normal vascular wall. After four days the suture line itself appears to be re-endothelialized completely. The flattening cells on the stitches get the aspect of ant hills. The boundaries of the cell are far beyond the central part, covered by numerous tiny microvilli, as a sign of increased metabolism.

16*

After seven days the vast majority of the stitches are covered by a substantial layer of endothelium. Not all the specimens are in the same phase. In some, after ten days, stitches are in full regeneration. In the same specimen re-endothelialized and populated stitches in construction can alternate. At some distance from the suture line sheets of

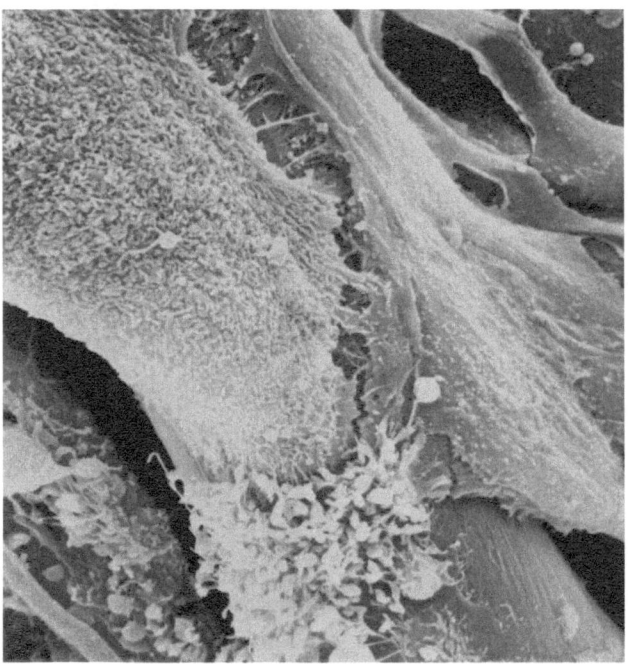

Fig. 2. Enlargement ×2,600. Large ant hill cell (macrophage?) top left, covering the basis of a stitch. Ten days after the operation

advancing endothelium can be seen growing over a blanket of platelets and fibrin.

After fourteen days the last phases of re-endothelialization are seen. Lettuce-like leucocytes are alongside regenerated endothelial cells. After 21 days re-endothelialization is complete, apart from a single mechanical injury made by the preparation. Even the most erect stitches are overgrown. Mostly the stitches can only be detected as small irregularities in the uniform layer of cells, forming a static picture of the flow properties of the blood.

Discussion

The normal arterial wall consists of three layers: the tunica intima (endothelium, basement membrane, internal elastic lamina), the tunica media (smooth muscle cells) and the tunica adventitia (connective tissue). According to Maximow and Bloom[15] the endothelial tissue has a

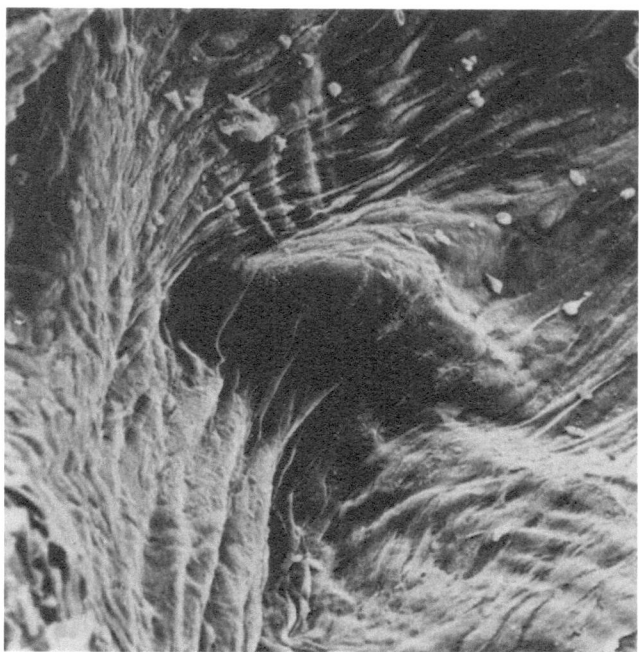

Fig. 3. Enlargement × 650. Completely re-endothelialized suture line and stitch. Fourteen days after operation

mesodermal origin, and is formed by the flattening of mesenchymal cells with the appearance of fibroblasts. Their longitudinal axis is adjusted to the direction of the flow of the blood stream[9]. The morphological characteristics of normal endothelium as seen by SEM have been recently described by Thurston[32] and O'Brien[18].

According to Björkerud[4] the reaction of the vascular wall to trauma is to be compared with that of the skin. Characteristic of the vessel wall is the phenomenon of the sub-endothelial thickening. Our few LM results did not justify the inclusion of this subject in this study.

There is no uniform relationship between endothelial injury, platelet reaction, and the blood clotting mechanism[26]. In the case of endothelial damage a platelet reaction is triggered mainly by collagen fibres from the deeper layers of the vascular wall[26, 27]. The platelet reaction consists of a platelet release reaction. The thrombocytes degranulate, and chemicals such as ADP and 5 HT are released in the blood[1]. Probably it is a positive feed-back mechanism, at which much energy is liberated, and a stabile lowenergy state develops[26].

Re-endothelialization is an important part in the phase of regeneration and repair of the vascular wall. Different theories are held about the actual source of new endothelial cells *in vivo*:

1. Re-endothelialization by advancing of cells from the edges of the defect. Poole *et al.*[20], employing the Häutchen technique, describe a platelet-fibrin blanket with monocytes as the endothelium advances from the edges to the centre of the defect. He discussed the different theories in 1971[21], and concluded that endothelium arises from endothelium. Other advocates of this theory are Florey[10], Nomura[17], Moseley[16], Fishman[11], and Thurston[32].

Stchelkounoff[29] suspected in 1936 on LM grounds a relation between smooth muscle cells and endothelial cells.

Björkerud[3] mentions the sub-endothelial cells and describes their origin from smooth muscle cells of the media. Buck[5] speaks of myo-intimal cells arising from smooth muscle cells by de-differentiation. Whissler[35] considers the arterial smooth muscle cell to be a multipotential mesenchymal cell, able to form collagen, elastin, smooth muscle fibres, and the basement membrane. Ts'ao[33] sees more resemblance between endothelial cells and neo-intimal cells than between the latter and smooth muscle cells. He has no doubts, however, that the former originate from smooth muscle cells and he speaks of a re-differentiation. Transmission Electron Microscopy (TEM) arguments a favor of this theory are brought by Rhoden[23], Still and Dennison[30], Nomura[17], Spaet *et al.*[28], Ts'ao[34], and Fishman[11].

3. The discussion about blood-borne cells as precursors of the endothelial cell has a long history[13]. It is very difficult to distinguish on LM grounds alone the different cells in their distinct manifestations. Ghani and Tibbs[13] use in their experiments long impermeable synthetic grafts. Stump[31] constructed hubs in the axis of the blood stream, inaccessible for the sedentary cells of the vascular wall. In diffusion chambers transformations from monocytes by way of macrophages and fibroblasts to endothelial cells were seen before. O'Neal *et al.*[19] notes a covering of three layers on a dacron hub floating freely in the blood stream. The outer one had, as seen by TEM, unmistakebly all the qualities of endothelium. Davies *et al.*[7] consider a haematogenic re-endothelialization as a possibility, as is the opinion of Pugatch[22].

Baumgartner and Spaet[2] observed, after the acute platelet reaction, adhesion of granulocytes within three hours on a denuded vascular segment and complete re-endothelialization within four days. They supported their observations with ^{3}H-thymidin labelling experiments.

Conclusion

From this study it appears that the possibility of the origin of endothelial cells from blood-borne elements is a tentative theory. Transformation from leucocytes, possibly monocytes, by way of macrophages and fibroblast-like cells to endothelial cells is a possible way by which denuded areas in the blood stream can be re-endothelialized.

Acknowledgments

The operations were performed in the Laboratory for Experimental Surgery, Department of Thoracic Surgery, State University Utrecht (head: Dr. G. A. Charbon). SEM studies were done with Dr. W. Berendsen, Department of Molecular Cellbiology, section Electronmicroscopy, State University Utrecht, the Netherlands.

References

1. Baumgartner, H. R., Tranzer, J. P., Studer, A., An electron microscopic study of platelet thrombus formation in the rabbit with particular regard to 5 HT release. Thromb. Diath. Haemorrh. *18* (1967), 592—604.
2. Baumgartner, H. R., Spaet, T. H., Endothelial replacement in rabbit arteries. Fed. Proceedings *29* (1970), 710 (Abstract 2627).
3. Björkerud, S., Reaction of the aortic wall of the rabbit after superficial, longitudinal, mechanical trauma. Virchows Archiv, Abteilung A, Pathologische Anatomie (Berlin) *347* (1969), 197—210.
4. Björkerud, S., Panel discussion following the survey of prof. Shimamoto. Angiology *25* (1974), 712—714.
5. Buck, R. C., Intimal thickening after ligature of arteries. An electron microscopic study. Circ. Res. *9* (1961), 418—426.
6. Clark, J. M., Glasgow, S., Luminal surface of distended arteries by scanning electron microscopy: eliminating configurational and technical artifacts. Brit. J. Exp. Pathol. *57* (1976), 129—135.
7. Davies, M. J., Woolf, N., Bradley, J. P. W., Endothelialisation of experimentally produced mural thrombi in the pig aorta. J. Pathol. *97* (1969), 589—594.
8. Davies, P. F., Bowyer, D. E., Scanning electron microscopy: arterial endothelial integrety after fixation at physiological pressure. Atherosclerosis *21* (1975), 463—469.
9. Flaherty, J. T., Pierce, J. E., Feerans, V. J., et al., Endothelial nuclear patterns in the canine arterial tree with particular reference to hemaodynamic events. Circ. Res. *30* (1972), 23—33.
10. Florey, H. W., Greer, S. J., et al., The pseudo-intima lining fabric grafts of the aorta. Brit. J. Exp. Pathol. *42* (1961), 236.

11. Fishman, J. A., Ryan, G. B., Karnovski, M. J., Endothelial regeneration in the rat carotid artery and the significance of endothelial denudation on the pathogenesis of myointimal thickening. Laboratory Investigations *32* (1975), 339—351.
12. Gertz, S. D., Rennels, M. L., Forbes, M. S., *et al.*, Preparation of vascular endothelium for scanning electron microscopy: a comparison of the effects of perfusion and immersion fixation. J. Microsc. (Oxford) *105* (1975), 309—313.
13. Ghani, A. R., Tibbs, D. J., Role of blood borne cells in organisation of mural thrombi. Brit. Med. J. *1* (1962), 1244—1247.
14. Gregorius, F. K., Rand, R. W., Scanning electronic observations of common carotid artery endothelium in the rat. Surg. Neurol. *4* (1975), 252—257.
15. Maximow, A. A., Bloom, W., A textbook of histology. Philadelphia and London: W. B. Saunders Comp. 1957.
16. Moseley, H. S., Connel, R. S., Krippaehne, W. W., Healing of canine aorta after endarterectomy: a scanning electron microscopic study. Ann. Surg. *180* (1974), 329—335.
17. Nomura, Y., The ultra structure of the pseudo-intima lining synthetic arterial grafts in the canine aorta with special reference to the origin of the endothelial cell. J. Cardiovasc. Surg. *11* (1970), 282—291.
18. O'Brien, B. McC., Microvascular reconstructive surgery. Edinburgh-London-New York: Churchill Livingstone. 1977.
19. O'Neal, R. M., Jordan, G. L., Rabin, E. R., *et al.*, Cells grown on isolated Dacron Hub for electron microscopic study. Exp. Mol. Path. *3* (1964), 403—412.
20. Poole, J. C. F., Sanders, A. G., Florey, H. W., The regeneration of aortic endothelium. J. Pathol. Bacteriol. *75* (1958), 133—143.
21. Poole, J. C. F., Cromwell, S. B., Bendit, E. P., Behavior of smooth muscle cells and formation of extracellular structures. Amer. J. Pathol. *62* (1971), 391.
22. Pugatch, E. M. J., The growth of endothelium and pseudo-endothelium of the healing surface of rabbit ear chambers. Proc. Roy. Soc. Med. *B 160* (1964), 412.
23. Rhoden, J. A. G., Ultrastructure of mammalian arterioles and precapillary sphincters. J. Ultrastruct. Res. *18* (1967), 181.
24. Rosenbaum, T. J., Sundt, T. M., Jr., Thrombus formation and endothelial alterations on microarterial anastomoses. J. Neurosurg. *47* (1977), 430—442.
25. Shimamoto, T., Yamashita, Y., Sunaga, T., Scanning electron microscopic observation of endothelial surface of heart and blood vessels. Proc. Jap. Academy *45* (1969), 507—511.
26. Spaet, T. H., Erichson, R. B., The vascular wall in the pathogenesis of thrombosis. Thromb. Diath. Haemorrh. (Suppl. 21) (1966), 67—86.
27. Spaet, T. H., Gaynor, E., Vascular endothelial damage and thrombosis. Adv. in Cardiology *4* (1970), 47—66.
28. Spaet, T. H., Stemermann, M. B., *et al.*, The role of smooth muscle cells in repopulation of rabbit aortic endothelium following balloon injury. Fed. Proc. *32* (1973), 219 (Abstr.).
29. Stchelkounoff, I., l' Intima des petits artères et des veines et le mesenchyme vasculaire. Archives d'Anatomie Microscopique *32* (1936), 139—194.

30. Still, W. J. S., Dennison, S. M., Reaction of arterial intima of the rabbit to trauma and hyperlipemia. Exper. Mol. Pathol. *6* (1967), 245.
31. Stump, M. M., Jordan, G. L., Jr., DeBakey, M. E., *et al.*, Endothelium growth from circulating blood on isolated intravascular dacron hub. Amer. J. Pathol. *43* (1963), 361—368.
32. Thurston, J. B., Bunke, H. J., Chater, N. L., Weinstein, P. R., A scanning electron microscopic study of microarterial damage and repair. Plast. and Reconstr. Surg. *57* (1976), 197—203.
33. Ts'ao, C., Myo-intimal cells as a possible source of replacement for endothelial cells in the rabbit. Circ. Res. *23* (1968), 671—682.
34. Ts'ao, C., Topographical and ultrastructural alterations of smooth muscle cells lining damaged rabbit aorta. Brit. J. Exp. Pathol. *56* (1975), 291.
35. Whissler, R. W., The arterial medial cell: smooth muscle cell or multifunctional mesenchyme? Circulation *36* (1967), 1.

Acta Neurochirurgica, Suppl. 28, 250—253 (1979)
© by Springer-Verlag 1979

Department of Neurosurgery, North Manchester General Hospital,
Manchester M8 6RB, and
Department of Pathology, Medical School, University of Manchester, England

Scanning Electron Microscopy of the Endothelial Surface of Small Diameter Vein Grafts in Rats Treated With Heparin

C. M. Bannister and S. A. Chapman

With 2 Figures

There are patients with cerebral ischaemia who would benefit from an extracranial-intracranial anastomosis but whose external carotid arteries are blocked and, therefore, do not have scalp arteries available for an anastomosis. In these cases a vein graft would seem to be the obvious choice to carry an extra supply of blood to the brain. However, at the point of anastomosis to the cerebral artery the vein graft would need to have a diameter of about 1 mm, and in rats vein grafts of this size have been shown to have a very poor patency rate (Bannister *et al.* 1977). The venous internal elastic lamina has a net-like construction, and lies over numerous collagen fibres in the subendothelial layer. Damage and loss of the endothelium during dissection and anastomosis exposes the collagen fibres to the blood stream, platelets and fibrin are deposited on them, and in less than an hour all the experimental grafts were occluded by thrombus. In spite of these findings vein grafts remain an attractive way of carrying blood to the ischaemic brain, and warrant further investigation for means of keeping them patent over long periods of time. Heparin was selected for investigation because of its anti-coagulant and anti-platelet adhesive actions.

· One cm lengths of veins were dissected fron the necks of albino rats and anastomosed upside down by two end-to-side junctions to the right common carotid arteries. Blood was allowed to flow through the grafts for 5, 15, 30, or 60 minutes before the grafts together with a few mm of the adjacent artery were excised. They were then fixed in buffered 2.5% glutaraldehyde, and prepared for scanning electron microscopy. The two grafts examined at 5 minutes were patent, at 15 minutes only one of three grafts was patent, at 30 minutes one of two grafts was patent, and at 60 minutes neither of two grafts was patent. Scanning electron microscopy of the patent grafts showed that few platelets and only small quantities of fibrin had been deposited on the arterial endothelium at any of the observation time in spite of endothelial

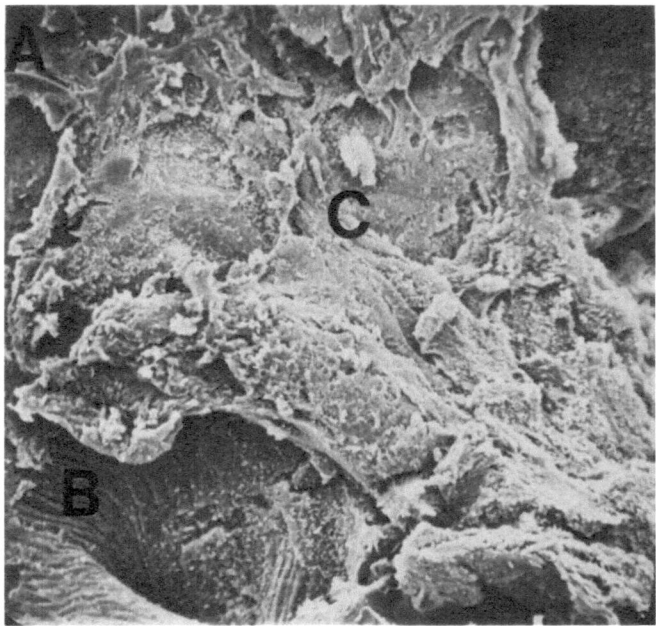

Fig. 1. Electron-micrograph of the endothelial surface of a vein graft in a rat which had not received heparin. The graft was examined 30 minutes after blood had started to flow through it. *A* suture, *B* arterial surface, *C* wads of fibrin on the anastomotic line and surface of the vein graft.
(Magnification = ×107)

damage, but at the anastomotic lines and at the sites of venous endothelial loss platelets and fibrin were deposited in increasing amount during the hour of observation (Fig. 1). Accumulation of the platelets and fibrin lead sooner or later within an hour to slowing of the blood flow through the grafts. Stagnant blood trapped in the graft clots and finally blocks the grafts.

Eight rats were given 10 units of heparin into a vein on the dorsum of the foot half an hour before the grafting procedure, and heparin

(25 units/ml) was also used to wash out the veins before they were anastomosed to the carotid arteries. The grafts were again examined 5, 15, 30, or 60 minutes after blood had started to flow through them. All the grafts were found to be patent, and after fixation in 2.5 % buffered

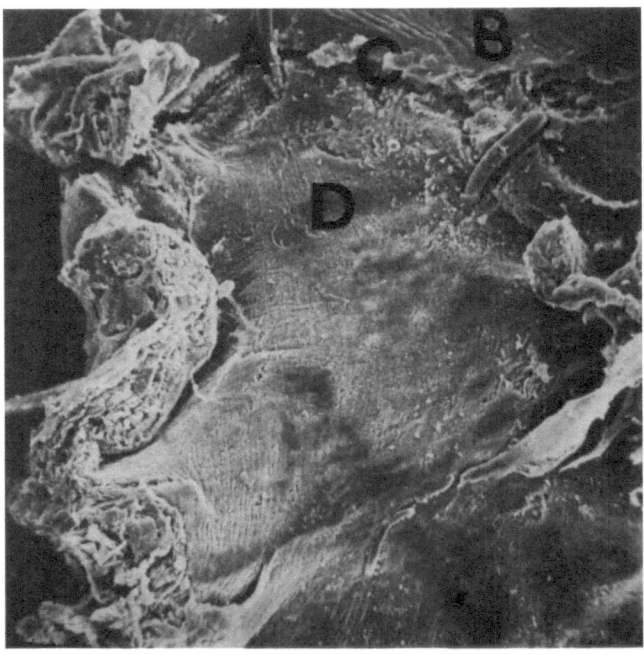

Fig. 2. Electron-micrograph of the endothelial surface of a vein graft after the rat had received intravenous heparin and the vein had been washed out with a solution of heparin before being grafted. The graft was examined 30 minutes after blood started to flow through it. *A* suture, *B* arterial surface, *C* and *D* suture line and venous surface of the graft almost free of platelets and fibrin. (Magnification = × 110)

glutaraldehyde they were prepared for scanning electron microscopy. There were significantly fewer platelets and smaller deposits of fibrin on the anastomotic lines and in the grafts where endothelium had been lost at all of the observation times (Fig. 2).

In the second part of the study the long term patency of vein grafts in rats treated with heparin was investigated. The grafting procedure was carried out in eight rats which had received heparin intravenously, and whose grafted veins had been washed out with a solution of heparin. The grafts were examined 1, 2, 3, 5, 7, 9, and 11 weeks later. All the grafts except the one examined at 7 weeks were patent. Scanning electron microscopy of the patent grafts showed that it took up to 5 weeks for the damaged arterial endothelium to re-endothelialize, and up to 10 weeks for the grafts' venous endothelium to heal. Throughout this time tissue other than endothelium was exposed to the blood stream but no new platelets or fibrin were deposited. The half-life of intravenous heparin is about $1^1/_2$ to 2 hours. During that time it seems likely that it alters the ability of collagen to attract platelets and promote the formation of fibrin.

We woundered whether washing out the veins only with heparin would be sufficient to keep the grafts patent. Therefore, in another 11 rats vein grafts were made after heparin had been used only to wash out the veins. The grafts were then re-examined at 1, 2, 3, 4, 5, 7, and 10 weeks. All the grafts except the 10-week one were patent. The scanning electron microscopic appearances of these grafts were very similar in all details to those of the grafts of the rats who received in addition intravenous heparin.

This study suggests that if it is necessary to use small diameter vein grafts to convey extra supplies if blood to the brain, the patency of the grafts can be maintained in a high proportion of cases by the use of heparin at the time of grafting. Heparin appears to act locally on the exposed subendothelial tissues, and it can be got to these tissues in effective quantities by washing out the veins with a solution of heparin before grafting.

Acknowledgments

We wish to thank Prof. Peter Yates for allowing us to carry out this work in his Department. One of us, C.M.B., receives a grant from Manchester Clinical Research Committee.

Reference

Bannister, C. M., Mundy, L. A., and Mundy, J. E., Comparative merits of autogenous arterial and venous bypass grafts as alternatives to direct arterial anastomosis. In: Microsurgery for Stroke (Schmiedek, P., ed.), pp. 105—118. New York-Heidelberg-Berlin: Springer. 1977.

Acta Neurochirurgica, Suppl. 28, 254—256 (1979)
© by Springer-Verlag 1979

The Department Sixto Obrador of Neurosurgery,
Centro Especial Ramón y Cajal de la Seguridad Social,
Ministerio de Sanidad, Madrid, Spain

Venous Patch in Arteries of 1 mm External Diameter

J. A. Gutierrez-Diaz, J. Iglesias, J. Silvela,
I. Nieto, and A. Córdoba

Introduction

The venous patch as a surgical technique was first described in the literature by Senning (1959) and by Crawford *et al.* (1959). This technique has demonstrated its value for the surgery of medium and large calibre arterial vessels. With the help of the surgical microscope it is possible to place venous patches in arteries with external diameters of approximately 1 mm. The technique of the venous patch may be of great help in several cerebrovascular affections.

In the present work it is intended to demonstrate the vascular permeability as observed both angiographically and histologically, as well as to show the structural evolution of the arterial wall following the implant of a venous patch with an external diameter of 1 mm, and followed for a period of six months. Also we have studied the possible functional or structural advantages of placing either the endothelium or the adventitia towards the lumen of the vessel.

Material and Methods

Using wistar rats and with the help of the operating microscope, the common carotid artery with an external diameter of approximately 1 mm, has been incised longitudinally for a distance of 6 to 8 mm. An autogenous venous patch taken from the external saphenous vein (external diameter 0.4 mm) has been sutured on the carotid wound by means of interrupted stitches with 10-0 nylon monofilament ($\varnothing$ 22). The stitches were placed every 0.3 mm. The artery was previously temporarily occluded with Scoville clips. In 20 animals (mean weight 200 g) the patch was placed with the endothelium towards the lumen of the artery, while in another 20 the adventitia was inwards. Follow-up was between one day and six months. In every case angiography was performed prior to the removal of the artery with the patch for biological study.

Results

Radiological Findings

First series. Endothelium towards the lumen. During the first week there is slight stenosis and deformity at the level of the implant as well as 1 to 2 mm above and below, producing a reduction of the arterial lumen by 0.1-0.2 mm. Later on, and after this first week, the stenosis and deformity slowly disappear, and the calibre of the artery and density of the contrast medium are similar to those seen in the contralateral artery of the animal that was taken as a control.

Second series. Adventitia towards lumen. The initial stenosis observed is less that described from the first series. Later on there are no angiographic differences from the first series.

Histological Findings

First series. Endothelium towards the lumen. Following surgery and during the first week a light deposit of fibrin is observed in the internal wall of the patch, as well as in the surrounding arterial wall. Fibrin reaches the adventitia of the patch through the collagenous fibres. When the patch has surface deformities or when there is a large number of stitches, the deposit of fibrin is larger. There is necrosis and loss of smooth muscle cells in the arterial wall proximal to the patch. After 24 hours of surgery there is a foreign body tissue reaction surrounding the stitch monofilament.

In the second week fibrin starts to disappear at the time that the great proliferation of cells from the patch endothelius is observed. This reaches its maximum in the third week. This proliferation does not produce stenosis of the lumen, and slowly disappears after the sixth week being substituted by collagenous fibres. The patch wall decreases in thickness.

Second series. Adventitia towards the lumen. The only difference in relation to the first series is that the cellular proliferation observed from the second week is larger in the external wall of the patch (venous endothelium) than in the internal one. From the fifth week the proliferation decreases, being substituted by collagenous fibres.

In both series and towards the six month period, small calcifications may be found. The arterial lumen always remains permeable.

Discussion

The study of both series has demonstrated that with the help of the surgical microscope it is possible to keep a full permeability of the artery following a venous patch implant in all cases. The initial stenosis may be the consequence of fibrin deposition. The sub-endothelial cellular proliferation seen after the second week does not interfere with the vascular calibre. From a technical point of view, the patch must be placed in such way that an equal tension is kept at every point of its surface, and the width of its medial part should not be larger than 0.4–0.5 mm. The space between stitches should never be smaller than 0.3 mm.

It does not seem to be matter which surface of the graft faces inwards. In both series the lumen is kept open, and the initial fibrin deposit seems to depend more on the surgical technique than on the fact of whether endothelium or adventitia is selected as the inner surface of the patch. Based on these results it is felt that the technique of the venous patch may be helpful in cerebrovascular microsurgery. The structural difference between the carotid arteries of the rat (3–4 elastic layers) and the human cerebral artery of a similar diameter should not be an important factor as it is felt that the cellular reactions depend more on the venous patch than the arterial wall.

References

Chatterjee, K. N., Warren, R., Gore, I., Autogenous arterial patch graft for arteriotomy closure. Surgery *52* (1962), 890—897.

Dale, W. A., Lewis, M. R., Lateral vascular patch grafts. Surgery *57* (1965), 36—47.

Senning, A., Strip grafting in coronary arteries. J. Thoracic Cardiovasc. Surg. *41* (1961), 542.

Acta Neurochirurgica, Suppl. 28, 257—259 (1979)

Riga Medical Institute, Riga Research Institute
for Traumatology and Orthopaedics, Riga, U.S.S.R.

Application of Magnetobiological Effects in Restorative Cerebral Angiosurgery

R. P. Kikuts, K. A. Treimanis, E. R. Zhilevich, and **E. A. Vitols**

With 2 Figures

Restorative operations on cerebral vessels are endangered by thrombus formation in the postoperative period.

Methods chosen for prevention of thrombosis are concerned with the use of special inert suture materials (silicones, fluoroplastics), special surgical or microsurgical techniques, and the administration of anticoagulants having local or general actions.

One of the factors causing thrombus formation is the change in local static bioelectric potentials of the vascular wall and the blood corpuscles.

For preventing electric triggers of thrombus formation, we have carried out experiments and clinical investigations into the use of continually acting polarized permanent magnetic fields (PMF) with the intention of providing conditions based on induced bioelectric phenomena.

We have elaborated silicone magnetic sleeves for covering the vessels during operation, so that the magnetic force lines cross the blood flow at right angles. The magnetic sleeve must be directed in such a way that the induced electromotive force provokes a potential difference in the blood with the negative potential on the side of the vessel injury or anastamotic suture.

We have studied the application of a magnetic sleeve with exactly orientated lines of magnetic force in a permanent field or an induction vector in 50 dogs after a measured mechanical bilateral injury of the carotid artery wall. The vectored magnetic silicone sleeve was applied on only one side.

The injury of the carotid wall caused, as a rule, complete thrombosis of the vessel, as was confirmed by angiographic and histological examinations.

On the other side, when silicone magnetic sleeves were applied after injury, we observed thrombosis in only three cases. Therefore, the results of our experiments encourage us to use vectored PMF for preventing vascular thromboses.

We have also proved the advisability of the application of silicone

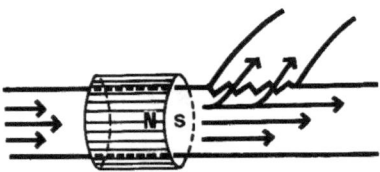

Fig. 1. Application of magnetic sleeves in microsurgical end-to-side sutures

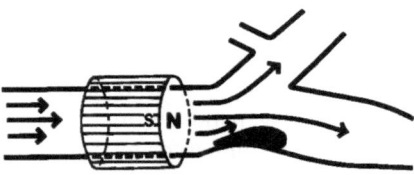

Fig. 2. Application of magnetic sleeves in intermittent deficiency of a carotis interna

magnetic sleeves in microsurgical manipulations. On animals we have carried out 20 microsurgical operations, performing arterial end-to-side anastomoses on 2 mm diameter vessels. As an additional adhesive material we have applied cyanoacrylate MK-6. For preventing thrombous formation we have applied a vectored silicone magnetic sleeve on the afferent vessel near the anastamosis.

Formation of a thrombus due to dysfunction of the sleeve was observed only once.

Our results justify the application of magnetic sleeves during the performance of extra-intracranial shunts (Fig. 1).

Magnetic silicone sleeves were also applied for preventing the formation of carotid thrombi in intermittent blood flow deficiency. In these cases magnetic sleeves have been applied to the common carotid arteries proximal to their bifurcations, where atherosclerotic plaques have usually been found. The sleeves were directed in such a manner that the negative potential would prevail on the side where the plaques were situated (Fig. 2). This method of treatment was applied in 25 patients followed up for 1.5 years. Use of magnetic sleeves in cases of partial obstruction of carotid arteries resulted in complete elimination of carotid bloodflow deficiency recurrences.

Conclusions

The value of magnetic silicone sleeves has been confirmed in 50 experimental observations on injuries of arterial walls. Exact orientation of the magnetic sleeves must be ensured.

In practical restorative angiosurgery this technique has been demonstrated during microsurgical manipulations for end-to-side connection of vessels.

The advisability of the application of magnetic sleeves was established also during operations on carotid arteries in cases of intermittent deficiency of these vessels.

The method is of great importance for the treatment of aged patients, when atherosclerotic plaques cannot be radically removed without serious danger.

The application of magnetic silicone sleeves must be considered an important and promising method for preventing thrombus formation in restorative cerebral angiosurgery.

Acta Neurochirurgica, Suppl. 28, 260—262 (1979)
© by Springer-Verlag 1979

Abteilung für Nuklearbiologie, Gesellschaft für Strahlen-
und Umweltforschung, Neuherberg (Leiter: Prof. Dr. H. Kriegel),
Augenklinik der Ludwig-Maximilians-Universität München
(Direktor: Prof. Dr. O.-E. Lund), Federal Republic of Germany

Microvascular Repair With Neodymium-YAG Laser

K. K. Jain and W. Gorisch

Introduction

Various techniques have been employed in the past for repair of accidental injuries and planned incisions of small blood vessels. Of these, microsuture is the most widely used. This method is time-consuming, and vascular occlusions may be required for periods longer than considered safe in the case of such organs as the brain. Bipolar coagulation has been occasionally used to repair a tear in a small vessel during surgery with the aim of preserving the lumen of the vessel. There is, however, no detailed laboratory study of the effect of this procedure on a vessel less than 1 mm in diameter.

Apart from planned incisions in small arteries for embolectomy, insertion of catheters, etc., there are accidental tears during routine neurosurgery. An example may be quoted of a tear in an internal carotid artery during removal of a parasellar meningioma. Then there are numerous small vessels (of unknown importance) which are cut here and there during tumour removal. Even the most meticulous neurosurgeon does not stop and try to repair each vessel, nor is it always possible to do so with the instruments and techniques available in the neurosurgical operating room.

We have investigated the use of Nd: YAG laser for repair of small blood vessels because it avoids instrumental contact with the vessel wall at the site of repair, and the radiating energy which is converted into the form of heat by absorption can be delivered precisely and in a short exposure time. We have compared its effectiveness with bipolar coagulation and microsuture technique.

Method

Over a period of months we have operated on 40 Wistar rats using various arteries and veins with diameters ranging from 0.3 mm to 1.1 mm. The Zeiss OPMI 6 operating microscope and microinstruments were used for preparation of vessels. Incisions were made in vessels to simulate various situations encountered in neurosurgery, both accidental and planned. Some vessels were repaired by suturing and bipolar coagulation. Most of the vessels, however, were subjected to laser repair. The Neodymium-YAG laser beam was transmitted through a flexible quartz fibre and focussed to a spot 0.5 mm in diameter. It was guided to the vessel incision by a pilot light, and adjusted by a micromanipulator.

The vessel to be repaired is occluded temporarily by microclips which were removed after the laser application. Usually one application was enough to seal a small incision. For larger incisions multiple adjacent exposures were needed. If the edge of the incision tended to gape, a small piece of muscle was placed over the incision, and the muscle was fused to the vessel wall. The contraction of the muscle plug was usually adequate to approximate the edges of the incision underneath.

Most of the experiments were done without the use of any anticoagulant. A thin film of blood over the incision facilitates the absorption of laser light. This procedure has also been tried on rats on anticoagulants and also after washing the vessel with heparin. It is possible to repair the vessel although it takes longer and requires multiple laser exposures. In most of the situations we can now complete laser repair of a vessel within a minute.

Some animals were sacrificed at intervals from immediately following surgery to periods as long as 10 weeks. The studies include:

1. Normal histology of the vessel wall,
2. SEM and TEM of the vessel wall, and
3. Angiography.

Results

The studies are not yet complete but no vessels between 0.7 mm and 1.1 mm in diameter became occluded after laser repair. Some vessels 0.3 mm in diameter thrombosed. This is partly due to vasospasm, and the results are improving with local applications of Eupaverine to the vessel.

Veins are easy to repair but are also the more susceptible to thrombosis, caused by temporary vascular clips. Washing the vein with heparin solution prevents this complication.

Tensile strength of the repaired vessel was measured once in an artery and once in a vein and there was no disruption with intraluminal pressures as high as 300 mm Hg. Histological studies indicate fusion of collagen of the vessel wall. SEM studies show a small clot at the site of repair. This clot is about the same as is seen associated with an arterial incision without application of laser and did not progress in size but rather regressed with healing. Control experiments with applications of laser alone to the vessel wall showed some alteration of the endothelium. No disruption of the vessel wall or aneurysm formation has been seen so far.

Discussion

The mechanism of action of laser is not clear. Heat is produced at the site of impact high enough to cause discoloration of vessel surface. Contraction and fusion of collagen is supposed to occur with heat.

Our results indicate that laser beam is superior to bipolar coagulation as heat is delivered faster and more precisely and there is no squeezing of the vessel wall by the tips of forceps.

Microscopic evaluation of the vessels repaired by laser shows much less trauma than in those treated by suturing and bipolar coagulation. For vessels as small as 0.3 mm diameter laser was the only technique that significantly enabled us to preserve the patency of vessels after repair. We recommend this technique for introduction into the neurosurgical operating room if proper technical facilities are available and safety requirements are met.

Acknowledgments

This study was partly supported by research grant MT-2715 by the Ministry of Research and Technology of the German Federal Government.

The authors would like to acknowledge the facilities provided for this work at: Zentrales Labor für Laser-Chirurgie, Abteilung für Angewandte Optik (Chief: Prof. W. Waidelich), Gesellschaft für Strahlen- und Umweltforschung.

The following have contributed to this publication:

1. Miss U. Imhof—histological studies,
2. Dr. U. Heinzmann—for Scanning Electron Microscope studies,
3. Ms. J. Byers—secretarial work.

Acta Neurochirurgica, Suppl. 28, 263—269 (1979)
© by Springer-Verlag 1979

Department of Neurosurgery* (Pr. R. Houdart),
Laribosière Hospital, Paris,
and Department of Vascular Surgery** (Pr. D. Guilmet,
Foch Hospital, Paris, France

Surgical Possibilities in the Third Portion of the Vertebral Artery (Above C 2)

Anatomical Study and Report of a Case of Anastomosis
Between Subclavian Artery and Vertebral Artery
at C 1-C 2 Level

B. George* and C. Laurian**

With 2 Figures

Operations on the vertebral artery (VA) below its entry into the foramen transversarium of C6 are well known[7, 15]. Above, in the foramina transversaria, exposure of the vertebral artery has been performed for arteriovenous fistula[4, 8, 12–14, 18, 19, 21], compressive unco-discarthrosis[9–17], or anastomosis from the external carotid artery[5, 6]. In the third portion, between C2 and the foramen magnum, the surgical route is much less well-known. A reappraisal of surgical possibilities in this portion of the vertebral artery has been performed after anatomical study. A simple route was defined and was used in one case.

Anatomical Study

Twenty anatomical specimens were used. The following points were studied. First, choice of the best route either between Sterno-cleido-mastoid muscle (SCM) and internal jugular vein or between trachea and oesophagus medially and jugulo-carotid tract laterally. Second, C1 and C2 transverse processes reached either by complete exposure of all the processes from C6 to C1 or directly. Third, elements crossing the route and hindering exposure of the artery. Fourth, disposition of the artery above C2.

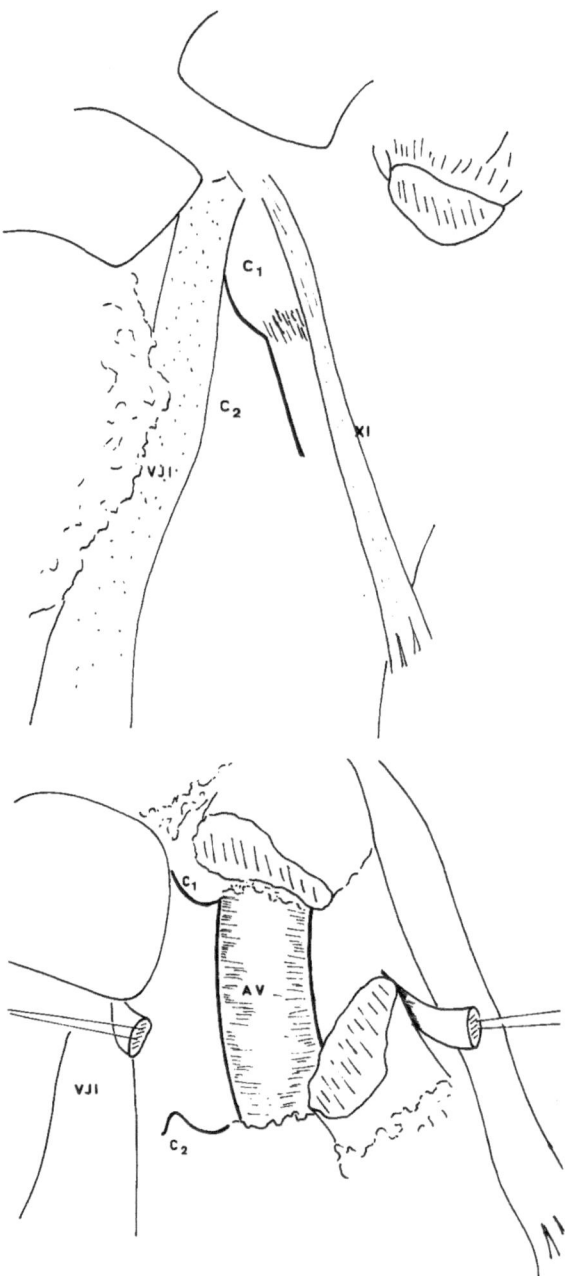

Figs. 1A, B. Drawings of the operative exposure. A. Transverse process of C1 between XI nerve and internal jugular vein (*VJI*). B. Vertebral artery (*AV*) under the transverse process of C1. Note the ends of the second cervical nerve divided and retracted

The skin incision starts behind the mastoid process, and then follows the anterior border of the sternomastoid muscle. The simplest route passes between SCM and internal jugular vein, after the mastoid attachment of the muscle has been divided. The sole element crossing this route is the XI nerve. This must be freed as high as possible and then be displaced laterally.

The transverse process of C1 is found one centimetre above and in front of the tip of the mastoid process. Hyper-extension and rotation of the head to the opposite side moves the transverse process of C1 anteriorly and superficially in such a way that it can be more easily exposed. On the contrary, the transverse process of C2, which does not turn with the head, remains deep, and its direct exposure is more difficult. It seems safer to expose C1, C3, and C4 before going to C2. This position not only brings C1 anteriorly, but also the posterior arch of atlas is widely exposed. Two muscles, Levator Scapulae and Superior Oblique, are inserted into the transverse process of C1 (Figs. 1A, B). To expose the VA between C1 and C2, these muscles must be divided close to the process. The artery lies just behind them. At least 1.5 centimetres of the vessel can be exposed. The anterior branch of the second cervical nerve usually crosses behind the artery. In rare cases it may cross anteriorly, and then must be cut.

Exposure of the VA above C1 is made after exposure below C1 and unroofing of the foramen. The posterior arch of atlas is freed first on its inferior edge and then on its superior. The VA is in a periosteal furrow up to its dural entry at the foramen magnum. It passes nearly vertically from C2 to C1, runs a little outwards, and then bends posteriorly to run horizontally backwards in the guttering on the posterior arch of atlas. Opening of the periosteal furrow shows the VA with its accompanying veins. It must be noted that the venous plexus is less developed between C2 and C1 than below or above.

Case Report

This approach has been used in a case of aneurysmal dysplasia at the C3 level on the left side (Figs. 2A, B). A primary direct surgical exposure had been done six months earlier by a postero-lateral route. Because of one further acute stroke after this incomplete procedure, a new operation was required.

On angiography, the right VA failed to fill the basilar trunk. So, under local anaesthesia, a balloon catheter was inflated on three occasions in the subclavian artery and the VA to test the patient's tolerance under clamping of the left VA.

The left VA was exposed by the above described technique without the unroofing of any foramen transversarium. The skin incision was prolonged down the anterior edge of SCM and laterally along the clavicle. The subclavian artery

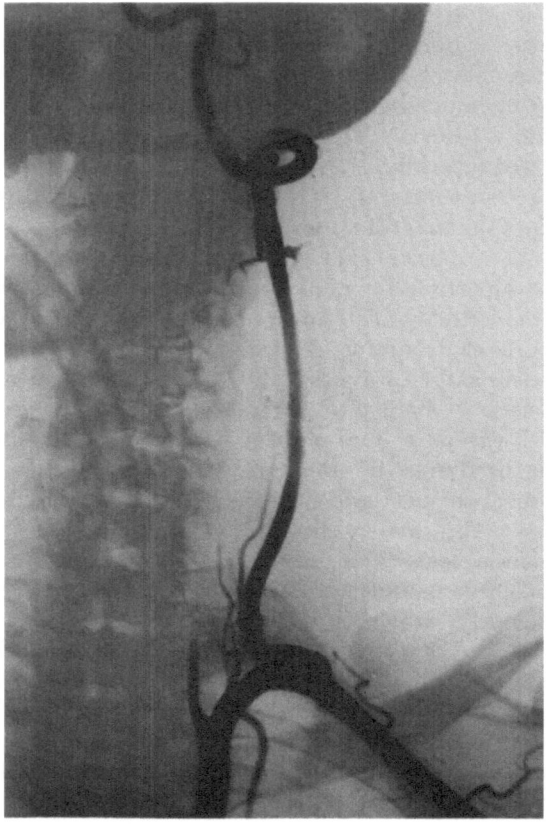

Figs. 2A, B. Operative aspects of the anastomosis with the clip below it.
A. Arteriographic control. Note the filling of the first part of the vertebral
artery. B. Photograph of anastomosis

was then controlled, and an autologous saphenous vein graft was interposed
between the subclavian artery and the VA by end-to-side anastomosis. Finally
the left VA was clipped below the anastomosis.

Discussion

Exposure of the VA in its third portion above the C2 level was done
by Matas in 1895 and also by Elkin in 1946, and by some others for
arteriovenous fistulas. More recently Clark and Corkill performed
anastomoses between the external carotid artery and VA at the C2
level, and Ausman has performed an anastomosis of VA to Pica. But in
this latter case a posterior approach was used.

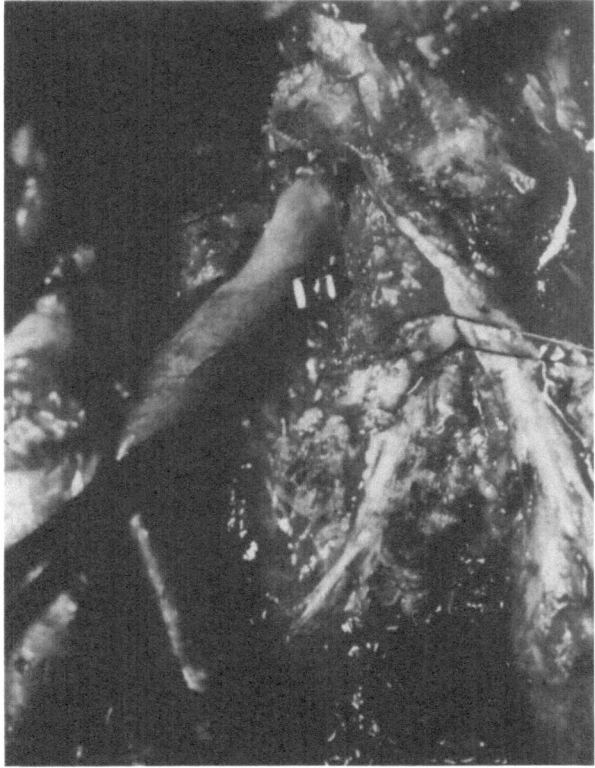

Fig. 2 B

The route described here is simple, without any vessel or nerve intervening. The XI nerve can be spared. In the extented and rotated position of the head, the transverse process of C1 becomes very superficial. The VA is then exposed under it. The less developed venous plexus at this level makes the approach more clear. One branch of the SCM must be cut, and sometimes the anterior branch of the second cervical nerve, without any ill-effect. The key is the head position and the highest possible freeing of the XI nerve.

Without unroofing the foramina of C1 and C2, about 1.5 centimeter of artery may be exposed. This is just sufficient to permit an anastomosis. Other surgical procedures may required opening of these foramina, and sometimes dissection of the VA on the posterior arch of atlas.

This approach may be used for lesions at the C1-C2 interspace:

dysplasia, arteriovenous fistulae. In this latter case primary control of VA surgically or by an inflated balloon under the lesion is useful because of the hypertrophied venous plexus. Revascularization of VA may be better done at this level either from the subclavian artery or the external carotid artery than from the posterior inferior cerebellar artery. Frequently after thrombosis the artery is recanalized at least from C2 to the vertebro-basilar junction; moreover the external carotid artery can be exposed by the same incision. Finally control of VA is likely to be required before an approach to the lesion in the foramen magnum or in the intervertebral foramina.

Summary

A reappraisal of surgical possibilities in the third portion of the vertebral artery (VA) above C2, has been done from an anatomical study on twenty autopsy specimens. A route passing between the internal jugular vein and the Sterno-cleido-mastoid muscle allows a simple approach to the transverse process of C1. After division of two muscles attached to this process, 1.5 cm of the VA can be exposed. For larger exposure of the artery, the foramen transversarium of C1 must be unroofed and the artery dissected in the guttering of the posterior arch of the atlas.

This surgical route was used in a case of aneurysmal dysplasia at the C3 level. An anastomosis between the subclavian artery and VA at the C1-C2 level was performed with an autologous saphenous vein graft.

The key points are the hignest possible freeing of the XI nerve and the head position. Rotation and extension move the transverse process and the posterior arch of the atlas superficially and anteriorly.

Key words: Vertebral artery; dysplasia; anastomosis; technique; anatomical study.

References

1. Ausman, J. I., Lee, M. C., Klassen, A. C., Seljeskog, E. L., Chou, S. N., Stroke: what's new? Cerebral revascularization. Minn. Med. *58* (1976), 223—227.
2. Ausman, J. I., Nicoloff, D. M., Chou, S. N., Posterior fossa revascularization: anastomosis of vertebral artery to PICA with interposed radial artery graft. Surg. Neurol. *9* (1978), 281—285.
3. Binkley, F. M., Wylie, E. J., A new technique for obliteration of cerebrovascular arterio-venous fistulae. Arch. Surg. *106* (1973), 524—527.
4. Chou, S. N., Story, J. L., Seljeskog, E. L., French, L. A., Further experience with arterio-venous fistulas of the vertebral artery in the neck. Surgery *62*, 4 (1967), 779—788.

5. Clark, K., Perry, M. O., Carotid vertebral anastomosis. An alternate technic for repair of the sub-clavian steal syndrome. Ann. Surg. *163*, 3 (1966), 414—416.
6. Corkill, C., External carotid vertebral anastomosis for vertebro-basilar insufficiency. Surg. Neurol. *7* (1977), 109—115.
7. Cormier, J. M., Laurian, C., Surgical management of vertebro-basilar insufficiency. J. Cardio-vasc. Surg. *17* (1976), 205—223.
8. Elkin, D. C., Harris, M. H., Arterio-venous aneurysm of the vertebral vessels. Report of ten cases. Ann. Surg. *124*, 5 (1946), 934—951.
9. Gortvai, P., Insufficiency of vertebral artery treated by decompression of its cervical part. Brit. Med. J. *2* (1964), 233—234.
10. Henry, A. K., Exposures of long bones and other surgical methods. Bristol: J. Wright and Sons Ltd. 1927 (Extensile exposure, Ed. 2), pp. 58—72. Baltimore: Williams and Wilkins Company. 1963.
11. Khodadad, G., Occipital artery posterior inferior cerebellar artery anastomosis. Surg. Neurol. *5* (1976), 225—227.
12. Kornmesser, T. W., Bergan, J. J., Anatomic control of vertebral arterio-venous fistulas. Surgery *75*, 1 (1974), 80—86.
13. Kuttner, H., Die Verletzungen und traumatischen Aneurysmen der Vertebralisgefäße am Halse und ihre operative Behandlung. Bruns. Beitr. Klin. Chir. *1* (1917), 108.
14. Jefferson, G., Bailey, R. A., Kerr, A. S., Suboccipital arterio-venous aneurysms of the vertebral artery. J. Bone Joint Surg. *38 B* (1965), 114—127.
15. Labauge, R., Thevenet, A., Peguret, C., Cesari, J. B., Résultats du traitement chirurgical des obstructions de l'artère vertébrale. 75° congrès Français de Chirurgie, pp. 150—160. Paris: Masson. 1976.
16. Matas, R., Traumatisms and traumatic aneurysms of the vertebral artery and their surgical treatment with the report of a cured case. Ann. Surg. *18* (1893), 477—517.
17. Pasztor, E., Decompression of vertebral artery in cases of cervical spondylosis. Surg. Neurol. *9* (1978), 371—377.
18. Sher, M. H., Meyer, N. I., Lenhardt, H. F., Trummer, M. J., Arterio-venous fistulas involving the vertebral artery. Report of 3 cases. Ann. Surg. *163*, 3 (1966), 408—413.
19. Shumacker, H. B., Campbell, R. L., Heimburger, R. F., Operative treatment of vertebral arterio-venous fistulas. J. Trauma. *6*, 1 (1966), 1—19.
20. Sundt, T. M., Whisnant, J. P., Piepgras, D. G., Campell, J. K., Holman, C. B., Intracranial bypass grafts for vertebral basilar ischemia. Mayo Clin. Proc. *53* (1978), 12—18.
21. Verbiest, H., Extracranial and cervical arterio-venous aneurysms of the carotid and vertebral arteries. Report of a series of 12 personal cases. John Hopkins Med. J. *12* (1968), 350—357.

Acta Neurochirurgica, Suppl. 28, 270—271 (1979)
© by Springer-Verlag 1979

III. Essential Investigations and Indications for Surgery

National Institute of Neurosurgery, Budapest, Hungary

Assessment of Regional Cerebral Blood Flow Using the XE-133 Inhalation Method in Patients Undergoing EIAB Surgery

I. Nyáry, J. Vajda, E. Pásztor, and M. Horváth

Since the advent of extra-intracranial arterial bypass (EIAB) surgery in the treatment of ischaemic cerebrovascular disease, few attempts were undertaken[1-3] to relate rCBF findings to the explanation of underlying pathology as well as to the selection of patients for operation, using the intracarotid injection method. Though non-invasive and repeatable, the Xe-133 inhalation technique was considered unfavourable for such studies. In spite of the indisputable superiority of the intracarotid injection method with respect to the more simple mathematical model, and lack of distortion due to recirculation and extracerebral contamination, the inhalation method has its points. Both hemispheres are readily accessible for comparison, and no problem emerges on how to label all regions of interest, since the isotope is distributed over the entire circulation. The recent innovation of new parameters such as Φ and S^4 may increase the sensitivity of the method, particularly in cases of impaired perfusion, thus overcoming the disadvantage of less power of spatial resolution inherent in this technique.

A clinical study was initiated applying the Xe-133 inhalation method to assess patients with stroke. Four collimated detectors were placed over both hemispheres in the temporo-central and parietal regions. In a patient with a history of vertebro-basilar insufficiency two detectors were placed symmetrically over the posterior fossa. Technical details were basically the same as described by Obrist et al.[5,6]. To facilitate the exploration of additional possible criteria in the selection of patients for EIAB surgery, functional activation tests also were included. By the inhalation of 7 per cent CO_2 in room air and induced arterial hypotension (Arfonad), two major determinants of CBF, CO_2 responsiveness, and autoregulation were studied. Hypotension was carried out under control of continuous systemic arterial blood pressure registration via a small polyethylene catheter placed into a peripheral (usually brachial) artery.

To date 24 stroke patients were investigated. Breakdown of this group, according to clinical diagnosis: 17 completed strokes, 4 PRINDs, 2 TIAs, and 1 vertebro-basilar insufficiency. Nineteen of these patients underwent microvascular anastomosis operation. Nine of them were studied postoperatively. We prefer later postoperative control, viz. 3–4 months after surgical intervention.

Our series was rather diverse with respect to the severity of symptoms, to the time elapsed between onset of symptoms and admission, and to the underlying pathology (19 patients presented with occlusion of one or both internal carotid arteries, 3 with occlusion of MCA, 1 with internal carotid stenosis, and 1 with occlusion of the right vertebral artery), and this variability was also reflected by rCBF patterns obtained from our measurements. Patterns of resting control CBF ranged from no interhemispheric difference (6 patients), mild but consequent depression of CBF (focal or hemispheric) on the affected side (14 patients), to marked interhemispheric difference (4 patients).

Functional analysis of CBF proved to be a sensitive indicator of impaired perfusion, because latent differences became enhanced due to activation tests. In case of good anastomosis, CBF increased compared to the preoperative state. However, slight interhemispheric difference in CO_2 responsiveness or autoregulation or both still persisted. On the other hand, in cases of angiographically proven patent anastomosis but with poor filling of intracranial vessels, patients might have benefited by the operation, according to improved CBF findings.

References

1. Heilbrun, M. P., Reichman, O. H., Anderson, R. E., et al., J. Neurosurg. 43 (1975), 706—716.
2. Schmiedek, P., Gratzl, O., Steinhoff, H., et al., Clin. Neurosurg. 23 (1976), 270—286.
3. Schmiedek, P., Gratzl, O., Spetzler, R., et al., J. Neurosurg. 44 (1976), 303—324.
4. Blauenstein, U. W., Halsey, J. H., Jr., Wilson, E. M., et al., Stroke 9 (1978), 57—66.
5. Obrist, W. D., Thompson, H. K., Jr., Wang, H. S., et al., Stroke 6 (1975), 245—256.
6. Nyáry, I., Pásztor, E., Advances in Neurol. 20 (1978), 517—520.

Acta Neurochirurgica, Suppl. 28, 272—274 (1979)
© by Springer-Verlag 1979

Service de Neuro-chirurgie B (Pr. B. Vlahovitch),
Centre Gui de Chauliac, Montpellier, France

Cortical Arterial Pressure in Extra-Intracranial Anastomosis *

J. M. Fuentes

With 2 Figures

The study of the blood pressure in the brain cortical artery of an extra-intracranial bypass permits examination of the angiographic picture of revascularization and tissue perfusion.

Methods

After dissection of the cortical artery and arteriotomy, the vessel is catheterized in two directions:

proximally to the dorsal or ventral branch of the Sylvian artery (against systemic blood flow) *i.e.*, RAP;

distally to the meningeal and cortical system (with the blood flow) *i.e.*, AAP.

During this catheterization, anterograde and retrograde blood is taken for gas analysis; peroperative sectorial angiography is obtainable as well as recordings of maximum and minimum instaneous pressures and average pressures.

Results (Fig. 1)

For an anaesthetized patient, head at the horizontal level, after craniotomy and without any arterial occlusion:

the RAP = 2/3 SAP (SAP = systemic arterial pressure) *i.e.*, if maximal SAP is 120 mm Hg ± 20 and minimal SAP is 70 mm Hg, the RAP (max.) is 80 mm Hg ± 15, and the RAP (average) is 75 mm Hg ± 5;

the AAP (max.) is 22 mm Hg ± 2;

the AAP (average) is 20 mm Hg;

the superficial temporal artery pressure (STAP) is equal to the SAP. STAP = SAP.

---

* Abbreviations: SAP = systolic arterial pressure; STAP = superficial temporal artery systolic pressure; RAP = retrograde arterial pressure; AAP = anterograde arterial pressure.

Basis. The haemodynamic work of an EICA depends on three pressure levels: STAP, AAP, RAP (see Fig. 2).

If EICA is indicated for carotid occlusion, RAP reflects the value of the circle of Willis, and AAP the meningeal and cortical system (retrograde revascularization). For Sylvian occlusion, RAP and AAP reflect the retrograde filling from the other Sylvian branches if the occlusion is incomplete, from the cortical areas of the anterior and posterior cerebral arteries if there is a complete occlusion.

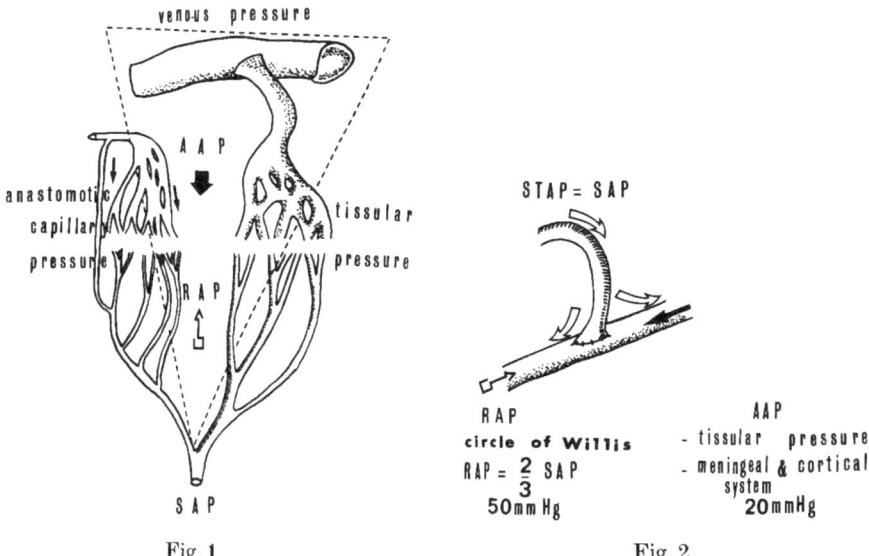

Fig. 1   Fig. 2

Statements and Cases (17)

In our experience, four possibilities may be encountered:

1. Patients with low RAP and normal AAP (RAP ≤ 50 mm Hg and AAP ≤ 25 mm Hg). Here is the best haemodynamic state. The low RAP allows a satisfactory retrograde filling of the cortical artery and adds several cerebral vascular sectors (filling of cortical arteries). This situation is mainly the result of Sylvian occlusion (six cases).

2. Patients with normal RAP and AAP (RAP $\simeq 80$ mm Hg, AAP $\simeq 22$ mm Hg ± 2). In this case, there is usually a carotid occlusion. A normal RAP means a good value of the circle of Willis and/or the external carotid (ophthalmic artery).

3. Patients with high AAP ($25 \leq$ AAP ≤ 40 mm Hg). If the AAP remains low, it is possible to revascularize two or three cortical arteries

in a retrograde way. However the tissue perfusion is bad, and if there is any brain oedema the AAP increases. If the AAP remains $\leq$ 40 mm Hg it is possible to do an EICA.

4. Patients with AAP > 50 mm Hg. In this condition there is always an brain oedema which contra-indicates any EICA, and leads sometimes to a surgical removal of a pseudo-tumoural softening of the brain (four cases).

Conclusion

After all these data, we think that the best pressure levels to indicate benefit from an EICA are the following:

$$RAP \leq 50 \text{ mm Hg}$$
$$AAP \leq 25 \text{ mm Hg}$$

(AAP max. = 22 mm Hg $\pm$ 2, AAP average = 20 mm Hg).

These values are based on a double point of view:

haemodynamic *i.e.* these levels allow retrograde vascularization of several cortical branches ($\geq$ 3);

physiological *i.e.* there is no brain oedema, and tissue perfusion is normal.

Acta Neurochirurgica, Suppl. 28, 275—277 (1979)
© by Springer-Verlag 1979

Neurosurgical Clinic, University of Düsseldorf
(Director: Prof. Dr. med. W. J. Bock), Federal Republic of Germany

Animal Experiments With Doppler Flow Transducers

H.-U. Thal and W. Leem

Introduction

In the microsurgery of vessels there exists the need for flow or pressure measurement or both in order to confirm proper reconstruction. Electromagnetic flow probes and Doppler transducers have been used in larger vessels. In arteries of small diameter up to now only reports on electromagnetic measurements have been given in the literature as well as some small remarks about Doppler flow transducers. We obtained some of the first commercially available Doppler flow transducers from 1 to 40 mm diameter with the Delalande apparatus. We investigated these transducers in the laboratory and tested them *in vitro* and *in vivo*.

Methods

At first we tried to control the calibration of the probes. For that reason we registered the flow in cm/sec in a closed loop system of 1 to 40 mm silicone and PVC-tubes produced by a pump, and counted the corresponding flow volume in ml/min. The flow volume was also measured with stopwatch and cylinder. The findings with human ACD-blood and other fluids were attached to the 1, 2, 3, and 4 mm probe.

The *in vivo* experiments were done in rats and dogs. The aortas of rats were cut and sutured for microsurgical training purposes. During these operations the measurements with the 1 and 2 mm probe were done. In the dogs autologous transplantations of the carotid artery were done. The transplants were taken from the femoral artery which again was sutured. The 3 and 4 mm probes gave us the security of having made a correct reconstruction.

Results

In tests the reproducibility of the closed loop tube and pump system had been found to be satisfactory within ± 10 % limits. The flow ranged from 15 to 150 ml/min. As is clear from the theoretical point of view, fluids without particles showed no reproducible flow pattern. A

18*

suspension of Indian ink gave only a qualitative and not a quantitative result. Some irregularities occurred with air bubbles in more viscous fluids such as glucose 10% and 20%, but not in Rheomakrodex[R] or human albumin. In human ACD-blood it soon became clear that the 1 mm probe showed a flow less than 10% of the real flow. This probe was neglected in further studies. In the other probes a constant flow of 65 ml/min was measured well with the 2, 3, and 4 mm probes when converting the Doppler flow velocity in the inner diameter of the tubes into flow volume. But one has to bear in mind that the result depends largely on the exact measurement of the inner diameter of the tube or the vessel. For example an inner diameter of 1.5 mm gives a flow volume of 55.8 ml/min when counting with a Doppler flow of 53 cm/sec. With the same Doppler flow and a smaller diameter of 0.3 mm, that is a diameter of 1.2 mm, one gets a flow volume of 34.8 ml/min, half the flow volume measured before. This example shows clearly the square function dependency of a secondary computing of the flow volume.

To get an impression of the linearity of the Doppler probes, flow volume had been increased stepwise from 15 to 150 ml/min. The mean velocity profile correlated well in the 2, 3, and 4 mm probes. This correlation between different flows and the velocity measured with the Doppler probes could be found in human ACD-blood down to a dilution of 1:5, which means a haematocrit of 20%. Below that value a visible reduction of about 10% occurred in the recording of the 1:6 dilution.

In the animal experiments it became clear that the 1 mm probe was too large for these small arteries, and it rotated after the wound closure when the rats began to move. Slightly better was the 2 mm probe, and satisfactory use was possible with the 3 and 4 mm probes. In 12 dogs the autologous transplantation of a small piece of the left femoral artery into the right carotid artery was performed. The results will be reported elsewhere.

Doppler flow measurements were done to control the postoperative blood velocity in correlation to the preoperative state. With this technique total obstruction could be detected and immediately corrected. No other signs were found in this condition; the artery was filled with blood distal and proximal to the sutures, and pulsated well. The re-anastomosis showed a normal flow velocity profile.

Discussion

Up to now mainly electromagnetic flow probes are in use. Some authors reject the Doppler method from the theoretical point of view, because of the uncertainty of getting the true velocity profile in the Doppler frequency shift signal, depending on vessel wall irregularities and turbulences. But who has experience with Doppler flow probes for interoperative use ?

Our findings show that the measurement of the flow velocity is qualitatively and quantitatively possible with 2, 3, and 4 mm Doppler flow probes. The 1 mm probe, which failed, may not be properly focussed.

In the range from 15 to 150 ml/min linearity and accuracy of flow velocity is well within the biological error of 10 %. Because of the square function between velocity and volume it is of no use to calculate the volume in ml/min from the Doppler signal in cm/sec. The inaccuracy of the measurement of the inner diameter of a vessel might give an error of about 50 % in volume, as shown in the check calculation.

The measurements with human ACD-blood give fair results down to a haematocrit of 20 %.

The usefulness of flow velocity measurement with Doppler flow probes was evident in our animal experiments, especially in carotid microsurgery in dogs.

Conclusion

A report on testing and application of Doppler flow probes has been given. Apart from the 1 mm probe, the 2, 3, and 4 mm probes gave fair results *in vitro* and *in vivo*. The Doppler flow velocity should not be transformed into flow volume because of the inaccuracy of measuring the inner diameter of a vessel or a tube.

One can say that flow measurements can be made not only with electromagnetic flow probes but with Doppler flow transducers as well.

Acta Neurochirurgica, Suppl. 28, 278—281 (1979)
© by Springer-Verlag 1979

Neurosurgical Department of Comenius University,
Bratislava, Czechoslovakia

The Role of Anastomoses in Brain Circulation

Study of Computer Model

P. Nádvorník and J. Ďuroš

With 1 Figure

In the last three years a suitable computer model of the brain circulation has been developed[1], for the study in detail of the significance and the efficiency of the natural and arteficial anastomoses in the brain vessel network.

Method and Results

One of our special interests is the change in regional CBF with various occlusions of the main brain arteries combined with some background factors, such as occlusive lesions of the communicating arteries of the Circle of Willis (CW), small vessel disease, and artificial extra-intracranial microanastomosis.

With the computer model, the normal configuration of the brain vessel network was simulated, and the following occlusions of afferent supply vessels to the CW were considered: 1. bilateral internal carotid artery (ICA) occlusion with or without unilateral vertebral artery occlusion; 2. unilateral ICA occlusion with or without bilateral or unilateral vertebral artery occlusion, and 3. bilateral or unilateral vertebral artery occlusion.

An additional occlusion of one of the communicating arteries of CW, namely the posterior communicating cerebral artery on the side of the main supply vessel occlusion, or the anterior communicating cerebral artery, has been imposed.

Complete occlusion of the main supply vessel has resulted in a decrease of CBF of less than 20% even in the most complicated case of bilateral ICA and unilateral vertebral artery occlusion. This value has been raised to 33% in the affected hemisphere and to 24% in the contralateral hemisphere with a combined occlusion of one posterior communicating cerebral artery.

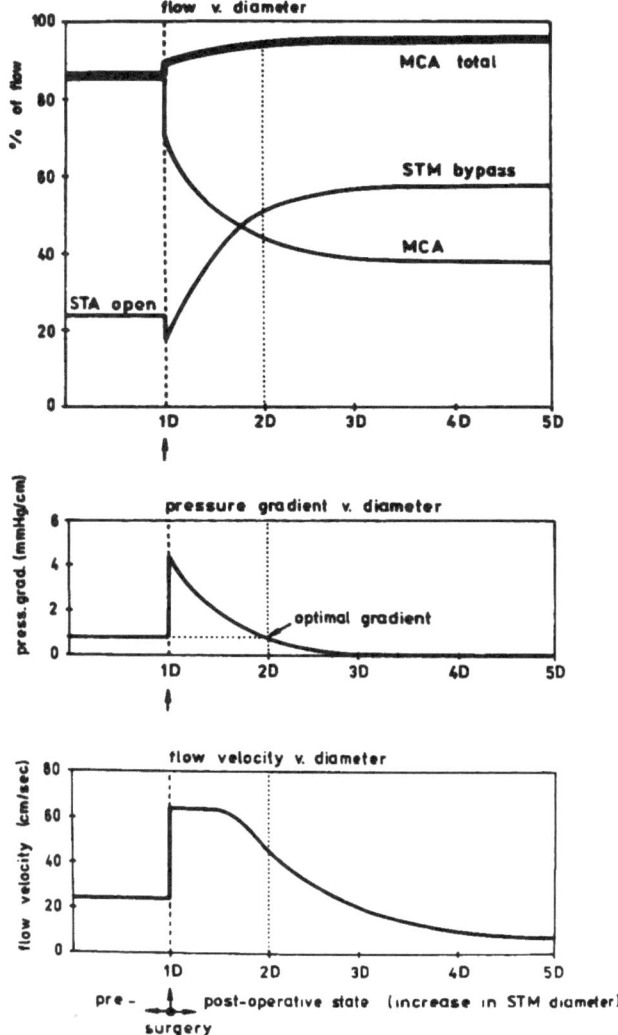

Fig. 1. Efficiency of STM anastomosis with 90 % MCA stenosis

The decrease in flow with a unilateral vertebral artery occlusion together with a the communicating brain artery occlusion has not reached 1%. This fact indicates a high degree of redundancy in the capacity of the vertebral system, since one vertebral artery alone is capable of providing the whole basilar flow and scarcely affecting the carotid flow.

In the study of efficiency of one extra-intracranial artificial anastomosis (STA) the computer model has been set to simulate the pre- and postoperative situation based on the measurements performed with the patients during extra-intracranial arterial bypass surgery. The blood flow in the open superficial temporal artery before the anastomosis seems to be up to 40 ml/min, which is 24% of the normal flow in middle cerebral artery. This flow decreases to 30 ml/min after the anastomosis, due to the vascular resistence of middle cerebral artery connected to the superficial temporal artery.

On a computer model a case with 90% middle cerebral artery stenosis in the first segment of vessel has been considered, and the pressure and velocity distribution along the middle cerebral artery before and after the extra-intracranial anastomosis has been calculated (Fig. 1).

The pressure gradient value of the anastomotic channel at the time of surgery increased to more than 4 mm Hg/cm with corresponding increase of the flow velocity. In the normal case the value of pressure gradient in arteries of the same size as the anastomotic channel is below 1 mm Hg/cm with an average value of 0.8 mm Hg/cm. In the postoperative period the anastomotic channel dilates, with adaptation to the new relations until the average value has been reached.

The flow through the segment of middle cerebral artery stenosis decreased to 46% of the normal flow during the postoperative period, but the total middle cerebral artery flow including the anastomotic channel flow reached a 94% value of the normal middle cerebral artery flow.

Discussion

Anastomoses in the brain vessel network are classified, from the anatomical point of view, into two basic groups: intracranial and extra-intracranial. According to the results on the computer brain circulation model it seems apparent that the anastomoses should be divided into three groups, according to their function.

The first group includes congenital anastomoses of CW, and cortical anastomoses. This group shows the steal effect, because the additional blood supply into the affected hemisphere is stolem from the unaffected one. These anastomoses act as parasitical phenomena in the collateral circulation.

The second group of anastomoses represents the congenital and artificial extra-intracranial anastomoses. The whole amount of additional blood supply is directed from the extracranial region.

The third special case of anastomosis is the connection of both vertebral arteries into the basilar artery. The computer modelling proved a high degree of redundancy in flow capability of this anastomotic system. The vertebrobasilar anastomosis creates a redundant system with sufficient blood supply for the function of the most important parts of the brain.

Summary

Anastomoses in the arterial system of brain investigated on the computer model can be divided into three basic groups. Parasitical anastomoses diverting blood into affected regions and stealing it from the unaffected parts, compensating anastomoses delivering blood from extracranial sources, and redundant anastomoses protected the vital parts of the brain.

References

1. Ďuroš, J., Nádvorník, P., Investigation of cerebral blood circulation on computer model. J. Neurosurg. Sci. *21* (1977), 4, 243—246.

Acta Neurochirurgica, Suppl. 28, 282—286 (1979)
© by Springer-Verlag 1979

Cerebral Revascularization With Extra-Intracranial Anastomoses for Vascular Lesions of Traumatic, Malformative, and Tumorous Origin

(Cooperative Study: 20 Cases)

M. Sindou*, P. Grunewald, Y. Guegan, A. Redondo,
and **A. Rey**

With 1 Figure

Besides the usual indications in chronic or acute insufficiencies of cerebral circulation, brain revascularization with extra-intracranial bypasses (EICB) can be useful in the treatment of vascular lesions of traumatic, malformative, and tumorous origin. This study demonstrates the interest in this kind of surgery from our experience in France, with consists of 20 cases (Drs. P. Grunewald, Y. Guegan, A. Redondo, A. Rey, and M. Sindou).

Summary of Cases and Operative Results

1. *1st Group: Traumatic Arterial Lesions* (nine cases).
This group includes one case of complete thrombosis of the internal carotid artery (ICA) treated with a simple EICB, and eight cases in which contusion of the sub-petrosal ICA had produced both severe stenosis and a false aneurysm inaccessible to any direct surgery. Three of them had also an embolus in the middle cerebral artery (MCA) which had migrated from the aneurysm. In two out of the eight cases—in which the stenosis was predominant—a simple EICB was performed. In the six others—in which the aneurysmal dilatation was quite considerable—an EICB followed by an ICA ligation at its origin were carried out.

In this group only one complication occurred which consisted of a transient neurological aggravation. At the arteriographic control the

---

* Dr. M. Sindou, Hopital Neurologique, 59 Bd Pinel, F-69003 Lyon, France.

anastomosis was patent in eight cases out of nine, and was found to vascularize the whole MCA territory on three occasions, half of this territory on four occasions, and only one or two cortical arteries on one occasion. Six of the eight patients with a pre-operative neurological deficit recovered a normal status after operation.

2. *2nd Group: Traumatic Carotido-Cavernous Fistulas* (five cases).

Five patients had an EICB prior to obliteration of their fistulas, which was undertaken on four occasions by means of an inflated balloon occluding the carotid lumen at the level of the arterio-venous communication, according to Prolo and Hanbery's method and, on one occasion, by a simple trapping.

In this group, no complications occurred. At the arteriographic control the five anastomoses were patent, and the territory they vascularized was extensive enough for carotid occlusion without danger.

3. *3rd Group: Intracranial Aneurysms* (five cases).

This group includes:

Two cases of giant aneurysm. The first one—situated at the intra-cranial carotid bifurcation on the right side—was treated with success as regards the malformation. However there was an increase in the hemiplegia caused by occlusion of the cervical ICA by a Selverstone's clamp after an EICB had been performed. The second one—located in the right MCA, was successfully treated by clipping the MCA trunk just above the malformation, after an EICB procedure.

One case of intracranial carotid bifurcation, associated with multiple aneurysms in the supraclinoid portion of the ICA. The first one was occluded by clipping its neck, the others were excluded by trapping the supraclinoid portion of the ICA after carrying out an EICB.

One case of aneurysm in the intracranial carotid bifurcation complicated by MCA embolism. After having clipped the neck of the aneurysm and made an unsuccessful attempt to perform an embolectomy, an EICB was successfully carried out in order to reinforce MCA vascularization.

And one case of MCA aneurysm. An operative accident led to the interruption of the artery, but an EICB performed without delay reestablished vascularization of the superficial MCA territory.

4. *4th Group: Arterial Lesions Secondary to Tumours* (one case).

The patient had a meningioma of the internal third of the sphenoidal ridge invading the ICA and the MCA on the right side. An EICB performed prior to removal of the tumour failed. This failure may be explained firstly, because a venous autograft had to be used to make the bypass between the occipital artery (too short) and the gyrus angularis artery, as the temporal superficial artery had unfortunately became occluded during therapeutic embolization of the tumorous afferent pedicles; secondly, because an unexpected cerebral herniation occurred during craniotomy secondary to the intracranial hypertension.

Discussion

The usefulness of the EICB procedure in the fields of traumatic, malformative, and tumorous vascular pathology is clearly demonstrated by the 20 cases in this series and by 15 others in the literature to date (see references). More than 85 % of the EICB's were patent and vascularized an extensive territory, generally equal or superior to half the superficial MCA territory. These results show that EICB's were justified at the hemodynamic level in these cases. Moreover, in 55 % of the cases, the EICB procedure was followed by an improvement in the neurological deficits although they had been considered stationary. If we cannot be certain that the EICB was entirely responsible for the neurological improvement we can, however, be almost sure that, without bypass, surgery would have made the patient's condition more serious and would have become impossible in most cases.

From a technical standpoint two remarks can be made. The first one concerns the timing of the ICA ligation when indicated. If there are good communicating arteries in the circle of Willis, ICA ligation can be performed immediately after the EICB. In these circumstances it is advisable to carry out a preoperative angiography in order to evaluate the patency of the anastomosis and the extent of its territory. Otherwise it seems preferable to use a Selverstone carotidian clamp and to check the development of the anastomotic supply arteriographically before complete occlusion. The second remark concerns the importance of respecting the superficial temporal artery when approaching any intracranial lesion which may eventually necessitate an EICB. However, if this artery has to be sacrificed the occipital or posterior auricular arteries may eventually be used, or a bypass with a venous autograft can be performed.

Fig. 1. Upper part: *A* stenosis and aneurysm of the sub-petrosal ICA of traumatic origin, *B* treated by cervical ligation preceded with EICB [STA, anastomosis (arrow), MCA]. Central part: *A* traumatic carotido-cavernous fistula (arrow), *B* occluded by means of a balloon inflated at the level of the arteriovenous communication (triangle), after an EICB procedure (arrow). Lower part: *A* giant aneurysm of the ICA bifurcation (the ICA vascularizes the middle cerebral art., the two anterior cerebral art. and the posterior cerebral art.), *B* treated with a progressive cervical carotid occlusion by means of a Selverstone clamp. *C* with half-reduction of the carotid lumen, the MCA territory is vascularized through the EICB and the flow coming from the ICA does not fill the aneurysm

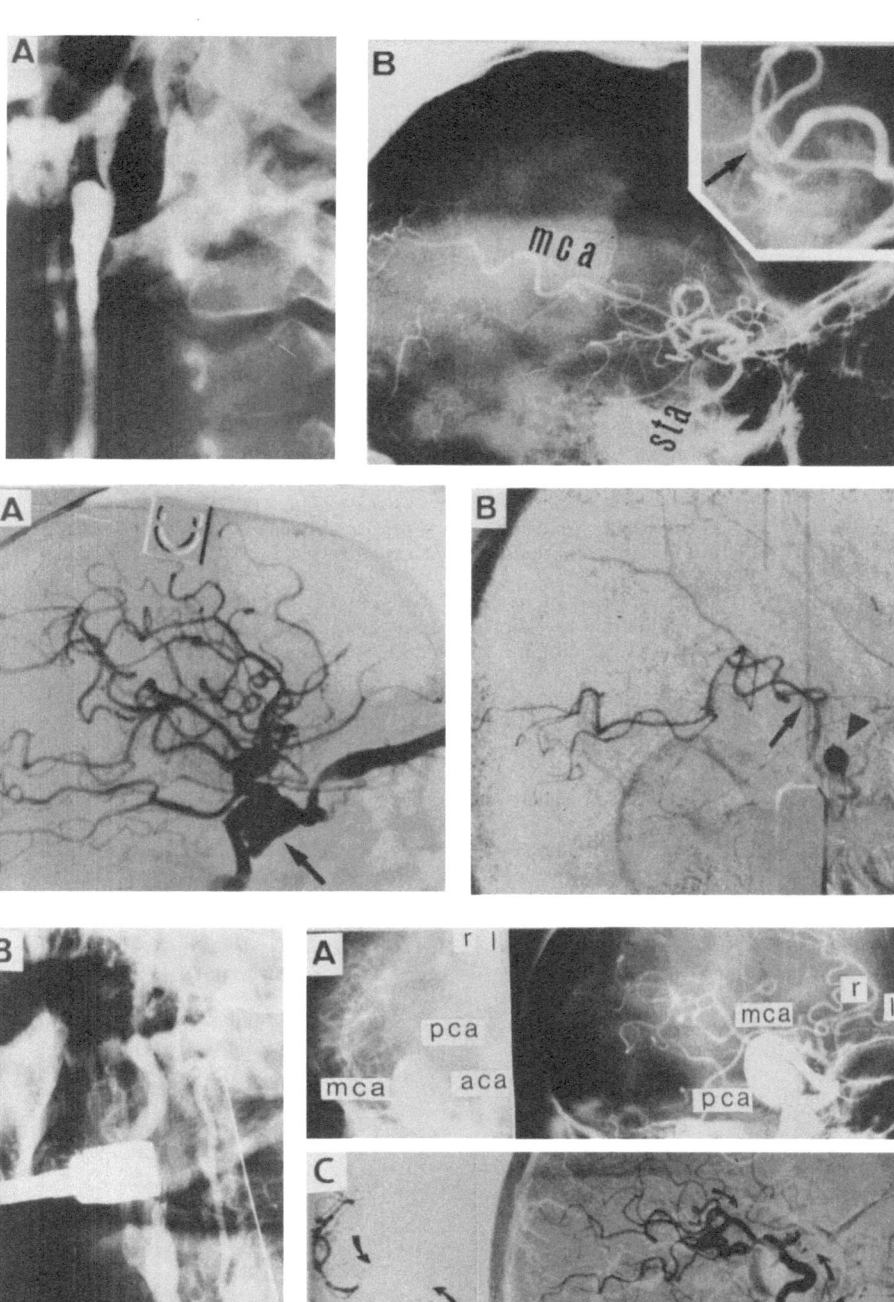

Fig. 1

References

Ammerman, B. J., Smith, D. R., Giant fusiform middle cerebral aneurysm: successful treatment utilizing microvascular bypass. Surg. Neurol. 7 (1977), 255—257.

Gratzl, O., Schmiedek, P., Steinhoff, H., Extracranial-intracranial arterial bypass in patients with occlusion of cerebral arteries due to trauma and tumour. Microneurosurgery (Handa, H., ed.), pp. 68—80. Baltimore: University Park Press. 1975.

Grunewald, P., Galibert, P., Anastomoses extra-intra-crâniennes. Communication à la IVè Rencontre Internationale de Microchirurgie du G.A.M., Lyon, Mai 1978.

Guegan, Y., Javalet, A., Eon, J. Y., Vallee, B., Pecker, J., Extra-intracranial anastomosis preliminary to treatment of carotid artery-cavernous sinus fistula. Surg. Neurol. 10 (1978), 85—88.

Redondo, A., Lebeau, J., Berthelot, J. L., Camena, M. C., Khouada, F., Aboulker, J., Ischémie cérébrale: traitement par micro-anastomoses vasculaires extra-intra-crâniennes. Nouv. Presse Méd. 7 (1978), 1625—1630.

Redondo, A., Aboulker, J., Anastomoses temporo-sylviennes. Communication à la IVè Rencontre Internationale de Microchirurgie du G.A.M., Lyon, Mai 1978.

Reichman, O. H., Selection of patients and clinical results following STA-cortical MCA anastomosis. Microneurosurgical anastomoses for cerebral ischemia (Austin, G. M., ed.), pp. 275—280. Springfield, Ill.: Ch. C Thomas. 1976.

Rey, A., Mamo, H., Thurel, C., Seylaz, J., Houdart, R., Extra-intracranial bypass. Communication à la IVè Rencontre Internationale de Microchirurgie du G.A.M., Lyon, Mai 1978.

Sindou, M., Brunon, J., Fischer, G., Goutelle, A., Mansuy, L., L'anastomose extra-intra-crânienne préalable à la ligature de la carotide. Neuro Chirurgie 23 (1977), 205—213.

Sindou, M., Brunon, J., Fischer, G., Goutelle, A., Mansuy, L., L'anastomose extra-intra-crânienne dans le traitement des anévrysmes du système carotidien. Communication à la IVè Rencontre Internationale de Microchirurgie du G.A.M., Lyon, Mai 1978.

Sundt, T. M., Siekert, R. G., Piepgras, D. G., Sharbrough, F. W., Houser, O. W., Bypass surgery for vascular disease of the carotid system. Mayo Clinic Proceedings 51 (1976), 677—692.

Yonekawa, Y., Yaşargil, M. G., Extra-intracranial arterial anastomosis clinical and technical aspects. Results. Advances and Technical Standards in Neurosurgery (Krayenbühl, H., ed.), Vol. 3, pp. 45—78. Wien-New York: Springer. 1976.

Acta Neurochirurgica, Suppl. 28, 287—290 (1979)
© by Springer-Verlag 1979

National Institute of Neurosurgery, Budapest
(Director: Prof. Emil Pásztor), Hungary

Prevention of Brain Stem Stroke
by Microvascular Anastomosis

M. Horváth, J. Vajda, and I. Nyáry

With 2 Figures

The vertebro-basilar arterial diseases are due to congenital vascular malformations and secondary circulation disturbances, such as arteriosclerotic stenoses and occlusions, cervical spondyloses, trauma, and thromboembolic mechanisms. If the morphological alteration is in the extracranial part of the arteries, in the neck, or in the subclavian artery, perhaps in the aortic arch, direct operation is possible. In some cases of occlusions of the vertebral artery, if this occlusion or stenosis does not extend beyond the level of the posterior inferior cerebellar artery (PICA), microarterial anastomosis between the occipital artery (OA) and the PICA could be indicated.

In a period of two and a half years we operated on 57 patients with vascular obstructive disease. We carried out 59 microarterial anastomosis operations, two because of vertebro-basilar arterial insufficiency.

Case Reports

1. PND (male), date of birth 1938. In May 1970 he suddenly lost consciousness for several minutes, became hemiplegic on the right side, and could not swallow four to six weeks later he recovered and could work again. There was no sign of arterial hypertension previously.

In Juli 1976 after a suboccipital haedache he had another similar stroke with severe right hemiparesis, left hypaesthesia, mild disturbances of swallowing and serious gait instability. We accepted him in October 1976 in a better condition. He had no paresis, and his gait and swallowing were normal. Right retrograde brachial angiography showed a narrow right vertebral artery without intracranial filling. Left retrograde brachial angiography showed no filling of the vertebral artery. Both internal carotid arteries and their branches were normal.

Operation, 8. November 1976. The day after surgery there was no numbness on the left side. The patient could walk on the 5th day and left the clinic on the 15th day.

Right carotid angiography six months later showed narrow filling of the anastomosis. The occipital artery was not enlarged. Two years follow-up: marked tendon reflexes on the right side, mild hypalgesia on the left. He can walk and swallow well, and has no further history of stroke.

2. GI (male), date of birth 1935. After five years of arterial hypertension, in May 1977 he had a cardiac infarct. Six months later there were sudden

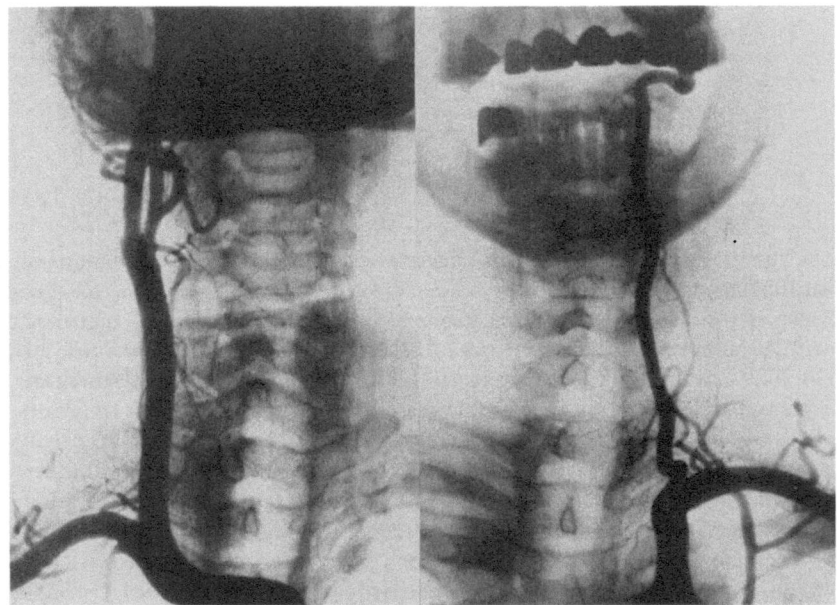

Fig. 1

dizziness, nasal speech, swallowing and gait problems, and spontaneous nystagmus. His blood pressure was 200 mm Hg. Slow improvement came after regular medical treatment with papaverine, aspirin, and antihypertensive drugs. He was accepted by our clinic in Budapest in July 1978. Right retrograde brachial angiography showed occlusion of the right vertebral artery, but refilling of the artery at the C2 level through muscular collateral branches. Left angiography showed significant narrowing of the first part of the left vertebral artery (Fig. 1). There was no alteration in the carotid arteries.

Operation, 14. June 1978. The patient had a CSF pool under the skin flap, but it disappeared two weeks later. He left our clinic three weeks after surgery in the same neurological state. Right brachial and carotid angiography four months later showed better filling of the right PICA through the artificial anastomosis (Fig. 2). Five month follow-up: his unstable gait became a little better, there had been no further stroke.

Both of our patients underwent an end-to-side microarterial anastomosis of the right OA to the PICA. The skin incision was made in the midline extending to an occipital skin flap. After preparing the OA and surrounding tissue one cm in diameter, we made suboccipital craniectomy, enlarging the bone removal to the right. The anastomosis

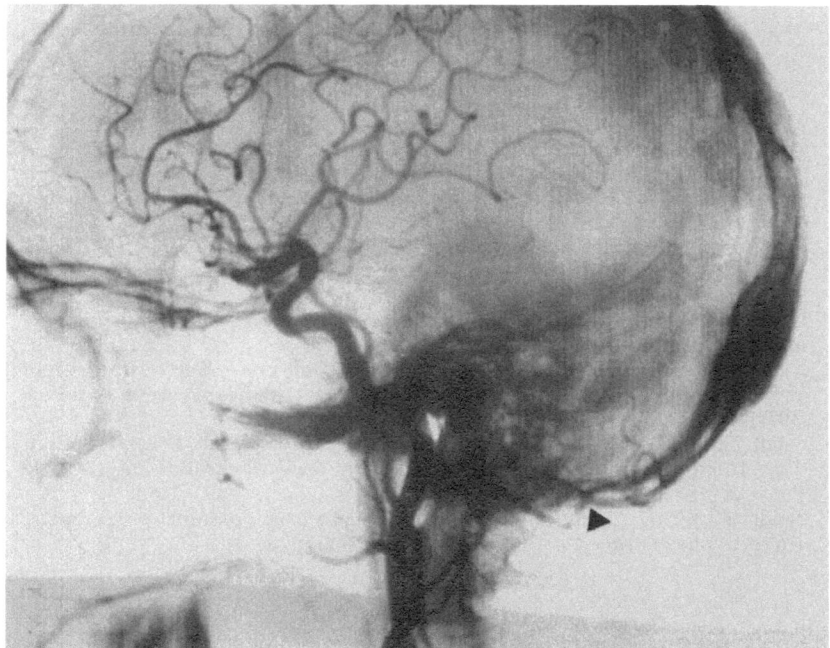

Fig. 2

was made with the tonsillar branch of the PICA, resulting in retrograde circulation in the proximal PICA. The operative procedure was similar to those of Khodadad (1976) and, later, Sundt and co-workers (1978).

We found that the sitting position is better (two patients) for the micromanipulation than the lying (one patient). The operation is not more difficult than that between the STA-MCA. Only the preparation of the muscular part of the OA needed more time, and there is a danger of a postoperative CSF pool. We have never seen such complication after STA-MCA anastomoses.

As far as the most exciting question, the indication is concerned, this is not quite clear. The most important points are:

Estimating the morphological and other circumstances in which the anastomosis between the OA and PICA can give protection against probale future stroke. The fact is well-known that patients with good natural collateral arterial supply are better after stroke. The artificial anastomosis could play this role in the prospective strokes. It is not worthwhile doing this operation on chronically disabled patients because their lesions are irreversible and operation can not ameliorate.

References

1. Ausman, J. I., Lee, M. C., Klassen, A. C., *et al.*, Stroke: What's new? Cerebral revascularisation. Minn. Med. *59* (1976), 223—227.
2. Cartlidge, N. E. F., Whisnant, I. P., Elveback, L. R., Carotid and vertebral-basilar transient ischemic attacks. A community study. Mayo Clinic Proc. *52* (1977), 117—120.
3. Horváth, M., Vajda, J., Microvascular anastomosis between the arteria occipitalis and arteria cerebelli posterior inferior. VI. Congress of Experimental Surgery, p. 80. Pécs, August 1977.
4. Khodadad, G., Occipital artery-posterior inferior cerebellar artery anastomosis. Surg. Neurol. *5* (1976), 225—228.
5. Khodadad, G., Singh, R. S., Olinger, C. P., Possible prevention of brain stem stroke by microvascular anastomosis in the vertebrobasilar system. Stroke *8* (1977), 316—321.
6. Sundt, T. M., Jr., Whisnant, I. P., Piepgras, D. G., Campbell, I. K., Holman, C. B., Intracranial bypass grafts for vertebral-basilar ischemia. Mayo Clinic Proc. *53* (1978), 12—18.
7. Sundt, T. M., Jr., Piepgras, D. G., Occipital to posterior inferior cerebellar artery bypass surgery. J. Neurosurg. *48* (1978), 916—928.

Acta Neurochirurgica, Suppl. 28, 291—293 (1979)
© by Springer-Verlag 1979

Department of Neurosurgery, University of Pécs, Hungary

The Importance of the Early Diagnosis of Preocclusive Carotid Artery Lesions

M. Bodosi, F. T. Mérei, and Gy. Gács

With 1 Figure

The rapid development of vascular surgery in recent years has created technical conditions for performing preventive reconstructive operations on cerebral arteries. This raises an urgent demand for the diagnosis of vascular lesions at an early phase of their development, when there has not yet been any irreversible damage of brain structure and function.

The present paper deals with the informative value of cerebral angiography for this purpose. The angiographic findings obtained in 840 cases with hemispheric ischaemic lesions are shown in Table 1. The most frequent findings were stenosis (318 patients), and occlusion (169 patients) of the internal carotid artery.

The summary of the clinical symptoms of the patients with internal carotid artery occlusion at the time of carotid angiography is given in Table 2.

It can be learned from this table that occlusion of the internal carotid artery results in irreversible brain damage of varying degree in about 80% of the cases. As for the remaining 20% of the patients, they are endangered in the sense that some haemodynamic disturbance (sudden drop of the blood pressure) will produce such damage in the future. The above data indicate that preserving or restoring the capability to work can be expected from vascular surgery in only one fifth of the patients with internal carotid occlusions. However, those with moderate or severe symptoms may be kept in good condition by a preventive operation, supposing it is performed in the preocclusive state.

No doubt the occlusions develop from stenoses. However, it is questionable whether every stenosis leads to occlusion. There is a noticeable difference between the angiographically detected distri-

19*

Table 1

Severe (over 66 %) stenosis of the internal carotid artery at the bifurcation of the common carotid artery (lesions suitable for direct surgery).	96 patients (11.4 %)
Severe (over 66 %) stenosis of the internal carotid artery in its distal portion (lesions inaccessible for the usual techniques).	42 patients (5.0 %)
Occlusion of the internal carotid artery.	169 patients (20.1 %)
Stenosis or occlusion of the middle cerebral artery.	64 patients (7.6 %)
Stenosis or occlusion of the anterior cerebral artery.	12 patients (1.4 %)
Occlusion of cortical branches of the middle cerebral artery.	102 patients (12.1 %)
Slight stenosis of the internal carotid artery.	180 patients (21.4 %)
So-called negative angiograms.	121 patients (14.4 %)
Others.	54 patients (6.4 %)

Table 2

TIA only.	13 patients (8 %)
Mild focal neurologic signs which have not influenced the patient in the everyday activity.	17 patients (10 %)
Mild or moderate neurologic symptoms.	62 patients (37 %)
Severe neurologic symptoms indicating cerebral infarction.	77 patients (45 %)

bution of occlusions of the internal carotid artery on the one hand, and that of stenoses, on the other. In 84 % of our patients the occlusion was found in the vicinity of the bifurcation of the common carotid artery (Fig. 1) whereas only two-third of the stenoses have the same localization. However, it should be stressed that angiography is able only to demonstrate the proximal, and in certain cases the distal, end of the occlusion, but not the exact site of its origin. As stated by Bernett, the internal carotid artery will be thrombosed nearly down to the bifurcation of the common carotid artery in a short time after an occlusion develops at the carotid siphon, and vice versa. In a previous paper we called attention to the fact that the contour of the proximal end of the occlusion can give some information about the site of its origin. Stenoses in the carotid siphon have the same chance of developing into occlusions as those situated at the bifurcation of the common carotid artery.

The initial clinical symptoms in our 169 cases with internal carotid artery occlusion were as follows:

completed stroke	81 patients (48%)
progressing stroke	21 patients (12%)
transient ischaemic attack	67 patients (40%)

It can be concluded from these data that, in a considerable proportion of the patients, the occlusion was preceded by a preocclusive

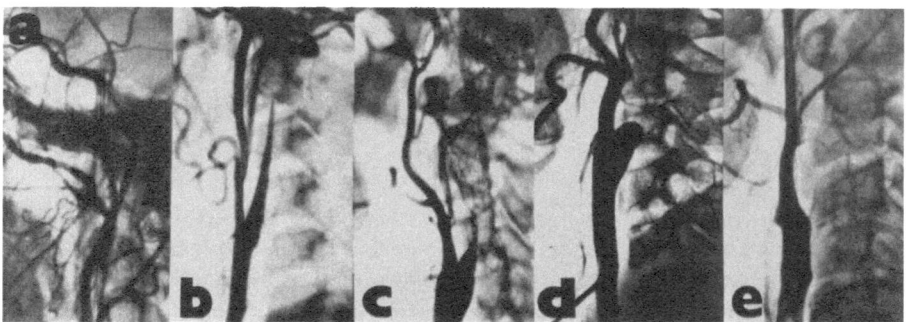

Fig. 1. The main types of the occlusion of the internal carotid artery.
a 10%, b 6%, c 28%, d 22%, e 34%

state with slight clinical signs, which could have been diagnosed angiographically as stenosis in the internal carotid artery.

Progression of a stenosis into an occlusion can proceed very quickly. In one of our cases it took place during angiography. The severe, ulcerated stenoses and the presence of fresh mural thrombus are the most dangerous conditions in this respect. Both can be easily demonstrated by angiography, and are indications for urgent surgery. In five such cases we have performed thromboendarterectomy with success.

When the sites of these lesions are inaccessible for direct surgical attack the occlusion cannot be prevented. However, the serious consequences of the occlusion might be avoided by means of an extra-intracranial bypass.

To sum up the matter, even slight signs of an ischaemic cerebral lesion are sufficient reason for a neurological evaluation and angiography in carefully selected patients. When this reveals pre-occlusive vascular lesions, adequate surgical intervention should be performed as soon as possible.

Acta Neurochirurgica, Suppl. 28, 294—297 (1979)
© by Springer-Verlag 1979

Postgraduate Institute of the Medical School
of Komenský University, Bratislava, Czechoslovakia

Microsurgical Approach to Bilateral Carotid Artery Occlusion

Š. Palkovič, P. Borák, and P. Nádvorník

With 1 Figure

Bilateral carotid artery occlusions occur not as rarely as was assumed in the past. In 200 patients suffering from occlusion of the carotid artery and treated by extra-intracranial microanastomosis[1], a 10% incidence of bilateral occlusions was observed.

Material

According to the angiographic examination these patients were classified in two different groups. The first group includes patients with complete occlusion of both carotid arteries; the second group includes patients with unilateral occlusion and a simultaneous stenosis of the contralateral carotid artery which might be presumed to develop later into complete occlusion. In both these groups, extra-intracranial microanastomosis, having a therapeutic and preventive character, was performed.

In patients with unilateral occlusion and contralateral stenosis of the carotid artery, an extracranial surgical procedure on the main arteries may also be considered[2]. However, from the neurosurgical point of view, we preferred microanastomosis as a method of treatment which is relatively free of risks.

The *indications for operative treatment* can be discussed on the grounds of two observations.

The first case is represented by a patient having a complete occlusion of the right carotid artery. Four vessel angiography showed that all the remaining main cerebral arteries participated in the collateral circulation through the communicating arteries, but only to a limited extent. The extra-intracranial microanastomosis was performed on the right side. The patient recovered and continued in his professional work. Ten months later, however, a state of mental confusion with speech disturbance developed, lasting for a period of some weeks. The angiographic examination of both carotid arteries showed a bilateral occlusion, the blood supply to both cerebral

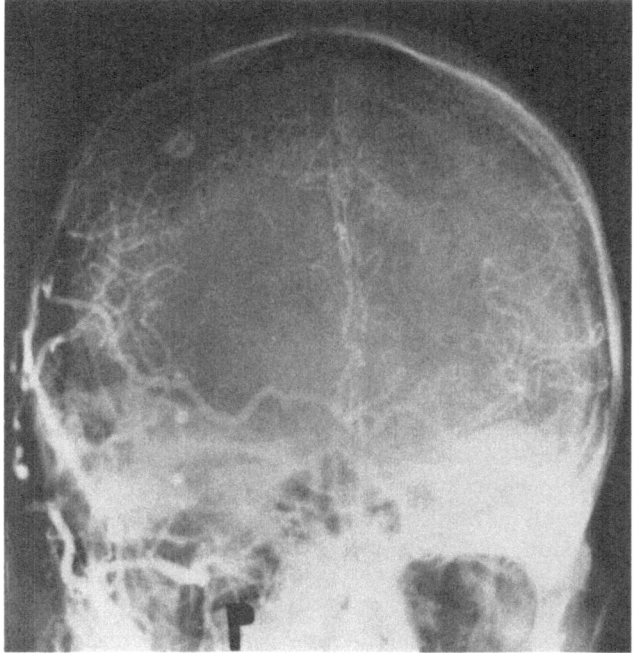

Fig. 1

hemispheres being preserved through the right extra-intracranial microanastomosis (Fig. 1). The occlusion of the left carotid artery apparently developed later and, due to the microanastomosis, the patient recovered without permanent sequelae.

For this reason, in other patients suffering from unilateral thrombosis and contralateral stenosis of the carotid artery we performed unilateral extra-intracranial microanastomosis, when an adequate collateral circulation through the anterior communicating cerebral artery developed. In patients with an insufficient collateral circulation we performed a bilateral extra-intracranial microanastomosis.

In the second group of patients who recovered from a bilateral occlusion of the carotid artery and who were recommended for surgical treatment, we proceeded in the same way. With these patients we gained a different important experience. With routine four vessel angiography of the cerebral arteries an during vertebral angiography a patient developed a severe general condition which resulted in the apallic syndrome despite the subsequently performed immediate extra-intracranial microanastomosis on the dominant side. Additional angiography showed that the microanastomosis provided an adequate blood supply to both cerebral hemispheres. In other patients we always started the angiographic examination with X-ray examination of the carotid arteries. When a bilateral thrombosis of the carotid artery was shown on X-ray, we did not performed vertebral angiography, and did the extra-intracranial microanastomosis exclusively on the basis of carotid angiography.

Discussion

Usually bilateral carotid thrombosis does not arise in both the arteries simultaneously. The occlusion arises first unilaterally and the occlusion of the contralateral artery develops after a delay. The patients present quite rarely for treatment with bilateral occlusion of the carotid artery. These different types of bilateral thrombosis of the carotid artery permit a choice of different sorts of microsurgical treatment as well as of examination. From our own experience in bilateral occlusion of the carotid artery it follows that the extra-intracranial microanastomosis is an effective procedure. Vertebral angiography in these cases is considered dangerous.

The experience gained from the microsurgical treatment of bilateral occlusions of the carotid artery contributes indirectly to the decision concerning the microanastomosis in cases when the patient recovered without sequelae from unilateral occlusion of the artery providing that the natural collateral circulation is apparently adequate. In such cases, the extra-intracranial microanastomosis is an effective means of securing the patient from a secondary occlusion of other main cerebral arteries. This approach is based on the experience that arteriosclerosis of cerebral arteries, which is the primary cause of occlusive disease, does not appear to be limited only to a single site in the arterial network of the brain.

Summary

Bilateral thromboses of the carotid artery present in the form of complete bilateral occlusion or in the form of unilateral occlusion associated with stenosis of the contralateral carotid artery. From our experience in a series of 20 patients extra-intracranial microanastomosis appears to be effective in both described groups.

References

1. Palkovič, Š., Nádvorník, P., Microanastomosis indication. J. Neurosurg. Sci. *21* (1977), 2—3, 199—201.
2. Patterson, R. H., Jr., Risk of carotid surgery with occlusion of the contralateral carotid artery. Arch. Neurol. *30* (1974), 188—189.

Acta Neurochirurgica, Suppl. 28, 298—301 (1979)
© by Springer-Verlag 1979

Department of Neurosurgery, University of Pécs, Hungary

Tandem Lesions of the Internal Carotid Arteries and Their Management

F. T. Mérei, M. Bodosi, and Gy. Gács

With 2 Figures

The significance of the combination of two or more vascular lesions (stenoses and occlusions) causing disturbances in the cerebral circulation has long been understood. Therefore, it is not surprising that, in one fifth of the patients with internal carotid occlusion a severe stenosis can be found in the contralateral internal carotid artery. This seriously influences the natural history of the disease.

Up to the early seventies the only surgical approach to the treatment of these cases had been endarterectomy of the stenosed internal carotid artery without any possibility of surgical intervention on the occluded side. In such cases even slight stenosis was accepted as an indication for extracranial vascular surgery.

The recent years the development of the extra-intracranial bypass operation has opened a direct way for the blood supply of the hemisphere on the side of the occluded internal carotid artery.

As revealed by CBF studies the artificial extra-intracranial anastomoses are capable of improving the circulation in contralateral hemispheres. Moreover, postoperative angiographic findings suggest that the artificial anastomoses can accommodate by dilatation to a gradual worsening of the blood supply through the contralateral internal carotid artery. Based on these observations, a single bypass operation on the occluded side without any surgical intervention on the symptomless opposite side has been preferred by the majority of surgeons during the past five years, even in patients with so called tandem lesions.

An accidental observation has made us change our opinion on this issue. In one of our tandem cases the stenosed internal carotid artery became occluded during preoperative angiography. A thrombo-endarterectomy was immediately performed on the freshly occluded

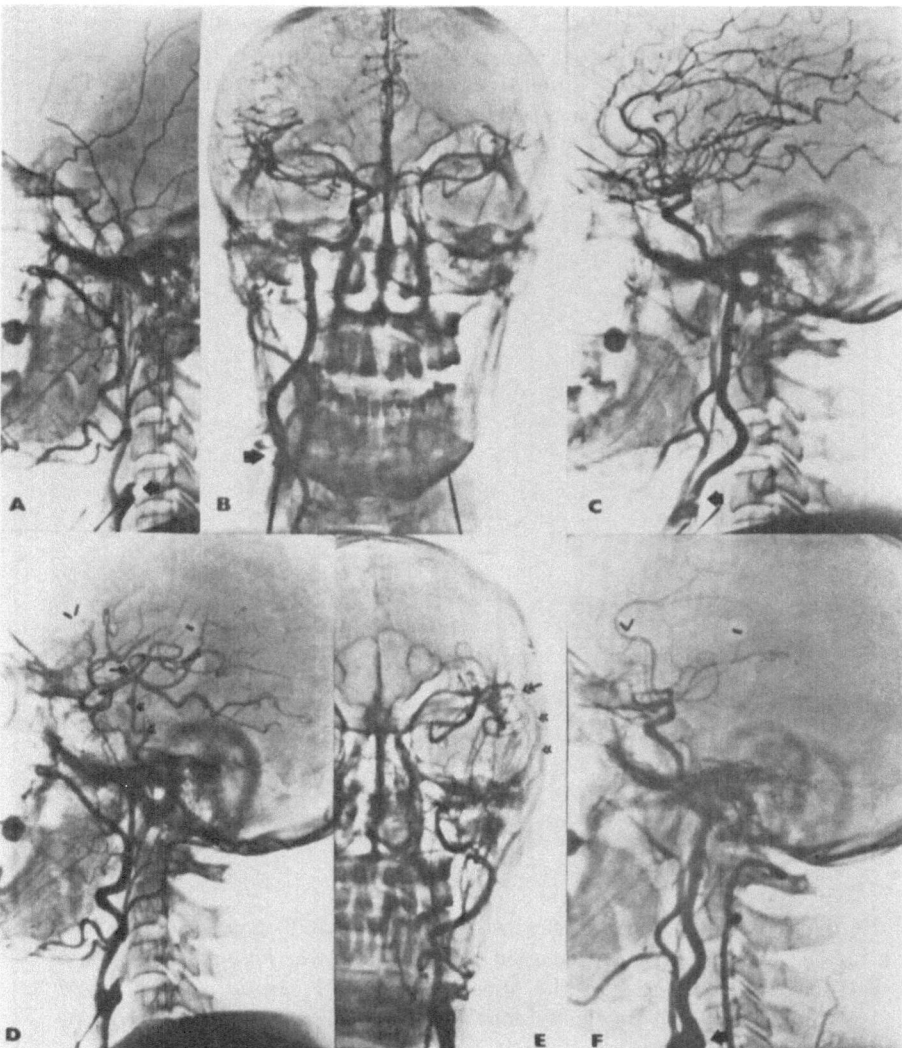

Fig. 1. 43-year-old male. Following several TIA's, paresis of the right arm and speech disorder developed. Angiography revealed a left-sided occlusion (arrow) of the internal carotid artery (*A*) and a slight stenosis (arrow) of the contralateral one (*B* and *C*), which supplied both hemispheres. After the anastomosis (arrow) between the superficial temporal artery (arrow-heads) and the middle temporal branch of the middle cerebral artery angiography (*D* and *E*) revealed that the territory of the middle cerebral artery is supplied by the new collateral system. One month later endarterectomy (arrow) of the right internal carotid artery was performed. The patency of the reconstructed artery was confirmed by brachial angiography (*F*)

side and two weeks later an extra-intracranial bypass operation was done on the other side.

This case calls the attention to the possibility of a sudden occlusion of the stenosed cerebral arteries. This is the reason why we now consider bilateral operations in each of our cases with tandem lesions.

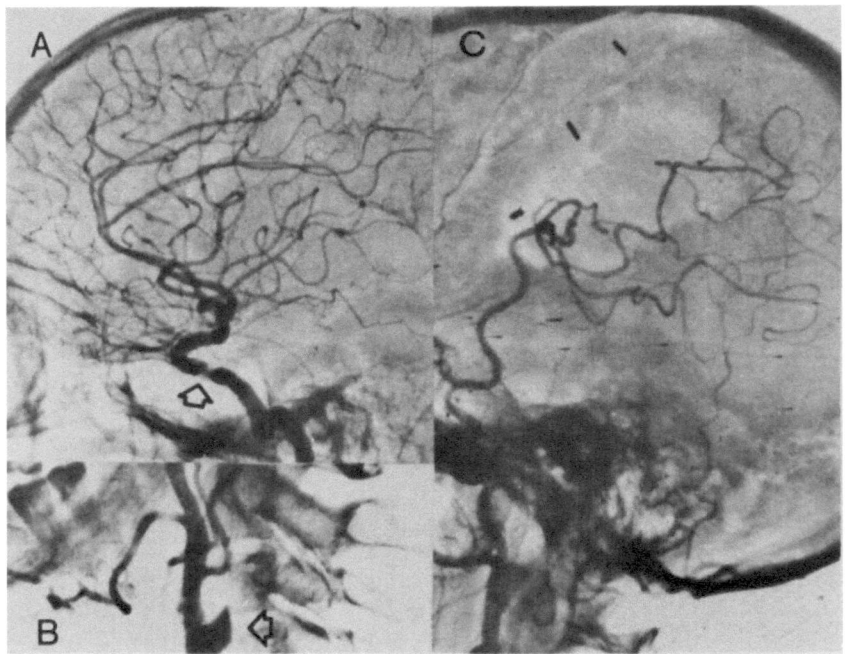

Fig. 2

During the last five years we have operated on 95 patients for internal carotid artery occlusion. This lesion was accompanied by a stenosis or occlusion in the opposite internal carotid artery in 27 patients. They can be classed into three groups according to the type and site of the lesions

Occlusion of both internal carotid arteries.   6 patients

Occlusion of one of the internal carotid arteries accompanied by a stenosis at, or distal to, the carotid siphon on the opposite side.   14 patients

Occlusion of one of the internal carotid arteries accompanied by a stenosis at the bifurcation of the common carotid artery on the opposite side.   7 patients

In the first two groups the sites of the vascular lesions are inaccessible to extracranial surgery. Therefore, no other possibility presents itself for the treatment of both lesions but the performance of extra-intracranial anastomoses on both sides, first on the side responsible for the clinical signs, and several weeks later on the other side.

In the third group of patients there are three questions to be answered:

1. Is it necessary to perform surgery on both sides or not? In disagreement with the prevailing opinion, our answer is "yes". The stenosis may cause severe haemodynamic disturbances or may be either the source of cerebral embolization or the site of thrombosis of the internal carotid artery. The latter results in completed stroke in 70 % of cases. As far as surgical intervention is concerned, we believe that doing an extra-intracranial anastomosis on the occluded side and endarterectomy on the other side should be considered.

2. The second question deals with the sequence of the two operations. It is known that during endarterectomy the internal carotid artery has to be closed while the endoluminal bypass is being inserted. This may cause irreversible damage in the brain because the other internal carotid artery also fails to function in these patients. Therefore, it seems reasonable to perform first the extra-intracranial anastomosis and the endarterectomy later (Fig. 1).

However, when arteriography reveals severe stenosis or fresh mural thrombus in the internal carotid artery indicating the risk that an occlusion will develop at the site of the stenosis before the second operation has been performed and cause completed stroke a reversed sequence of the operations seems reasonable.

3. The third question to be considered is the optimum length of the intervall between the two surgical manoeuvres. Our experiences concerning this point are insufficient to enable a firm answer because, in our cases, this intervall varied between two and six weeks according to the clinical conditions of the patients. However, the one month period recommended by the Extra-Intracranial Bypass Study appears, in general, to be right.

Acta Neurochirurgica, Suppl. 28, 302 (1979)

Department of Neurosurgery, Ospedale Maggiore Niguarda, Milano, Italy

Multiple Angiographic Studies and Tri-Dimensional Assessment of Regional Cerebral Perfusion on Patients Treated by EC-IC Bypass

M. Collice

Angiographic Studies: Sixty postoperative angiographies of 40 consecutive patients treated by EC-IC bypass were reviewed. Major results can be expressed as follows. Total patency rate (early and late controls) in approx. 95% of cases, with patency increasing on subsequent studies. Enlargement of donor artery in 50%. Intracranial steal reduction in 10%. Enlargement of pre-existing collaterals in 6%.

As for the intracranial filling via the shunt two parameters have been considered: A. the revascularization of the proximal segment of MCA as index of Sylvian triangle vascularization (41% of cases); B. the number of MCA cortical areas supplied by the shunt (1 area in 26.7%, 2 areas in 23.3%, 3 areas in 26.7%, and 4-6 areas in 23.3% of cases).

In 15 patients where intraoperative blood pressures have been measured, postoperative intracranial filling degree only partialy reflected the pressure gradient between donor and recipient arteries.

Postoperative angiographic findings have been also compared to pre-operative arteriographic and clinical conditions and clinical course.

Tri-Dimensional Assessment of Regional Cerebral Perfusion: This was obtained by intracarotid infusion of 81-m Kripton and single photon Emission Computed Tomography. Patients were selected for this study according to postoperative angiographic results in order to investigate the revascularization patterns usually obtained after such an operation. So, patients showing 1, 2, 3, and 4 cortical areas supplied by the bypass have been studied.

Detailed information on the flow distribution and redistribution inside the hemispheres has been obtained.

Acta Neurochirurgica, Suppl. 28, 303 (1979)
© by Springer-Verlag 1979

CHU Beaujon, France

Extra-Intracranial Cerebral Anastomosis Operation in Acute Ischaemia as an Emergency

A. Redondo, R. Deruty, A. Rey, J. Lagarrigue, and P. Grunewald

Cerebral revascularization in acute cerebral ischaemia may be a valuable procedure.

Fifty-nine patients have been operated on within two weeks following the ictus. In each case an extra-intracranial anastomosis was performed supplying the middle cerebral artery territory, except for one patient who was operated upon with a double anastomosis in the basilar territory.

Cerebro-vascular obstructions responsible for cerebral ischaemia were situated at different levels:

internal cervical carotid artery (21 cases),

middle cerebral artery (21 cases),

intracranial carotid artery (12 cases),

basilar artery (1 case).

Before surgery 46 patients out of 59 had a severe deficit, 8 a moderate deficit, 5 a slight deficit.

Postoperative results seems fair:

the patency rate of the anastomosis is 69%,

clinical postoperative recovery is observed in 87% of cases when the anastomosis is patent.

The clinical recovery varies according to the preoperative clinical status and the level of arterial obstruction.

This surgical cerebral revascularization is a new possibility for the treatment of acute cerebral ischaemia, and seems more efficient than spontaneous revascularization.

Acta Neurochirurgica, Suppl. 28, 304—305 (1979)
© by Springer-Verlag 1979

CHU Rennes, France

EICA in Transient Ischaemic Attacks and Neurological Deficits

R. Guegan, R. Deruty, A. Rey, and J. Lagarrigue

From the French cooperative study (300 cases in October 1978) 76 cases of TIA or PRIND were collected. Sixty-three cases only were included in this review: 60 men, 3 women—mean age 55—(from 26 to 71 years).

Forty-nine cases were of TIA, 20 cases of PRIND; in six cases TIA and PRIND were associated.

The lesions responsible were unilateral in 29 cases and bilateral in 34. Total obstruction was found in 38 cases (36 carotid artery, 2 middle cerebral artery). Total carotid obstruction on one side was frequently associated with a controlateral stenosis (23 cases).

Risk factors were: HTA 24 cases, diabetes mellitus 7 cases, myocardial infarction 8 cases, hypercholesterolaemia 2 cases.

Cerebral revascularization by EICA was performed with a single anastomosis (57 cases), a double anastomosis (3 cases), bilateral EICA (3 cases).

The patency rate assessed by angiography (39 patients) or Doppler (32 patients) was 92%.

Postoperative morbidity (7 cases) was: acute subdural haematoma in one case, transient neurological deficit in five cases, scalp necrosis in one case.

The mortality rate in the immediate postoperative period is low (1.5%—2 cases): intracerebral haemorrhage (one case): myocardial infarction 24 hours following surgery (one case).

Later on, two patients died from myocardial infarction (5 and 14 months after surgery).

The follow-up period is 16 months (mean value—from 4 to 71 months).

Out of 63 patients 57 are asymptomatic, with a good result in 91% of cases.

Twenty-two patients had more than one transient ischaemic attack before surgery. Some had several attacks a day. These patients were totally relieved of their ischaemic attacks in 95 % of cases.

Our results are similar to those reported in the literature (Reichman 83 %, Austin 85 %, Chater 92 %, Gratzl and Schmiedeck 100 %, Yaşargil 81 %).

Surgery seems mainly indicated in arterial extra- or intracranial total obstruction, because in these cases the haemodynamic factor is preponderant.

When the lesion responsible is stenosis of the intracranial arterial system, revascularization is more questionable. The indication for surgery must be balanced with medical therapy because microembolization is the main factor. Revascularization may lower the embolic risk by modification of the local circulation pattern.

Acta Neurochirurgica, Suppl. 28, 306—307 (1979)
© by Springer-Verlag 1979

Extra-Intracranial Anastomosis in Patients With Completed Strokes

P. Galibert and P. Grunewald, Amiens, France

A round table conference on EICA of the Société Française de Neurochirurgie took place in October 1978.

One hundred and ninety cases from 17 Neurosurgical Centres (Amiens: Galibert-Grunewald 43; Bordeaux: Cohadon-Castel 4; Clermont Ferrand: Redondo 3; Guadeloupe: Lemaistre-Galibert 1; Limoges: Bokor 4; Lyon: Deruty 31; Lyon: Sindou 23; Montpellier: Fuentes 6; Nantes: Lajat 6; Paris: Lebesnerais 8; Paris: Merienne-Recoules 3; Paris: Porta 4; Paris: Redondo 20; Paris: Rey 16; Rennes: Pecker-Guegan 8; Toulouse: Lagarrigue 5; Tours: Santini 5) were collected, but only 151 could be studied further.

The term Completed Stroke signifies for us the neurological syndrome stabilized after 15 days.

1. We have divided, arbitrarily, the completed stroke into four groups:

Complete hemiplegia	74 cases
Partial hemiplegia without autonomy	34 cases
Partial hemiplegia with autonomy	34 cases
Isolated aphasia	9 cases

2. Angiographic findings were essentially occlusive lesions (internal carotid, middle cerebral artery) and multifocal stenosis unapproachable by direct surgery.

Some cases were fibrous dysplasia, dissecting aneurysms, and Moya Moya disease.

3. Gamma scintigraphy was done 59 times. Thirty-one local lesions were shown.

When there was complete hemiplegia, 69% of cases had local increased uptake.

4. Seventy-seven per cent of cases were operated on before the fourth month.

5. Anatomical results. Control of EICA was by angiography or the Doppler procedure.

Eighty-nine per cent of the patients had a patent bypass.

6. Clinical results. In terms of Neurological syndrome:

	Complete hemiplegia	Partial hemiplegia with autonomy	Partial hemiplegia without autonomy	Isolated aphasia
Excellent (recovery)	1	12	1	1
Fair (improvement)	30	10	22	5
Poor	42	10	9	3

Remark. When the anastomosis was closed the clinical result was always poor.

There was no correlation between clinical result and operation date.

7. Death rate. The global mortality was 12%, divided into:

Early (1st month) 5%.
Delayed (from 2 to 15 months) 7%.

The early mortality was attributable to the surgical procedure in only 2% of cases (bleeding, pulmonary embolism).

8. Morbidity. The morbidity rate was less than 2% (acute subdural haematoma 1 case, haemorrhagic softening 1 case).

9. Global study of results (in living patients).

	France 146 cases	Chater 36 cases	Schmiedeck 28 cases	Reichman 13 cases
Recovery and improvement	56%	50%	28,5%	69,2%
Poor	44%	50%	71,5%	30,8%

It would be necessary to compare these numbers with those of natural history of completed stroke.

In conclusion. Without histological proof it is difficult not to advise this technique of revascularization in patients with completed strokes.

Acta Neurochirurgica, Suppl. 28, 308 (1979)

Neurochirurgische Universitätsklinik, Bonn, Federal Republic of Germany

Effect of Extra-Intracranial Arterial Bypass (EIAB) on Cerebral Circulation and EEG

K. H. Holbach and H. Wassmann

An EIAB (superficial temporal to middle cerebral artery) was carried out in about 100 stroke patients with occlusive lesions in the internal carotid or middle cerebral artery. Angiographic, neurological, and EEG analytical follow-up examinations were regularly performed in these patients following surgery.

Follow-up angiography indicated that the superficial temporal artery (STA) and the cerebral cortical arteries close to the shunt can enlarged considerably, that new collateral vessels can develop at the site of the craniotomy—a phenomenon described as encephalo-myosynangiosis—and that the new collateral channel is able to take over a steadily increasing part of the cerebral circulation. The follow-up EEG analyses indicated that the cerebral blood supply from the new collateral channel was usually associated with an increase in electrical brain activity, and that the persistence of the level of EEG improvement was dependent on the increase of cerebral blood supply from the STA. The postoperative bilateral increases in electrical brain activity indicated that not only the mainly affected operated side benefits from the blood supply but also the contralateral hemisphere. Consequently, redistribution in the cerebral circulation or reversal of intracerebral steal appears to play an important role following EIAB surgery.

Acta Neurochirurgica, Suppl. 28, 309 (1979)
© by Springer-Verlag 1979

Neurochirurgische Universitätsklinik, Bonn, Federal Republic of Germany

Advantage of Using Hyperbaric Oxygenation (HO) in Combination With Extra-Intracranial Arterial Bypass (EIAB) in the Treatment of Completed Stroke

K. H. Holbach and **H. Wassmann**

One hundred and twelve stroke patients with persisting neurological deficits due to occlusive lesions in the internal carotid or middle cerebral artery were studied. They were randomy assigned to a surgical or a medical treatment group. Each of the 112 patients underwent hyperbaric oxygenation (HO) treatment (consisting of a series of 15 single HO-sessions given daily) before either surgical treatment, *i.e.* extra-intracranial arterial bypass (EIAB), or medical treatment. Long term follow-up neurological and EEG analytical examinations were regularly carried out.

The results indicated that the percentage of improved patients was significantly higher in the surgically treated group while the percentage of worsened and dead patients was significantly higher in the medically treated control group, and that nearly all the patients with a favourable electroencephalographical or neurological response, or both, to HO showed a positive response to EIAB surgery, while in patients where HO treatment was considered to be ineffective there was little or no change in impaired neuronal functions following EIAB surgery. Consequently, the evaluation of the effect of HO treatment on post-stroke alterations of the brain can be helpful in differentiating between reversible and irreversible changes, and thus response to HO treatment may be used as a criterion for the prognosis of the cerebrovascular lesion and also for selection of patients for EIAB surgery.

Acta Neurochirurgica, Suppl. 28, 310—311 (1979)

IV. Balloon Techniques

Six Hundred Endovascular Neurosurgical Procedures in Vascular Pathology

A Ten-Year Experience

F. A. Serbinenko, Moscow, U.S.S.R.

In the Burdenko Neurosurgical Institute of AMS of the U.S.S.R. there has been developed a method of catheterization and vessel occlusion with the help of a detachable balloon catheter. The method appeared to be very effective and has been used extensively in the leading neurosurgical clinics of the country. Today it is being further developed in thoracic and abdominal surgery.

In the Burdenko Neurosurgical Institute there have been more than six hundred endovascular constant and more than five hundred temporary functional brain vessel occlusions in vascular pathology such as arteriovenous and arterial aneurysms. Surgical procedures have been carried out under local anaesthesia or intubation anaesthesia in infants. The age of the patients is between 11 months and 72 years.

The experience we have obtained, allows us to draw definite conclusions.

1. The method appears to be a most effective mode of treatment when we deal with caroticocavernous fistulae. In such cases destructive and reconstructive procedures may be carried out. There have been about 56 destructive operations. The advantage of such procedures over trapping is that the ophthalmic artery is preserved and may take part in brain collateral blood supply.

In most cases reconstructive operations are now carried out. There have been 110 operations of this kind. Reconstruction of the cavernous part of the carotid artery is achieved by means of balloon occlusion of the channel through which arterial blood passes from the carotid artery into the cavernous sinus. If the latter is a large single cavity, reconstruction is achieved by means of occlusion with several balloons (maximum 14 in 1 case). Such surgical procedures have been carried out successfully, and in all of our patients with carotid-cavernous fistulae we observed complete recovery.

2. The endovascular method has been used in 88 patients with radical inoperable arteriovenous aneurysms fed by many channels from several sources. More than 300 large feeding vessels have been occluded, as many as 8 in one patient. Sometimes aneurysms were completely without any blood supply. In most cases we observed considerable reduction in the size of the malformation (about 75% compared to the initial size). Remote results of treatment were studied in 50 patients. Anaverage follow-up observation is about 4.5 years. Successful results have been achieved in 27 patients out of 31 suffering from epileptic seizures. Recurrent haemorrhage was observed in only 3 patients, out of 40 who had it before operation. In many cases headache disappeared completely.

3. Arterial aneurysms are difficult for carrying out reconstructive procedures because of the anatomo-topographical structure of the neck and body the of aneurysm itself. Today we can speak arterial aneurysm cavity occlusion with blood flow preserved in eight patients. Carotid artery occlusion has been carried out at the level of the neck on aneurysm in 30 patients. In 10 patients with traumatic pseudo-aneurysms accompanied by nasal bleeding, the operations were very successful. In such cases the cavernous part of the carotid was occluded with the balloon at the level of the artery rupture. The possibility of a reconstructive operation is demonstrated.

4. The endovascular method greatly contributed to the treatment of fistulae between dural arteries and sinus, together with superselective catheterization and embolization of small vessels. In such pathology we have carried out occlusions of the ophthalmic artery, internal maxillary artery, stem and branches of the middle meningeal artery, and also occlusions of fistulae in carotid-jugular aneurysms, and vertebral artery-neck muscle venous plexus fistulas.

5. The functional occlusion of brain vessels gave the opportunity to carry out physiological brain function study, and to evaluate adequacy of brain collateral blood supply with the help of clinical and angiographical findings and quantitative methods of blood flow measurement. Hydrogen clearance technique allowed us to determine the extreme level of blood flow (16-19 mg/100 g a minutes) in which distinct clinical symptoms of brain circulation insufficiency are observed.

6. The development of the catheter occlusion technique allowed us to carry out selective contrasting and demonstration of intracerebral tumours. The opportunity of chemotherapy by means of introducing antiblastic agents through the balloon catheter to the neoplasm is being studied.

Acta Neurochirurgica, Suppl. 28, 312—315 (1979)
© by Springer-Verlag 1979

Research Institute of Neurosurgery, Kiev, U.S.S.R.

Endovascular Method of Excluding From the Circulation Saccular Cerebral Arterial Aneurysms, Leaving Intact Vessels Patient

A. P. Romodanov and V. I. Shcheglov

With 3 Figures

Recently special attention has been attracted to intravascular interventions using the Serbinenko balloon catheter. This method allows new endovascular operations for various malformations of the cerebral vessels including saccular cerebral artery aneurysms. The detachable balloon catheter permits exclusion of the saccular cerebral artery malformation from the circulation leaving intact the patency of the aneurysm-bearing vessel (F. A. Serbinenko 1971, 1974, 1976; Yu. N. Zubkov 1973; A. P. Romodanov et al. 1975; Yu. A. Zozulia, V. I. Shcheglov 1976). This relatively simple method opens new horizons in reconstructive surgery of brain vessels. It also proved to be effective in occluding saccular aneurysms considered inoperable by the routine intracranial technique (carotid cavernous aneurysms, large-sized aneurysms).

Material and Methods

This communication is based on an analysis of 65 intravascular interventions performed in 57 patients with saccular cerebral artery aneurysms at the Kiev Research Institute of Neurosurgery during 1974-1978. Location of the aneurysms: supraclinoid—33; cavernous carotid—6; middle cerebral artery—11; anterior communicating artery—7. Seven of the 57 patients had giant aneurysms. The most frequent clinical manifestations of the disease were subarachnoid haemorrhages (42 cases), visual and endocrine disorders, increased sellar size (8 cases), in one case aneurysm was suspected due to paresis of the oculomotor nerve in one patient it was accidentally found during examination for a head injury.

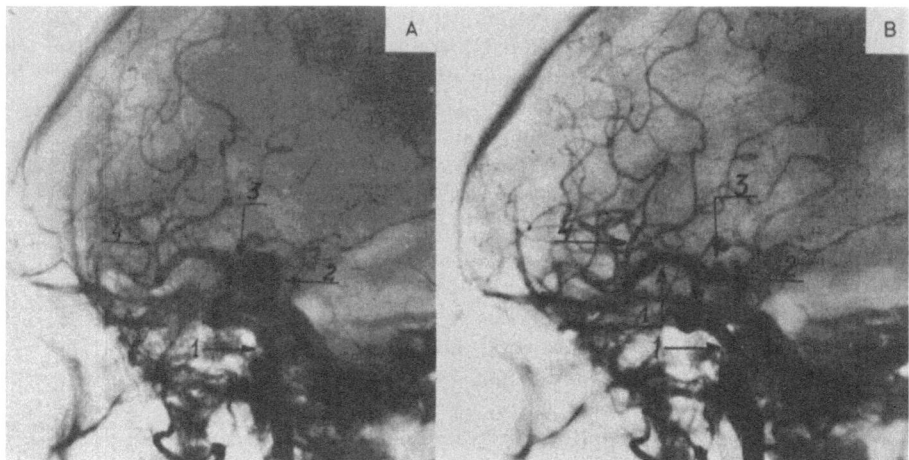

Fig. 1. A. Before operation. Carotid angiogram. *1* internal carotid artery; *2* saccular aneurysm; *3* neck of aneurysm; *4* middle cerebral artery. B. After operation. Carotid angiogram. *1* internal carotid artery; *2* working end of balloon; *3* main part of balloon filled with contrast medium (verografin) and silicone; *4* middle cerebral artery. Saccular aneurysm excluded from circulation. Intact patency of intracranial vessels

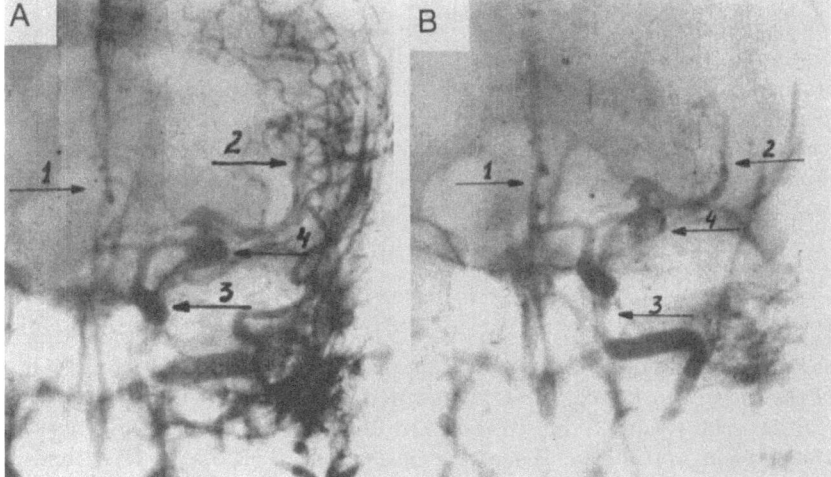

Fig. 2. A. Before operation. Carotid angiogram. *1* anterior cerebral artery; *2* middle cerebral artery; *3* internal carotid artery; *4* saccular aneurysm of middle cerebral artery. B. After surgery. Carotid angiogram. Saccular aneurysm excluded by balloon which is filled partially by verografin, partially by silicone. The balloon has a silver mark. Intact patency of intracranial vessels

All patients were operated on during the cold period following careful analysis of EEG, EchoEG, coagulographic, and other data. Angiography is a confident method of assessing the location, size, and neck of the aneurysm as well as of estimating the capacities of the circle of Willis in the collateral circulation.

Of major importance is the preoperative period which includes intensive drug treatment with the purpose of improving the microcirculation, rheological properties of the blood, prevention of vascular spasm (vasodilating agents, anticoagulants, dextran). The preoperative period with carotid artery aneurysms also included training of the collateral circulation by compressing the carotid artery at the side of the aneurysm. Such preparation creates favourable conditions for successful intravascular exclusion of saccular aneurysms from the circulation by means of a balloon catheter.

The operation was performed by the Serbinenko method under local anaesthesia which was supplemented by sedative and pain-killing cocktails. Heparin was used in the course of intervention for thromboembolism prophylaxis. Of prime importance was the manufacture of a balloon catheter related to the size, form, and location of the aneurysm. Introduction of the balloon into the aneurysm cavity under the control of an X-ray television screen presented no difficulties in 41 of 57 patients. In 10 cases, for introduction of the balloon into the aneurysm cavity, various non-standard techniques have been employed with two or three balloon catheters. In six cases repeated trials to introduce the balloon failed. After being introduced into the aneurysm cavity the balloon was filled with optimum amounts of contrast medium necessary to exclude the aneurysm. Then, instead of the contrast medium, silicone was introduced into the balloon catheter. Following detachment of the catheter from the balloon the operation was terminated by control serial angiography.

Results

In 51 of 57 patients we introduced the balloon into the aneurysm cavity and excluded it from the circulation. The patency and function of the aneurysm-bearing artery remained intact in 47 of these 51 cases (carotid artery aneurysms—32 cases; middle cerebral artery—10 cases; anterior communicating artery—5 cases, Figs. 1, 2, 3). In five cases exclusion of the aneurysm was parallelled by occlusion of the internal carotid artery. In the course of surgery or immediately after it transient (29 cases) or persistent (4 cases) functional disorders of the brain were observed. Of the 57 patients 53 were operated upon by the balloon catheter technique, and 51 of them were discharged in a satisfactory condition; 46 resumed work or studies; 3 showed a mild and 2 a marked hemiparesis after the operation. Two patients died after endovascular surgery, one on the third postoperative day due to acute ischaemic stroke, and the second on the 22nd day due to rupture

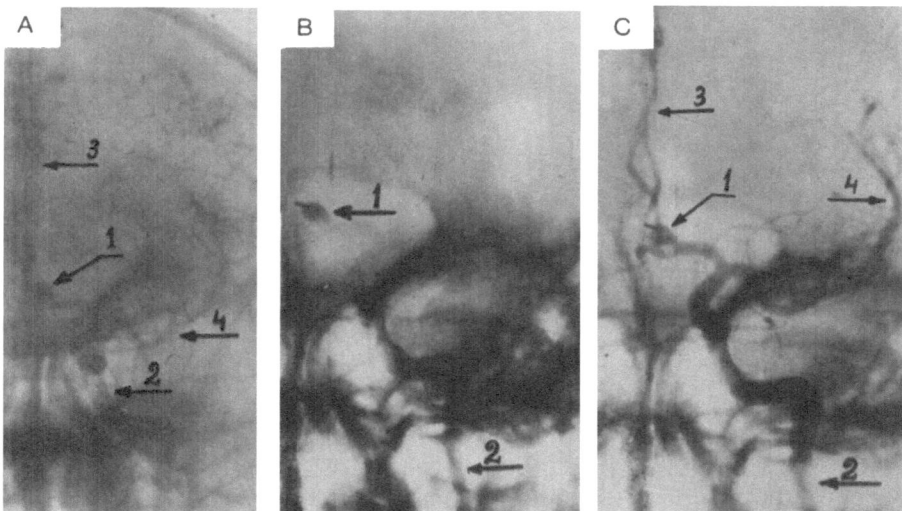

Fig. 3. A. Before surgery. Carotid angiogram. *1* saccular aneurysm of anterior communicating artery; *2* internal carotid artery; *3* anterior cerebral artery; *4* middle cerebral artery. B. After surgery. Carotid angiogram. Early arterial phase; contrast medium only in internal carotid artery *2*; the aneurysm cavity shows a balloon partially filled with verografin and silicone *1*. C. After surgery. Carotid angiogram of the same series. Late arterial phase. *1* saccular aneurysm of the anterior carotid artery excluded by a balloon; *2* internal carotid artery; *3* anterior cerebral artery; *4* middle cerebral artery

of the aneurysm which could not be completely obliterated because of a preoperative complication. Control angiography was performed in 19 patients one year after operation, revealing partial filling of the aneurysm with contrast medium in one case.

Our experience indicates that the endovascular method of excluding saccular cerebral arterial aneurysms from the circulation is efficient, and may be considered the method of choice in most patients with aneurysms of the carotid artery system. We hope that this method will find wide application.

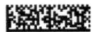